Some Aspects of Speech and the Brain

SUSANNE FUCHS/HÉLÈNE LŒVENBRUCK,
DANIEL PAPE/PASCAL PERRIER
(eds.)

Some Aspects of Speech and the Brain

PETER LANG
Frankfurt am Main · Berlin · Bern · Bruxelles · New York · Oxford · Wien

Bibliographic Information published by the Deutsche Nationalbibliothek
The Deutsche Nationalbibliothek lists this publication in the Deutsche Nationalbibliografie; detailed bibliographic data is available in the internet at <http://www.d-nb.de>.

Cover illustration by
courtesy of iStock Internantional Inc.
www.istockphoto.com.

ISBN 978-3-631-57630-4

www.peterlang.de

Content

About the editors vii
Contributors ix
Preface 1

1 N100 component: An electrophysiological cue of voicing perception 5
Ingrid Hoonhorst, Cécile Colin, Emily Markessis, Monique Radeau, Paul Deltenre, and Willy Serniclaes

2 Direct brain-feedback and prosody processing 35
Grzegorz Dogil and Giuseppina Rota

3 Phonetotopy within a neurocomputational model of speech production and speech acquisition 59
Bernd J. Kröger, Jim Kannampuzha, Anja Lowit, and Christiane Neuschaefer-Rube

4 Some aspects of language plasticity in epileptic patients as assessed by functional MRI 91
Monica Baciu and Emilie Cousin

5 Functional neuroimaging of speech production in Parkinson's disease: Towards a better understanding of dysarthria physiopathology 115
Serge Pinto, Gaelle Fillatre, and Alain Ghio

6 The neurobiological correlates of developmental dyslexia 141
Sylviane Valdois, Carole Peyrin, and Monica Baciu

7 Brain imaging and cortical excitability in persistent developmental stuttering 163
Martin Sommer, Nicole Spindler, Kathrin Knappmeyer, Evke Jane Hunter, Veronika Gutmann, Alexander Wolff von Gudenberg, and Walter Paulus

8 The sensory-motor theory of semantics: Evidence from functional imaging 177
Uta Noppeney

9 Pointing is 'special' 211
Hélène Lœvenbruck, Marion Dohen, and Coriandre Vilain

10 How special is speech? 259
Rudolph Sock and Béatrice Vaxelaire

11 Pre-lexical speech processing in the brain 295
Georg Meyer, Sophie Wuerger, and Elvira Perez

12 The role of syllabification in the lexical segmentation of German and Slovak 331
Adriana Hanulíková

13 From production to perception and back: An analysis of two pitch accents 363
Barbara Gili Fivela

About the editors

Susanne Fuchs is a senior researcher at the Zentrum für Allgemeine Sprachwissenschaft (ZAS) in Berlin. She obtained her PhD at QMUC in Edinburgh, Scotland. The main interest of her work is to link phonetics / phonology and motor control in order to understand general biological principles shaping individuals' sound production. She used a variety of techniques to study speech production and aerodynamics.

Hélène Lœvenbruck became a CNRS Research Associate at former ICP (now Speech & Cognition Department, GIPSA-lab) in 1998. Her research areas include the neural circuits of deixis (pointing), the acoustic, articulatory and perceptual correlates of prosody, language acquisition and the physical correlates of non-audible speech, in healthy subjects and schizophrenic patients. She is editor-in-chief of *In Cognito - Cahiers Romans de Sciences Cognitives*, an international quadrilingual journal of Cognitive Science.

Daniel Pape is currently working at the Zentrum für Allgemeine Sprachwissenschaft Berlin (ZAS, Germany) and at the Instituto de Engenharia Eletrónica e Telemática de Aveiro (IEETA, Portugal). He obtained his PhD at the Humboldt University in Berlin. His current research focuses on the relationship between speech production and perception, in particular on pitch phenomena in a cross-linguistic context.

Pascal Perrier is a Professor at the INP Grenoble and a researcher at the Speech and Cognition Department of GIPSA-lab (CNRS, Grenoble, France), where he is the head of the „Acoustics, Aeroacoustics, Biomechanics and Control" research group. His research interests are the analysis and the modelling of speech production, with a special focus on physical models of speech articulators and of their motor control.

Contributors

Monica Baciu
Laboratoire de Psychologie et Neurocognition & CNRS, Université Pierre-Mendès-France, Grenoble, France

Cécile Colin
Unité de Recherche en Neurosciences Cognitives, Université Libre de Bruxelles (U.L.B.), Belgium

Emilie Cousin
Laboratoire de Psychologie et Neurocognition & CNRS, Université Pierre-Mendès-France, Grenoble, France

Paul Deltenre
Clinique de Neurophysiologie, Hôpital Brugmann, Brussels, Belgium

Grzegorz Dogil
Institute for Natural Language Processing, Universität Stuttgart, Germany

Marion Dohen
Département Parole et Cognition (ex ICP) de GIPSA-lab, CNRS, INPG, UJF, U. Stendhal, Grenoble, France

Gaelle Fillatre
Laboratoire Parole et Langage, CNRS & Université Aix-Marseille, Aix-en-Provence, France

Alain Ghio
Laboratoire Parole et Langage, CNRS & Université Aix-Marseille, Aix-en-Provence, France

Barbara Gili Fivela
University of Salento, Lecce, Italy

Alexander Wolff von Gudenberg
Institut der Kasseler Stottertherapie, Bad Emstal, Germany

Veronika Gutmann
Department of Clinical Neurophysiology, University of Göttingen, Germany

Adriana Hanulíková
Institute for German Language and Linguistics, Humboldt Universität, Berlin, Germany

Ingrid Hoonhorst
Unité de Recherche en Neurosciences Cognitives, Université Libre de Bruxelles (U.L.B.) & FNRS, Belgium

Evke Jane Hunter
Department of Clinical Neurophysiology, University of Göttingen, Göttingen, Germany

Jim Kannampuzha
Department of Phoniatrics, Pedaudiology, & Communication Disorders, Medical Faculty, RWTH Aachen University, Germany

Kathrin Knappmeyer
Department of Clinical Neurophysiology, University of Göttingen, Göttingen, Germany

Bernd J. Kröger
Department of Phoniatrics, Pedaudiology, & Communication Disorders, Medical Faculty, RWTH Aachen University, Germany

Hélène Lœvenbruck
Département Parole et Cognition (ex ICP) de GIPSA-lab, CNRS, INPG, UJF, U. Stendhal, Grenoble, France

Anja Lowit
University of Strathclyde, Division of Speech and Language Therapy, Department of Educational and Professional Studies, Glasgow, United Kingdom

Emily Markessis
Faculté de Médecine, Université Libre de Bruxelles (U.L.B.), Belgium

Georg Meyer
School of Psychology, University of Liverpool, Liverpool, United Kingdom

Christiane Neuschaefer-Rube
Department of Phoniatrics, Pedaudiology, & Communication Disorders, Medical Faculty, RWTH Aachen University, Germany

Uta Noppeney
Max-Planck-Institute for Biological Cybernetics, Tübingen, Germany

Walter Paulus
Department of Clinical Neurophysiology, University of Göttingen, Göttingen, Germany

Elvira Perez
School of Psychology, University of Liverpool, Liverpool, United Kingdom

Carole Peyrin
Laboratoire de Psychologie et Neurocognition & CNRS, Université Pierre-Mendès-France, Grenoble, France

Serge Pinto
Laboratoire Parole et Langage, CNRS & Université Aix-Marseille, Aix-en-Provence, France

Monique Radeau
Unité de Recherche en Neurosciences Cognitives, Université Libre de Bruxelles (U.L.B.), Belgium

Giuseppina Rota
Institute for Natural Language Processing, Universität Stuttgart, Germany

Willy Serniclaes
Laboratoire Psychologie de la Perception, CNRS & Université René Descartes, Paris 5, France

Rudolph Sock
Institut de Phonétique de Strasbourg, Université Marc Bloch, Strasbourg, France

Martin Sommer
Department of Clinical Neurophysiology, University of Göttingen, Göttingen, Germany

Nicole Spindler
Department of Clinical Neurophysiology, University of Göttingen, Göttingen, Germany

Sylviane Valdois
Laboratoire de Psychologie et Neurocognition & CNRS, Université Pierre-Mendès-France, Grenoble, France

Béatrice Vaxelaire
Institut de Phonétique de Strasbourg, Université Marc Bloch, Strasbourg, France

Coriandre Vilain
Département Parole et Cognition (ex ICP) de GIPSA-lab, CNRS, INPG, UJF, U. Stendhal, Grenoble, France

Sophie Wuerger
School of Psychology, University of Liverpool, Liverpool, United Kingdom

Preface

EEG, MEG, fMRI, PET, TMS... These days the literature on speech and language research is full of these abstruse abbreviations, which actually refer to marvellous and powerful experimental tools that have opened the doors to the observation of the human brain in action. Thanks to these brain imaging techniques, today those times seem prehistoric in which students of speech and language sciences were taught that speech communication was essentially associated with two areas of the left hemisphere around the Sylvian fissure: Broca's area, which is located in the inferior frontal gyrus and was considered to be responsible for speech production, and Wernicke's area, which is located in the posterior temporal lobe and was considered to be responsible for speech perception. In reality, this was not really that long ago, less than 15 years in any case, but it was a time when brain imaging techniques were in their infancy, rare, quite inaccurate, and extremely complex to use. Since then, the tremendous development of their capacities and the emergence of highly specialized experimentalists and physicists have allowed the acquisition of an impressive amount of new information about the brain in action, and particularly about the speaking and hearing brain. Classic neurophysiological models of language and speech have been shattered and new concepts have emerged.

The first neuroimaging study of language functions in the brain was published in the journal *Nature* by Petersen et al. (Petersen et al., 1988)[1]. With a PET scan (Positron Emission Tomography) these authors measured brain blood flow in right-handed volunteers listening to or repeating isolated frequent English nouns presented either acoustically or visually. They compared the results with the activations observed when non-speech stimuli were presented or when non-speech movements of the lips or the jaw were produced. As expected from the classic model, they observed a specific left lateralization of the language processing when stimuli were presented acoustically; however, during speech production they found a bilateral activation around the Sylvian

1 Petersen, S.E., Fox, P.T., Posner, M.I., Mintun, M.A., & Raichle, M.F. (1988). Positron emission tomographic studies of the cortical anatomy of single-word processing. *Nature* 331(6157), 585-589.

fissure that was also observed in non-speech movements. Thus they showed that the brain activity associated with language is more complex than the classic Broca-Wernicke model would have predicted. They hypothesized that multiple brain areas structured in networks with different parallel paths were involved in the processing of language. Full of hope in the development of brain imaging techniques, they concluded, extrapolating beyond the specific issue of language processing, that thanks to *"the combination of cognitive and neurobiological approaches,"* of which their study is an example, *"solutions to the problem of mind-brain inter action that have intrigued us for so long should be illuminated"*! (p. 589)
Since then, a considerable number of brain imaging studies have been carried out. The ultimate goal of Petersen et al. has (fortunately?) not yet been reached, but substantial new knowledge about the production and the processing of speech and language has been acquired. In the majority of the studies, the left-lateralization of language in the brain tends to be confirmed, but it is not systematic. In addition, evidence has been found of the contribution of a number of brain areas, including, in addition to Broca's and Wernicke's areas, the anterior temporal lobe, the inferior parietal lobe, the cerebellum, the left superior median frontal lobe, the supplementary motor area, and the anterior insula, among others.
With the goal of gaining an overview of these recent developments and of their specific implications for speech communication research, and in order to grasp the methodological problems associated with their use (time and spatial resolution, complexity of the protocols, statistical data post-processing, etc.), we organised a summer school entitled *"Cognitive and Physical Models of Speech Production, Speech Perception and Their Interactions. Part II: Brain and Speech"* in September 2007, in the mountains surrounding Grenoble in France.[2] Ten invited speakers presented tutorials about various aspects of speech production and perception and the brain, and 45 participants presented their own research work. The present book is a collection of a subset of the presentations of the invited speakers and the participants. We selected

2 The summer school was supported by the French Centre National de la Recherche Scientifique (CNRS), the German Research Council (DFG), Grenoble INP, the city of Grenoble, the Region Rhône-Alpes, and the Association Francophone de la Communication Parlée.

some of the best contributions from the summer school and asked the authors to submit a paper for the book. Each chapter underwent a peer-review process with two reviewers[3].

A best student paper award was given to **Ingrid Hoonhorst** at the summer school for her presentation of work carried out in collaboration with C. Colin, E. Markessis, M. Radeau, P. Deltendre, and W. Serniclaes. Their paper opens the book. It raises the question as to the nature of the neurophysiological correlates of voicing contrast perception in speech. Using Electroencephalography (EEG), Hoonhorst et al. suggest that the late auditory cortical evoked-potential N100 could be a good candidate, and address issues related to the link between the acoustic and the phonological levels of speech perception.

Real time functional Magnetic Resonance Imaging (rtfMRI) is at the centre of **Dogil and Rota**'s chapter. rtfMRI can be used to elicit desired behavioural effects by regulating specific brain region activations through neurofeedback. **Dogil and Rota** study how modulating the right inferior frontal gyrus influences the processing of prosodic features.

"Phonetotopy" is the new concept introduced by **Kröger et al.**, who propose a neurocomputational model of speech production and acquisition. They suggest that speech production control is based on a phonetic neural map which is structured in such a way that the ordering of the phonetic states matches the well-known phonetic classification.

Baciu and Cousin study the cerebral plasticity associated with language processing in adult patients with temporal lobe epilepsy. Using fMRI they note atypical lateralization of language with an intersubject variability of the cerebral reorganisation due to extrinsic factors.

Pinto et al. present a literature review and a discussion of the possible implications of neuroimaging studies for the understanding of Parkinsonian dysarthria and of the fact that motoric improvements due to subthalamic nucleus stimulation do often not extent to speech.

Valdois et al. suggest that developmental dyslexia results from two main disorders. Atypical functioning in left perisylvian regions provides evidence of a phonological processing disorder, while atypical parietal activations are consistent with a visual attention span disorder.

---

3 Special thanks to the reviewers for their very constructive and helpful work.

Sommer et al. provide an overview of neuroimaging studies suggesting that persistent developmental stuttering originates from peculiarities in brain structure, motor cortex excitability and inter-hemispheric inhibition. They propose a framework integrating these findings and psychological factors to explain this speech disease.
Noppeney studies how semantic concepts are represented and processed in the human brain. In the framework of the sensory-motor theory of semantic memory, results of functional imaging studies are presented suggesting that semantic processing of tools and actions is associated with activations within the visuo-motor system.
Lœvenbruck et al.'s chapter is the merging of two original papers, which explain its length. It is observed that the ocular, digital and prosodic pointing used in human communication present common patterns of left parietal activation, which could originate from the *'special'* role of index finger pointing in language acquisition. Syntactic pointing is different, probably due to a grammaticalization process.
Sock and Vaxelaire observe differences in kinematics and vocal tract configurations in speech as compared to other biological gestures. They argue that these specificities arise from the necessity for speech to preserve linguistic identity and phonological contrast, while ensuring the viability of motor strategies.
Meyer et al. present theoretical models of prelexical speech perception and evaluate their predictions on the basis of experimental fMRI and EEG data, while demonstrating potential limitations of these brain imaging techniques.
Hanulíková considers German and Slovak, two languages which have different syllabification rules. She studies how native speakers of these languages divide bisyllabic non-words in a syllable reversal task. She observed different results for both languages and concludes that syllabification preferences do not influence speech segmentation.
Gili Fivela investigates the perceptual distinction of two pitch accents in Pisa Italian. She observes that they are not perceived categorically, and she raises general issues about the use of the Categorical Perception paradigm for intonation.

Susanne Fuchs, Hélène Lœvenbruck, Daniel Pape, Pascal Perrier

1

The N100 component: An electrophysiological cue of voicing perception

INGRID HOONHORST
CECILE COLIN
EMILY MARKESSIS
MONIQUE RADEAU
PAUL DELTENRE
WILLY SERNICLAES

Abstract: In many languages the voicing distinction between stop consonants in initial position depends on laryngeal timing. The time interval between closure release and voicing onset (Voice Onset Time) has been extensively investigated since it is the major acoustic correlate of voicing. This chapter reviews the literature on the neurophysiological correlates of voicing perception with an emphasis on the basic auditory sensitivity common to human newborns and animals. Since it has been shown that the acoustic level of perception is indexed by late cortical evoked-potentials, we recorded the N100 component in French-speaking subjects, for whom the phonological boundary corresponds to none of the acoustic ones. We hypothesized that in French, the basic acoustic boundaries should be revealed by the N100 characteristics without any contamination by the phonological one. This hypothesis was confirmed by the results, which open the way to a better understanding of the link between the acoustic and the phonological levels of speech perception.

1. INTRODUCTION

1.1. VOICING

In 1977, Abramson opened the way to a wide field of research by defining Voice Onset Time (VOT) as the *"temporal relation between the onset of glottal pulsing and the release of the initial stop consonant" (p. 296)* and by underlining the importance of the temporal order between these two events, i.e. the temporal order between voicing onset and closure release. Voicing lead was used to characterize productions in which periodic energy precedes closure release, while voicing lag described the inverse pattern.

The huge number of subsequent studies conducted on VOT can certainly be explained by the peculiarly straightforward relation between the perception of voicing and VOT, which is the most important cue for voicing perception, at least in initial position (Lisker et al., 1978). In medial position, it is combined with other temporal cues related to laryngeal timing (Saerens et al., 1989). These other acoustic cues, such as the value of the fundamental frequency, formant transition duration and the frequency value of F1, only affect voicing perception when the VOT is ambiguous and they are therefore considered as secondary cues (Summerfield & Haggard, 1977; Hillenbrand, 1984).

There are multiple reports showing that the VOT perceptual boundary shifts as a function of place of articulation (Abramson & Lisker, 1970b; Sharma et al., 2000) and vocalic context (Summerfield & Haggard, 1974). This provides supplementary degrees of freedom for the design of experiments on voicing perception in various contexts.

1.2. TWO OR THREE LEVELS OF SPEECH PERCEPTION?

Based on their empirical findings showing an effect of inter-stimulus-interval (ISI) on discrimination performances, Werker and Logan (1985), followed by other authors (Burnham, 1986; Flege, 1988; 1992), developed a three-factor model of speech perception in which the acoustic, phonetic and phonological levels of speech processing are dissociated. They showed a correlation between the ISI and the complexity of the level of perception reached: ISIs of 250, 500 and 1500 ms were respectively associated with the acoustic, phonetic and phonological levels of perception. The acoustic level was related to the ability to discriminate acoustic contrasts that are not phonological in any language of the world; the phonetic level was tied to the ability to discriminate contrasts which are phonological in languages not spoken by the subject, and the phonological level was linked to the capacity to discriminate phonemes belonging to his/her own language. The key finding of this study was the demonstration that the experimental setting may influence the subject's discrimination and lead him/her to perceive contrasts that are phonological neither in his/her language nor in any of the other languages.

This study raised two main issues in the field of the development of perceptual abilities. First, by underlining the impact of experimental conditions on the ability to discriminate fine-grained contrasts, one must accept the existence of successive levels of speech processing which we may expect to correspond to a hierarchical functional organization of the perceptual system. Secondly, even though Werker and Logan (ibid) postulated a phonetic level of perception, they did not specify its nature and cautiously concluded *"it is not clear whether phonetically relevant perception is a function of a specific linguistic processor or the result of second-order auditory factors [...]" (p. 43).*

The suggestion of an intermediary phonetic mode of perception comes from the observation that human perceptual boundaries are built up as a combination of trade-off between acoustic cues, which Werker and Logan (1985) called *"second-order auditory factors"*. Indeed, some authors have shown that categories of voicing come from the combination of VOT and first formant (F1) transition (Simon & Fourcin, 1978) or that categories for place of articulation arise from the second and third formant (F2 and F3) combination. Since the resolution of this debate remains unclear, we will use a simplified scheme with two levels of speech perception: an acoustical and a phonological one. The acoustic level is characterized as non-speech specific and is common to non-human animals and human babies before six months of age. As for the phonological level of perception, it is both speech- and language-specific. Combined results gathered with diverse methods (Multi-Unit-Activity, Current Source Density, intra-cortical and scalp recordings of cortical activity) have provided evidence of the neurophysiological correlates of these two levels of voicing perception. Single-unit activity recordings in the cat auditory nerve (Sinex & McDonald, 1988; 1989), in the inferior colliculus (Chen et al., 1996; Chen & Sinex, 1999) and in the primary auditory cortex of monkeys (Steinschneider et al., 2003) and of humans (Liégeois-Chauvel et al., 1999) have provided some support for a hierarchical functional organization of the perceptual system.

Behavioural experiments have demonstrated that animals (Kuhl & Miller, 1975; 1978) and infants below six months of age raised in diverse linguistic backgrounds (Eimas et al., 1971; Lasky et al., 1975) share common voicing categories delineated by -30 ms and +30 ms VOT boundaries (Abramson & Lisker, 1970a). By analogy with the "language-universal" categories of Miller and Eimas (1996), defined as the initial categories according to which the initial acoustic space is partitioned, we will use "universal boundaries" throughout the chapter to refer to the initial boundaries (-30 and +30 ms VOT) that delineate the voicing continuum, i.e. the acoustic boundaries to which animals and infants before six months of age are sensitive.

Other behavioural and electrophysiological studies have found evidence of the maturation from a universal and acoustic mode to a phonological mode of perception (e.g. Werker & Tees, 1984; Hoonhorst et al., submitted) according to rules of the mother tongue. Indeed, it has been shown for voicing that the two universal boundaries (-30 and +30 ms) are used in Thai (Donald, 1978), whereas in English (Lisker & Abramson, 1967), only the +30 ms VOT boundary remains relevant. In French, Spanish, Polish, Dutch, Hebrew and Arabic (Serniclaes, 1987; Williams, 1977; Flege & Eefting, 1986; Maassen et al. , 2001; Horev et al., 2007; Yeni-Komshian et al., 1977), none of the universal boundaries are relevant. Indeed, a new phonological boundary located at 0 ms VOT emerges, just midway between the two universal predispositions for perceiving voicing. The emergence of this new boundary centred on 0 ms VOT is the most commonly used mechanism in two-category languages. With its single boundary at +30 ms, English appears as an exception among the languages with two VOT categories. It is nevertheless on English that the vast majority of studies have been conducted.

1.3. CATEGORICAL PERCEPTION

Categorical perception (CP), which allows the definition of a finite percept on the basis of an infinite number of acoustic realizations, is the major characteristic of the hierarchical system for speech processing. The study of perceptual boundaries and their mechanisms is therefore at the heart of research on speech perception.

Categorical perception is frequently presented as a transform by which continuous physical variations are encompassed into discrete perceptual categories, i.e. there is an analog-to-digital transformation (Harnad, 1987). Identification and discrimination tasks have been extensively used to find evidence of CP. While identification requires labelling auditory stimuli, discrimination requires the subject to determine whether pairs of stimuli are identical or different. Categorical perception is often presented as the fact that we are only able to discriminate stimuli that do not have the same labelling. However, according to Liberman et al.. (1957), who first defined this phenomenon, CP does not imply an all-or-none capacity but refers to the observation that the contrasts between sounds separated by the same acoustic distance and belonging to different phoneme categories are more easily discriminated than those inside categories (Liberman et al., 1957). Carney et al. (1977) reinforced this relative nature of the CP phenomenon by emphasizing *"the improved discrimination of stimuli near a category boundary" (p. 969).*

Although the hierarchical organization as well as the categorical mode of speech perception is firmly established, their physiological correlates remain to be better delineated. Determining the link between basic auditory mechanisms and the perception of voicing is the core interest of the research presented below.

1.4. NEURAL ENCODING OF VOICING

The comparison between humans and non-human animals suggests that VOT universal boundaries, located at -30 and +30 ms, have developed according to constraints imposed by the auditory system. Several studies have been devoted to the understanding of the physiological correlates underlying these boundaries.

In 1959, Hirsh distinguished two psychoacoustical abilities: one was the minimal delay that must separate two sounds in order for each of them to be perceived independently and the other concerned the minimal delay necessary to allow the determination of their temporal order (i.e. which one appears first). The conclusions of the various experiments conducted with different stimuli presented in Hirsh's study were that while only two ms are sufficient for a subject to distinguish the presence of two sounds, about 20 ms are needed to determine the temporal order of the same two sounds. This difference by a factor of 10 is, according to Hirsh, related to the involvement of two different mechanisms, i.e. *"more central structures for the anatomical and physiological correlates" (p. 767)* must be involved in the second task. This higher threshold of the perceptive system which determines the temporal order between two successive events is not specific to auditory stimuli, since Piéron (1964) reached similar conclusions for the visual modality. Considering that temporal order is the critical cue to perceive the sign of VOT or TOT[1] (Pisoni, 1977) and that at least 20 ms are needed to determine temporal order between two sounds, several studies have sought to find a correlate of the corresponding neural code.

The neural code is defined by Eggermont (2001) as the link between behaviour (discrimination performances, for our purpose) and neural activity. Because by definition discrimination implies two percepts, it is expected that discrimination between two stimuli occurs as soon as their two neural representations are sufficiently different as to evoke different percepts.

Regarding the +30 ms VOT boundary, several studies have suggested that the neural code for VOT values greater than 30 ms is a double-peaked *("double-on")* response time-locked to closure release and voicing onset as opposed to a single-peak *("single-on")* response for shorter VOT values. In this respect, it is worth noting that the majority of the world's languages make the most of this neurophysiological signature by producing voiced and voiceless phonemes with VOT values strategically positioned with respect to the single- vs double-on response boundaries.

---

1 Tone Onset Time is the non-speech analogue of VOT and corresponds to the time elapsed between two tone onsets.

The following section presents some of the key results in the field of neural encoding of voicing.

1.4.1. DATA ON ANIMALS

Testing the discrimination abilities of Macaque monkeys on a /bae-dae-gae/ continuum, Kuhl and Padden (1983) showed that they were sensitive to the same boundaries as human beings, demonstrating in this way that neither categorical perception nor the sensitivity to acoustic contrasts are human-specific. Acoustic boundaries were therefore associated to natural psychophysical boundaries (Kuhl & Miller, 1975) and attributed to auditory constraints that could serve as natural markers to shape the perceptive map.

Further evidence of the contribution of universal boundaries to categorical perception was given by Sinex and McDonald in numerous studies (e.g. 1988; 1989) in which they recorded the discharge pattern of the auditory nerve fibre responses in chinchillas. Results of these studies highlighted the role of neural variability in perceiving acoustic categories. Indeed, Sinex and McDonald (ibid) showed that neural representations of voicing in the auditory nerve are non-linear since the variance in the latency of neural responses is far more important for within-category exemplars of a stimulus than for between-category exemplars. This high degree of uncertainty within categories was responsible for weaker discrimination performances.

This non-linear neural encoding of linear acoustic changes was also shown by Chen et al. (1996) in the discharge pattern of the inferior colliculus of chinchillas and by Steinschneider et al. (1994; 1995) and Steinschneider et al. (2003) in the primary auditory cortex of monkeys. More specifically, Steinschneider et al. (1995) described two patterns of neuron discharge responses when animals were submitted to stimuli varying in VOT values from 0 to 60 ms with 20 ms VOT steps. Stimuli like /da/, with a VOT value shorter than 20 ms, elicited a *"single-on response"* time-locked to closure release whereas /ta/ stimuli elicited a *"double-on response"* time-locked to both closure release and voicing onset. Interestingly, this differential pattern of responses according to the VOT values is the same as that observed by Sinex and McDonald (1988) in the auditory nerve fibres but is different from the one recorded in thalamocortical fibres (Steinschneider et al., 1994). Responses recorded in the primary auditory cortex are indeed characterized by transient time-locked responses on both closure release and voicing onset whereas neural responses in thalamocortical fibres are characterized by a time-locked response on closure release followed by a phase-locked repetitive response during vocal fold vibrations. This led Steinschneider et al. (1994) to state that the transformation of the pattern of response between the thalamus and the auditory cortex, i.e. the accentuation of the transient onset components, is at the root of the voiced-voiceless distinction.

Whatever the relative roles of auditory nerve and cortical mechanisms in the build-up of the single- vs double-on neural code of VOT categories, the fact that it is expressed in the time-locked response pattern of many cortical neurons allows it to be studied by means of non-invasive scalp recordings.

1.4.2. DATA ON HUMANS

Dealing this time with the perception of human beings, Steinschneider et al. (1999) presented /ba-da-ga/ and /pa-ta-ka/ stimuli to English-speaking epileptic subjects while recording intra-cortical activity (Multi Unit Activity, Current Source Density, Auditory Evoked-Potentials – AEP) from the Heschl's gyrus, the planum temporale and the superior temporal gyrus. Results showed a differential pattern of results according to the VOT value: stimuli characterized by a VOT of 0 or 20 ms elicited a single-on response whereas a VOT of 40, 60 or 80 ms generated a double-on response time-locked to closure release and voicing onset. Results led these authors to suggest that a 20 ms refractory period after closure release is at the root of this differential response pattern. Only stimuli with a VOT longer than at least 20 ms would be able to elicit the second transient response associated with voicing onset. These results stressed the link between the psychoacoustical boundary (+30 ms in English), typically obtained with identification and discrimination tasks, and the auditory constraints that underlie this sensitivity. Simos et al. (1998a; 1998b) also highlighted this link by showing a non-linear decrease in the N100 magnetic response amplitude when subjects were presented with TOT stimuli with values increasing from +20 to +40 ms. Simos et al. (1998) showed the same positive correlation between the amplitude of evoked N100 magnetic field (N100m) and VOT values with /ga-ka/ stimuli.

Regarding the representation of voicing in the auditory cortex, Steinschneider et al. (1999; 2005) showed that categorical perception of voicing relies in particular on primary and secondary auditory cortical fields. They found evidence that the anterior portion of Heschl's gyrus, which corresponds to the primary auditory cortex, is more specialized than the posterior portion in the representation of the two transient events of VOT, i.e. closure release and voicing onset. More specifically, electrodes localized in the lateral sites of the anterior portion of Heschl's gyrus provided larger responses time-locked to voicing onset relative to responses time-locked to closure release than electrodes localized in central and medial sites. Using surface recorded cerebral evoked magnetic fields, Simos et al. (1998a; b) demonstrated a more medial localization of the N100m for stimuli with VOT values of 40 and 60 ms than for those with 0 and 20 ms VOT values. Although they used quite different methods, these two studies suggest that the detailed representation of voicing is different between different cortical regions.

As far as hemispheric lateralization is concerned, Liégeois-Chauvel et al. (1999) demonstrated the specialization of the left Heschl's gyrus for processing transient acoustic information contained in voiced and voiceless syllables in human beings while general temporal processing in animals is treated bilaterally in the primary auditory cortex. Trébuchon-Da Fonséca et al. (2005) reached the same conclusions with /ba-pa/ stimuli. This left hemispheric dominance for the processing of VOT was, however, not supported by Steinschneider et al. (2005), who obtained the same results when recording neural responses in the right Heschl's gyrus. Given the possible role of the preexisting epileptogenic lesions in the subjects participating in the latter two studies, one must remain cautious before drawing definite conclusions on lateralization of the VOT-related double-on response.

Concerning the correspondence between intra-cortical recordings and scalp recordings, Trébuchon-Da Fonséca et al. (2005) compared both methodologies and obtained comparable results. As different locations in

the Heschl's gyrus respond differently to the transient events contained in voiced and voiceless stimuli, one must be prepared when performing scalp recordings to obtain, as stated by Steinschneider et al. (2003), *"a composite wave that reflects activation of multiple auditory cortical fields, each with its own capacity to follow temporal features of complex sounds" (p. 318).*
Sharma and Dorman (1999) recorded scalp auditory evoked-potentials and found a single-on response with short VOT values (perceived as /da/) as opposed to a double-on response pattern (perceived as /ta/) for longer VOT values. The first peak, labelled N100', was evoked by the closure release, and the second, labelled N100, by voicing onset. Although this result led Sharma and Dorman to suggest that the morphology of the N100 component was a neurophysiological correlate of voicing perception, they later provided evidence for a different view (Sharma & Dorman, 2000). In the latter study, they presented syllables with different places of articulation. When performing identification and discrimination tasks, English-speaking subjects showed a VOT perceptual boundary centred on 27.5 ms for the /ba-pa/ continuum and on 46 ms for the /ga-ka/ continuum. This well-known shift of the VOT boundary according to the place of articulation (the consonants with more back articulation display longer VOTs: Lisker & Abramson, 1967; for the trade-off between F1 and VOT associated with this shift, see Summerfield & Haggard, 1977; Parker, 1988) was not associated with a corresponding shift in the neurophysiological boundary between the double- and single-on patterns. It was therefore concluded that the N100 morphology (single vs double-peak) was not a reliable indicator of voicing contrast. Although a correspondence between the psycho-acoustic boundary and the physiological one was found by Stein-schneider et al. (2005) with intra-cortical recordings when varying place of articulation, they acknowledged that the matching between these two types of boundaries was not perfect, showing in this way the complexity of the trade-offs between acoustic events involved in the perception of voicing.
As to the N100 morphology, Eggermont and Ponton (2002) concluded that it does not reflect cortical correlates of voicing perception but rather intrinsic properties of the auditory cortex that *"may have been exploited by speech production mechanisms and tailored to the various temporal contrasts that are found around the 30- to 50-ms range" (p. 95).* This could mean that

the appearance of a double-peak indexes the threshold of VOT values that can be reliably evaluated in terms of relative temporal order (Hirsh, 1959). Whereas VOT processing by the auditory cortex accounts for the universal acoustic boundaries, the perceptual boundaries in a phonological framework are language-specific and depend on the relationship between different features (Carden et al., 1981; Serniclaes & Wajskop, 1992).

It is therefore not surprising that several examples of the discrepancy between the N100 morphology boundary and the phonological boundary have been reported in different languages. An example of such dissociation was given by Sharma and Dorman (2000), who showed that Hindi- and English-speaking adults, who do not have the same phonological boundary for voicing, do however share the same N100 pattern of results. This result was replicated for Hebrew, a language for which neither the -30 nor the +30 ms universal boundary is relevant (Horev et al., 2007). Horev et al. (ibid) showed that /ba-pa/ stimuli with VOT values of -15 and +15 ms, which belonged to different phonological categories in Hebrew, evoked similar N100 components.

Understanding of the neurophysiological correlates of voicing perception in languages such as Hebrew, in which the phonological boundary is located around 0 ms, is particularly of interest. The emergence of this new phonological boundary, just midway between the two universal ones, is reputed to be based on mechanisms derived from our basic ability to determine the temporal relationships between two different acoustic events. Indeed, the 0 ms boundary corresponds to the perception of the temporal order between events with simultaneity as a boundary, not as a category. The mere accumulation of the outputs of the negative and positive VOT detectors would give rise to poor categorical perception: the 0 ms boundary is positioned in the middle of a 60 ms region (i.e. between -30 and +30 ms) in which neither negative VOT nor positive VOT are detected. The perception of temporal order would be completely ambiguous for the stimuli located inside this region if the outputs of the negative and positive VOT detectors were simply cumulated. Some kind of integration between VOT detectors must therefore be necessary for the categorical perception of temporal order, and behavioural data collected with adult French listeners support this assumption (Serniclaes, 1987; 2000). Labelling data collected with stimuli generated by factorial variation of negative and positive VOT suggest that outputs of the two VOT detectors interact in such a way that their boundaries converge to 0 ms, a process which has been referred to as "coupling". The higher complexity of temporal order perception is congruent with the fact that the neural correlates of the 0 ms VOT boundary are not reducible to those found for the processing of the universal VOT boundaries. Understanding these correlates is therefore of special interest.

2. THE PRESENT STUDY

We are not aware of any study having explored the electrophysiological N100 morphology over a single VOT continuum encompassing both the negative and the positive universal boundaries. Our study capitalized on the fact that the phonological boundary is centred on 0 ms in French to explore whether evidence can be found of the two universal boundaries by recording AEP. Should these neurophysiological correlates be available, insight into the mechanism by which they contribute to the phonological boundary could be gained by manipulating them.

The aim of this study was to determine whether /də-tə/ syllables with VOT values varying from -75 to +75 ms presented to French-speaking subjects would show an N100 correlate of the two universal boundaries. As the N100 component reflects the encoding of the successive events that compose the stimuli, it was expected that for positive VOT values greater than +30 ms, the N100 component would be composed of two peaks, the first evoked by closure release and the second by voicing onset. For negative VOT values longer than -30 ms, the N100 component should also be double-peaked but with the first peak evoked by voicing onset and the second by closure release. Finally, for VOT values between -30 and +30 ms, the N100 should be single peaked.

This study involves two specific features that set it apart from other studies, one pertaining to the selection of French-speaking subjects and another pertaining to the stimuli used. French is indeed characterized, in contrast to English, by a mismatch between the acoustic (-30 and +30 ms VOT) and the phonological (0 ms VOT) boundaries. This discrepancy enabled us to unambiguously dissociate the effects of the acoustic and phonological boundaries on the morphology of the N100 component. As to the stimuli, the use of symmetrical positive and negative VOT values encompassing the -75 to +75 ms range allowed us to investigate both universal VOT boundaries.

Our working hypothesis was that if the N100 morphology is the neurophysiological correlate of basic acoustic mechanisms implied in voicing perception, we should observe a double-peak response along the acoustic universal boundaries, even though the phonological boundary to which French-speaking subjects are sensitive does not correspond to either of these boundaries. Indeed, even though the universal boundaries are no longer phonologically relevant in French after six months of age (Hoonhorst et al., submitted), the demonstration that there still exist neurophysiological correlates of the ability to discriminate these initial voicing boundaries would give some support to the assertion that the phonological mode of perception corresponds to a higher level of perception which is based on basic auditory mechanisms of which we can still find evidence in adult subjects.

2.1. METHODS

2.1.1. PARTICIPANTS

Five native French speakers (four women and one man) aged 22–35 years (mean: 28 years and 5 months) volunteered to participate in the study. All were right-handed according to the Edinburgh Handedness Inventory (Oldfield, 1971) questionnaire and reported normal hearing.

2.1.2. STIMULI

Speech stimuli were synthesized syllables composed of the apical stop consonant /d/ or /t/ followed by the neutral vowel /ə/ so as to limit contextual effects (Serniclaes, 2005). Six syllables with VOTs varying from -75 ms to +75 ms with a 30 ms acoustic step were created.

Stimuli were generated by a parallel formant synthesizer (Klatt, 1980) provided by R. Carré (http://www.tsi.enst.fr/~carre/). The onsets of the

initial frequency transitions of F1, F2 and F3 were 200, 2200 and 3100 Hz, respectively. Steady state formant frequencies were 500, 1500 and 2500 Hz, respectively. The F0 value was 120 Hz, and the transitions lasted 20 ms. The overall duration of all syllables was 200 ms (Figure 1). Negative VOT was synthesized with periodic energy (60 dB), F1 bandwidth at 50 Hz, and F2 and F3 bandwidths both at 600 Hz. Positive VOT was synthesized with aperiodic energy (30 dB), with F1 bandwidth at 600 Hz, and F2 and F3 bandwidths at 70 and 100 Hz, respectively. The voiced vocalic segment was synthesized with periodic energy (60 dB) and with F1, F2 and F3 bandwidths at 50, 70 and 100 Hz, respectively.
Results of research conducted by Medina and Serniclaes (2006) with the same stimuli showed that French-speaking adults' identification boundary was centred on 0 ms VOT and that adults' AX discrimination scores peaked for the contrast straddling this boundary.

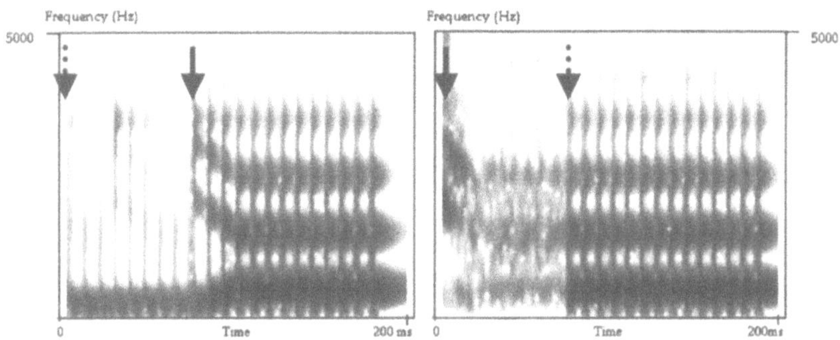

Figure 1: /də/ and /tə/ stimuli with -75 ms VOT (left) and +75 ms VOT (right). The solid black arrow represents closure release and the dotted black arrow the onset of voicing.

2.1.3. Procedure

Threshold measurement: Subjects were tested in a sound-attenuated booth using an adaptive three-alternative forced choice procedure, with a three-down, one-up decision rule using Tucker-Davis Technologies (TDT) hardware and software (System III ; PsychRP 1.05). The target stimulus used for measuring the auditory threshold was one of the six

stimuli used in the experiment, a /də/ syllable characterized by a VOT value of -45 ms. The inter-stimulus-interval (ISI) lasted 500 ms.
Each trial, composed of three intervals marked by lights, one containing the target sound, was initiated by the subject. Intensity was first reduced in 5 dB steps until the fourth reversal occurred and then by 2 dB steps. The procedure stopped after 12 reversals and the first four reversals were excluded from the calculation of the average threshold. The threshold was measured two to three times. The final threshold corresponded to the mean threshold separated by less than 2 dB, i.e. the reference used for delivering the stimuli 50 dB above the individual threshold in the electrophysiological recordings.

EEG recording: Subjects were seated in a comfortable armchair. They passively listened to auditory stimuli while reading a book of their choice. They could take a break whenever they wished.
Stimuli were presented in 30 blocks of 360 stimuli, each lasting +/- seven minutes depending on the ISI, which was randomized and fluctuated between 500 and 1500 ms. Each block was composed of 60 exemplars of each stimulus delivered in a pseudo-randomized order at 50 dB SL, binaurally through insert earphones (ER-1 TUBEPHONE, Etymotic Research) connected to eartips (12 mm) placed in the ear canal through a 280 mm long silicon tubing. The pseudo-randomized sequence was created on an Eevoke device (ANT Software, The Netherlands) and interfaced with TDT hardware (System III), the former to control for presentation order and the latter to provide digital-to-analog conversion and to control for intensity.
Brain electrical activity was recorded using the 32-channel ASA EEG/ERP system (ANT). Thirty-two electrodes were embedded in a waveguard cap (ANT) based on the 10-20 system. The tip of the nose was taken as the reference and an electrode placed on the forearm served as ground. Electro-ocular activity (EOG) was monitored from two bipolar pairs of Bluesky electrodes located at the outer lateral canthi and the infra- and supra-orbital areas of the left eye. Impedances were kept below 5 kΩ.

2.1.4. DATA ANALYSIS

The signal was amplified (x20 for EEG and EOG channels), band-pass filtered (0.1–30 Hz) and continuously digitised with a sampling rate of 512 Hz. Continuous EEG was segmented in 1000 ms epochs including a 200 ms pre-stimulus onset baseline on which baseline correction was carried out. Responses exceeding +/-100 μV were excluded from averaging. An averaged waveform for each of the six stimuli was computed for each subject and across subjects to obtain grand averaged waveforms. Data analysis consisted of a visual examination for the presence of a single- or a double-peak pattern. Two time windows were delineated, the first one lasting from 0 to 120 ms to search for the first peak and the second one from 120 to 200 ms to search for the second peak (Sharma et al., 2000). A double-peak pattern was acknowledged only if two peaks were segregated between the two pre-defined time windows covering their respective expected latencies. Owing to the small number of subjects (five) involved in this pilot study, no statistical analyses were performed.

2.2. RESULTS

The N100 component was observed for each VOT value (e.g. for +75 ms VOT stimuli, Figure 2). Its scalp distribution showed the classic polarity reversal across the Sylvian fissure.

Two distinct N100 morphologies can be dissociated relative to the VOT value: VOT values between -30 ms and +30 ms gave rise to one single N100 peak while VOT values outside the -30 ms to +30 ms range evoked a double-peaked N100, at least for temporo-parietal localizations. For the sake of clarity, we will label single peaks as N100 and designate the two components of double-peaked waveforms as N100c or N100v, according to which acoustic event (closure release or voicing onset), on the basis of the peak latency, evoked the component.

For most electrodes on the scalp convexity (see Figure 2), a double-on response, composed of N100c followed by N100v, was easily observed for +45 and +75 ms VOT stimuli whereas single-on responses were associated with -15 and +15 ms VOT stimuli. For long negative VOT values (-75 and -45 ms), double-on responses composed of N100v followed by N100c were observed at parietal (Pz) and temporal (T7, T8) electrodes only. For +75 ms VOT stimuli, a more complex pattern, composed of three negative peaks, was observed at the T7 and T8 electrodes.

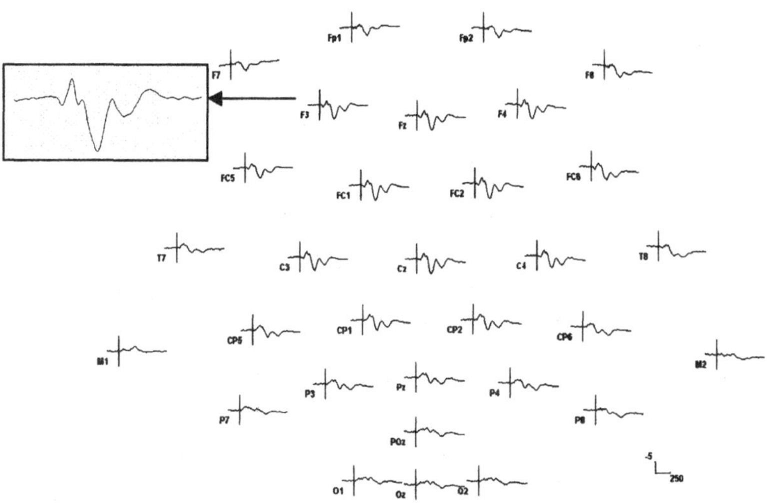

Figure 2: Grand averaged AEP evoked by +75 ms VOT stimulus. The vertical black line represents stimulus onset.

Since we did not notice any difference according to electrode lateralization and because the double-peak pattern was only observed for parietal and temporal electrodes in the negative VOT region, only waveforms recorded at the Cz, Fz , Pz, T7 and T8 electrodes (Figures 3, 4, 5, 6 and 7) are shown.

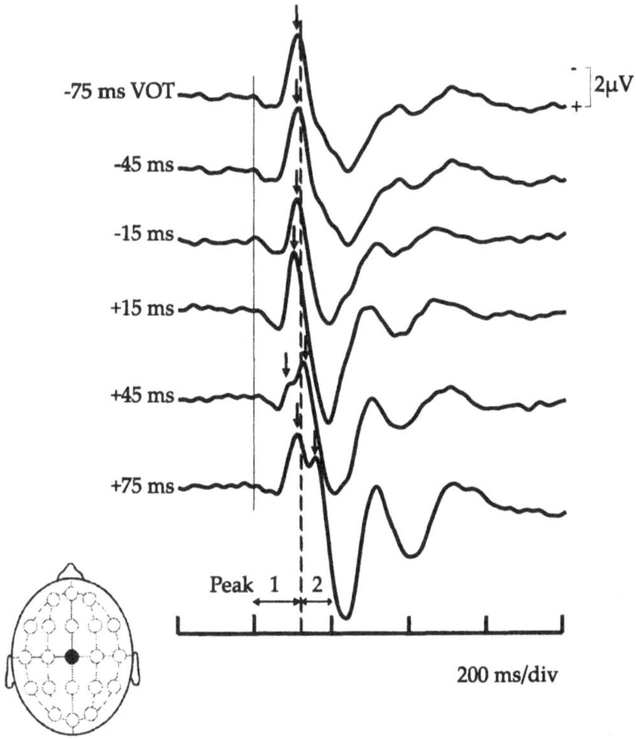

Figure 3: Grand averaged AEP recorded at the Cz electrode for -75, -45 and -15, +15, +45 and +75 ms VOT stimuli. The thin vertical black line represents stimulus onset. The dashed vertical black line delineates the limit between the two temporal windows (from 0 to 120 ms and from 120 to 200 ms, respectively) used to locate the first and the second peaks, marked by arrows.

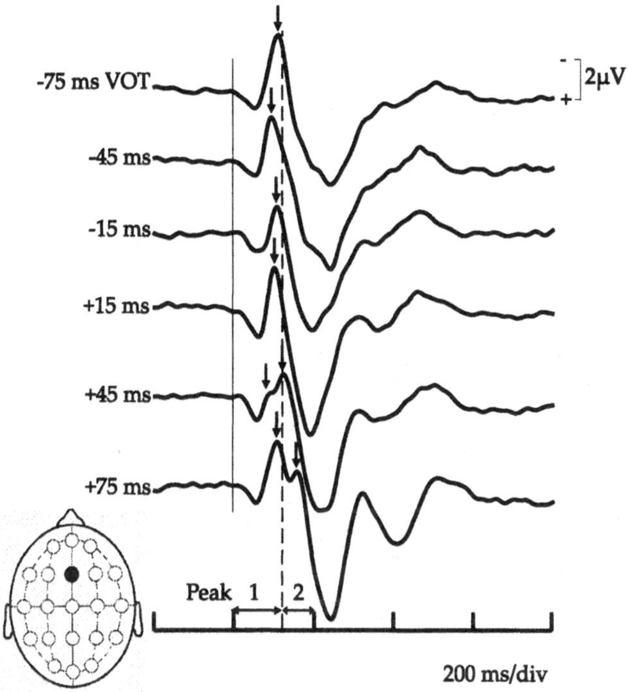

Figure 4: Grand averaged AEP recorded at the Fz electrode for -75, -45 and -15, +15, +45 and +75 ms VOT stimuli. The thin vertical black line represents stimulus onset. The dashed vertical black line delineates the limit between the two temporal windows (from 0 to 120 ms and from 120 to 200 ms, respectively) used to locate the first and the second peaks, marked by arrows.

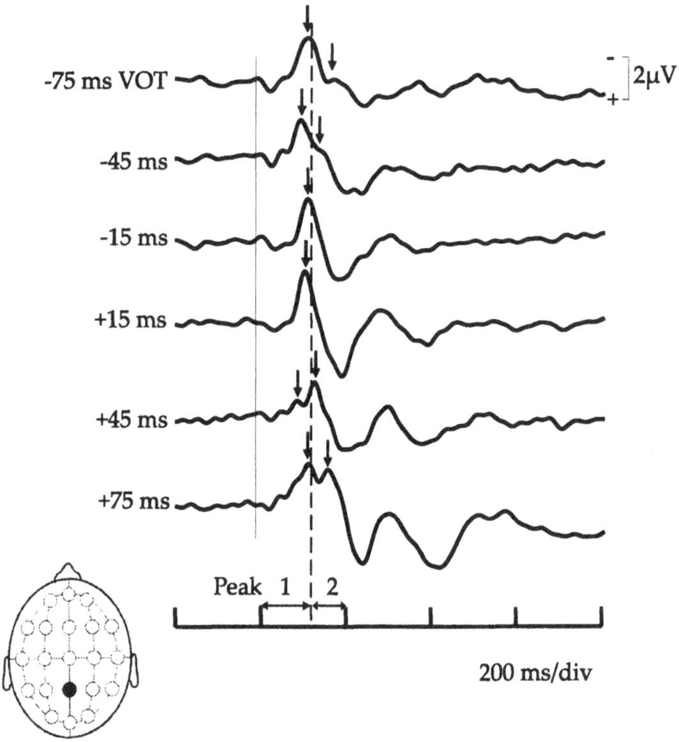

Figure 5: Grand averaged AEP recorded at the Pz electrode for -75, -45 and -15, +15, +45 and +75 ms VOT stimuli. The thin vertical black line represents stimulus onset. The dashed vertical black line delineates the limit between the two temporal windows (from 0 to 120 ms and from 120 to 200 ms, respectively) used to locate the first and the second peaks, marked by arrows.

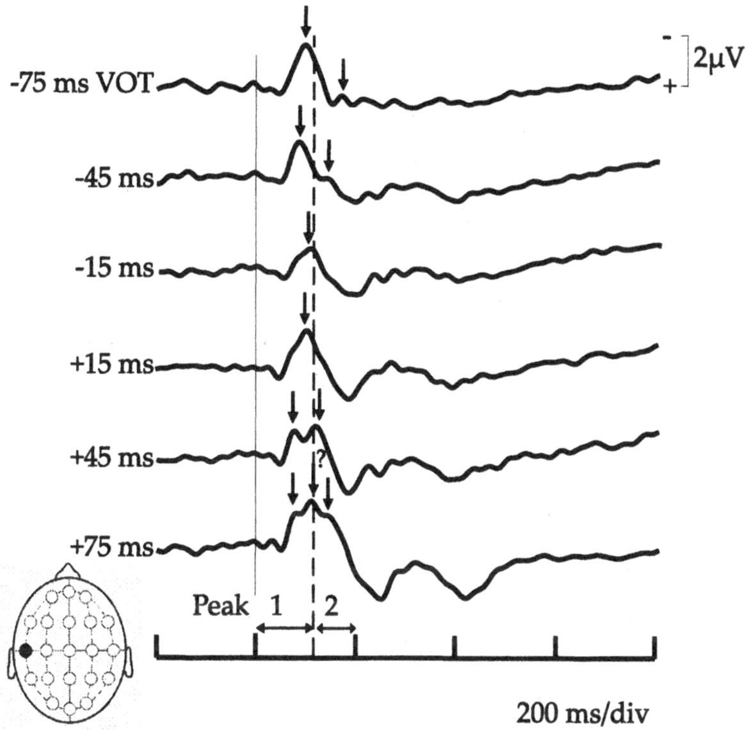

Figure 6: Grand averaged AEP recorded at the T7 electrode for -75, -45 and -15, +15, +45 and +75 ms VOT stimuli. The thin vertical black line represents stimulus onset. The dashed vertical black line delineates the limit between the two temporal windows (from 0 to 120 ms and from 120 to 200 ms, respectively) used to locate the first and the second peaks, marked by arrows. An unexpected middle peak (arrow with a question mark) is present for +75 ms VOT.

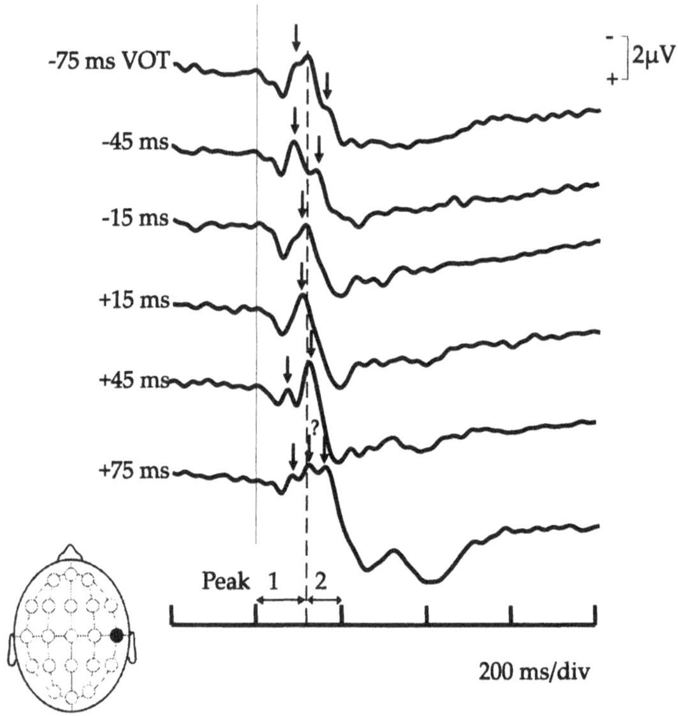

Figure 7: Grand averaged AEP recorded at the T8 electrode for -75, -45 and -15, +15, +45 and +75 ms VOT stimuli. The thin vertical black line represents stimulus onset. The dashed vertical black line delineates the limit between the two temporal windows (from 0 to 120 ms and from 120 to 200 ms, respectively) used to locate the first and the second peaks, marked by arrows. An unexpected middle peak (arrow with a question mark) is present for +75 ms VOT.

2.3. Discussion

The results presented above clearly show that, for French-speaking subjects, whose phonological boundary is distinct from the universal acoustic ones, there is still a clear evoked-potential correlate of the acoustic boundaries. This trace takes the common form of a double-on N100 wave appearing when VOT values exceed both the positive and negative universal boundaries. The expression of the double-on pattern on the scalp is, however, more widespread for positive than for negative VOT values. In the latter case, the double-on pattern is restricted to temporo-parietal electrodes.

The results obtained in the positive VOT region replicate, for French-speaking subjects, what has already been shown for English-speaking subjects. This adds weight to the demonstration that the double-on effect is independent of the phonological percepts (Sharma & Dorman, 2000). To the best of our knowledge, this is the first time that a scalp-recorded double-on boundary effect has been demonstrated at the level of the negative acoustic boundary. The results therefore confirmed our working hypothesis, according to which there remains a N100 trace of the basic neurophysiological mechanism from which phonological percepts are developed. Also, it is worth noting that whatever the region of the VOT continuum exploited by productions of a particular language, the voiced-voiceless opposition is associated with the single- vs double-on responses. Indeed, the opposition between long-lead (with VOT productions between -125 and -75 ms; Lisker & Abramson, 1964) and short-lag voicing distributions (with VOT productions between 0 and +25 ms; ibid) in French is echoed by differential double- vs single-on peaks of N100. English-speaking subjects benefit from the same correspondence. The short-lag distribution with VOT productions between 0 and +30 ms (associated with voiced phonemes; Kessinger & Blumstein, 1997) is coded by a single-peaked N100 waveform whereas the long-lag distribution with VOT productions between 50 and 170 ms (associated with voiceless phonemes; ibid) is coded by double-peaked N100.

An unanticipated finding was the differential scalp topography of the double-on response between the positive and the negative VOT regions. The underlying reason for this peculiar distribution remains to be

investigated. A first hypothesis that can be put forward is that there is a difference in the relative contributions of the several cortical areas engaged in the perception of voicing (primary auditory cortex, anterior auditory field, secondary auditory cortex as showed by Eggermont, 2000) and of the different portions of the anterior part of the Heschl's gyrus (lateral, central and medial as showed by Steinschneider et al., 2005). This difference in the cortical contributions is likely to be due to different interactions between the successive acoustic events according to their temporal order. For consonants characterized by a positive VOT value, the first formant transition plays an additional significant role (Burnham et al., 1991) while for consonants characterized by a negative VOT value the forward masking effect between the voicing bar and the closure release is larger. These acoustical interactions contribute to the greater psychoacoustic saliency described by Stevens and Klatt (1974) for phonemes with a positive VOT value.
As regards the forward masking effect, Eggermont (1995) showed that the characteristics (frequency, duration, amplitude) of the first feature that evokes the first N100 have a direct influence on the amplitude of the second response evoked by the second feature. Eggermont (1995) pointed out *"a strong interaction, reminiscent of forward masking, between the efficacy of the voiceless burst* [i.e. closure release] *in evoking neural activity and the size of the subsequent response to the onset of response" (p. 919).*
Whatever the genuine mechanism underlying the difference in the scalp topography for symmetrical positive and negative VOT values (-75 vs +75 ms and -45 vs +45 ms), the results suggest that it reflects the neural code for determining the VOT sign.
The differential contribution of the different cortical areas engaged in the perception of voicing (Eggermont, 2000) and of the different portions of the auditory cortex (i.e. lateral, central and medial; Steinschneider et al., 2005) in the perception of voicing could also explain the unanticipated pattern of three negative responses obtained at the T7 and T8 electrodes for the +75 ms VOT stimulus. One hypothesis for the appearance of the middle peak could be that this response is the result of the algebraic sum of different neuronal subpopulations with slightly different latencies.
Finally, the fact that we did not notice any lateralization effect reinforced the conclusions drawn by Shtyrov et al. (2000), who stated that *"P1, N100 and P2 responses, being non-specific responses to acoustic stimuli, are*

insensitive to the speech context of the sound and cannot be used for determining the brain's hemisphere dominant in speech perception" (p. 2896). These preliminary results open the perspective of assessing how the acoustic boundaries are integrated to give rise to the phonological boundary. The idea is to manipulate the acoustic boundaries either by studying pathologies such as acquired sensory hearing loss (Tremblay et al., 2003), simulated hearing loss (Martin et al., 1997), and auditory-based learning disorders (Cunningham et al., 2000) in which they may be modified or by using auditory training techniques (Tremblay & Kraus, 2002).

3. CONCLUSION

In this chapter, we have summarized research aimed at cracking the neural code of voicing perception. The core idea underlying the present work was to seek neurophysiological correlates of the initial and universal basic auditory sensitivity that we share with animals and which underlies our ability to process the temporal order between two events. No matter whether our mother tongue has selected one of these initial acoustic boundaries for phonological use (e.g. English) or has built an entirely new phonological boundary (e.g. French), our data show that it remains possible to non-invasively record a neurophysiological signature of this primary ability from the scalp.

The single- vs double-on N100 recorded in our experiment with French-speaking subjects for either positive or negative VOT values seems a promising tool to investigate the encoding of voicing. A logical next step is to investigate how modifications of the basic acoustic boundaries influence the phonological percepts.

REFERENCES

Abramson, A.S. (1977). Laryngeal timing in consonant distinctions. *Phonetica* 34, 295-303.

Abramson, A.S. & Lisker, L. (1970a). Discriminability along the voice onset time continuum: Cross-language tests. In B. Hala, M. Romportl and P. Janota (eds.) *Proceedings of the 6th International Congress of Phonetic Sciences, Prague 1967*, 569-573, Prague: Academia.

Abramson, A.S. & Lisker, L. (1970b). Voice timing perception in Spanish word initial stops. *Journal of Phonetics* 1, 1-8.

Burnham, D.K. (1986). Developmental loss of speech perception: Exposure to and experience with a first language. *Applied Psycholinguistics* 7, 207-240.

Burnham, D.K., Earnshaw, L. J., and Clark, J. E. (1991). Development of categorical identification of native and non-native bilabial stops: Infants, children and adults. *Journal of Child Language* 18, 231-260.

Carden, G., Levitt, A., Jusczyk, P.W., and Walley, A. (1981). Evidence for phonetic processing of cues to place of articulation: Perceived manner affects perceived place. *Perception and Psychophysics* 29, 26-36.

Carney, A.E., Widin, G.P., and Viemeister, N.F. (1977). Non categorical perception of stop consonants differing in VOT. *Journal of the Acoustical Society of America* 62, 961-970.

Chen, G.D., Nuding, S.C., Narayan, S.S., and Sinex, D.G. (1996). Responses of single neurons in the chinchilla inferior colliculus to consonant-vowel syllables differing in voice-onset-time. *Auditory Neuroscience* 3, 179-198.

Chen, G.D. & Sinex, D.G. (1999). Effects of interaural time differences on the responses of chinchilla inferior colliculus neurons to consonant-vowel syllables. *Hearing Research* 138, 29-44.

Cunningham, J., Nicol, T., Zecker, S., and Kraus, N. (2000). Speech-evoked neurophysiologic responses in children with learning problems: Development and behavioral correlates of perception. *Ear & Hearing* 21, 554-568.

Donald, S.L. (1978). *The perception of voicing contrasts in Thai and English.* University of Connecticut at Storrs : Dissertation.

Eggermont, J.J. (1995). Representation of a voice onset time continuum in primary auditory cortex of the cat. *Journal of the Acoustical Society of America* 98, 911-920.

Eggermont, J.J. (2000). Sound-induced synchronization of neural activity between and within three auditory cortical areas. *Journal of Neurophysiology* 83, 2708-2722.

Eggermont, J.J. (2001). Between sound and perception: Reviewing the search for a neural code. *Hearing Research* 157, 1-42.

Eggermont, J.J. & Ponton, C.W. (2002). The neurophysiology of auditory perception: From single-units to evoked-potentials. *Audiology & Neuro-Otology* 7, 71-99.

Eimas, P.D., Siqueland, E.R., Jusczyk, P., and Vigorito, J. (1971). Speech perception in infants. *Science* 171, 303-306.

Flege, J. (1988). The production and perception of speech sounds in a foreign language. In H. Winitz (ed.). *Human communication and its disorders: A review.* Norwood, NJ: Ablex, 224-401.

Flege, J. (1992). The intelligibility of English vowels spoken by British and Dutch talkers. In R. Kent (ed.). *Intelligibility and Speech Disorders: Theory, Measurement and Management*. Amsterdam: Benjamins, 157-232.

Flege, J. & Eefting, W. (1986). Linguistic and developmental effects on the production and perception of stop consonants. *Phonetica* 43, 155-171.

Harnad, S. (1987). *Categorical perception: The groundwork of cognition*. New York: Cambridge University Press.

Hillenbrand, J. (1984). Perception of sine-wave analogs of voice onset time stimuli. *Journal of the Acoustical Society of America* 75, 231-340.

Hirsh, I.J. (1959). Auditory perception of temporal order. *Journal of the Acoustical Society of America* 31, 759-767.

Hoonhorst, I., Colin, C., Markessis, E., Radeau, M., Deltenre, P., and Serniclaes, W. (submitted). French native speakers in the making: When a phonological boundary does not match universal predispositions.

Horev, N., Most, T., and Pratt, H. (2007). Categorical perception of speech (VOT) and analogous non speech (FOT) signals: Behavioral and electrophysiological correlates. *Ear & Hearing* 28, 111-128.

Kessinger, R., & Blumstein, S. (1997). Effects of speaking rate on voice-onset time in Thai, French, and English. *Journal of Phonetics 25*, 143-168.

Klatt, D.H. (1980). Software for a cascade/parallel formant synthesizer. *Journal of the Acoustical Society of America* 67, 971-995.

Kuhl, P.K. & Miller, J.D. (1975). Speech perception by the chinchilla: Voiced-voiceless distinction in alveolar plosive consonants. *Science* 190, 69-72.

Kuhl, P.K. & Miller, J.D. (1978). Speech perception by the chinchilla: Identification functions for synthetic VOT stimuli. *Journal of the Acoustical Society of America* 63, 905-917.

Kuhl, P.K. & Padden, D.M. (1983). Enhanced discriminability at the phonetic boundaries for the place feature in macaques. *Journal of the Acoustical Society of America* 73, 1003-1010.

Lasky, R.E., Syrdal-Lasky, A., and Klein, R.E. (1975). VOT discrimination by four to six and a half month old infants from Spanish environment. *Journal of Experimental Child Psychology* 20, 215-225.

Liberman, A.M., Harris, K.S., Hoffman, K.S., and Griffith, B.C. (1957). The discrimination of speech sounds within and across phoneme boundaries. *Journal of Experimental Psychology* 54, 358-368.

Liégeois-Chauvel, C., de Graaf, J.B., Laguitton, V., and Chauvel, P. (1999). Specialization of left auditory cortex for speech perception in Man depends on temporal coding. *Cerebral Cortex* 9, 484-496.

Lisker, L. & Abramson, A.S. (1967). Some effects of context on voice onset time in English stops. *Language and Speech* 10, 1-28.

Lisker, L., Liberman, A.M., Erickson, D.M., and Dechovitz, D. (1978). On pushing the voice onset time boundary about. *Language and Speech* 20, 209-216.

Maassen, B., Groenen, P., Crul, T., Assman-Hulsmans, C., and Gabreëls, F. (2001). Identification and discrimination of voicing and place of articulation in developmental dyslexia. *Clinical Linguistics and Phonetics* 15, 319-339.

Martin, B.A., Sigal, A., Kurtzberg, D., and Stapells, D.R. (1997). The effects of decreased audibility produced by high-pass noise masking on cortical event-related potentials to speech sounds /ba/ and /da/. *Journal of the Acoustical Society of America* 101, 1585-99.

Medina, V. & Serniclaes, W. (2006). Late development of the categorical perception of speech sounds in pre-adolescent children. *ZAS Papers in Linguistics* 42, 13-32.

Miller, J.L. & Eimas, P.D. (1996). Internal structure of voicing categories in early infancy. *Perception & Psychophysics* 58, 1157-1167.

Oldfield, R.C. (1971). The assessment and analysis of handedness: The Edinburgh inventory. *Neuropsychologia* 9, 97-113.

Parker, E. (1988). Auditory constraints on the perception of voice-onset time: The influence of lower tone frequency on judgments of tone-onset simultaneity. *Journal of the Acoustical Society of America* 83, 1597-1607.

Piéron, H. (1964). *La sensation. Que sais-je?*: Presses Universitaires de France.

Pisoni, D.B. (1977). Identification and discrimination of the relative onset time of two-component tones: Implications for voicing perception in stops. *Journal of the Acoustical Society of America* 61, 1352-1361.

Saerens, M., Serniclaes, W., and Beeckmans, R. (1989). Acoustic versus contextual factors in stop voicing perception in spontaneous speech. *Language and Speech* 32, 291-314.

Serniclaes, W. (1987). *Etude expérimentale de la Perception du Trait de Voisement des Occlusives du Français.* Université Libre de Bruxelles: Unpublished Doctoral Thesis.

Serniclaes, W. (2000). La perception de la parole. In P. Escudier & J.L. Schwartz (eds.). *La parole: Des modèles cognitifs aux machines communicantes.* Paris: Hermes, Science Publications, 159-190.

Serniclaes, W. (2005). On the invariance of speech percepts. *ZAS Papers in Linguistics* 40, 177-194.

Serniclaes, W. & Wajskop, M. (1992). Phonetic versus acoustic account of feature interaction in speech perception. In J. Alegria, D. Holender, J. Junça de Morais, and M. Radeau (eds.) *Analytic Approaches to Human Cognition,* Proc. of the

Conference in Honour of Paul Bertelson, Brussels, June 1991. Amsterdam: North-Holland, 77-91.

Sharma, A. & Dorman, M.F. (1999). Cortical auditory evoked-potential correlates of categorical perception of voice onset time. *Journal of the Acoustical Society of America* 106, 1078-1083.

Sharma, A. & Dorman, M.F. (2000). Neurophysiologic correlates of cross-language phonetic perception. *Journal of the Acoustical Society of America* 107, 2697-2703.

Sharma, A., Marsh, C., and Dorman, M.F. (2000). Relationship between N1 evoked-potential morphology and the perception of voicing. *Journal of the Acoustical Society of America* 108, 3030-3035.

Shtyrov, Y., Kujala, T., Lyytinen, H., Ilmoniemi, R.J., and Näätänen R. (2000). Auditory cortex evoked magnetic fields and lateralization of speech processing. *NeuroReport* 11, 2893-2896.

Simon, C. & Fourcin, A.J. (1978). Cross-language study of speech-pattern learning. *Journal of the Acoustical Society of America* 63, 925-935.

Simos, P.G., Breier, J.I, Zouridakis, G., and Papanicolaou, A.C. (1998a). Magnetic fields elicited by a tone onset time continuum in humans. *Cognitive Brain Research* 6, 285-294.

Simos, P.G., Breier, J.I., Zouridakis, G., and Papanicolaou, A.C. (1998b). MEG correlates of categorical-like temporal cue perception in humans. *NeuroReport* 9, 2475-2479.

Simos, P.G., Diehl, R.L., Breier, J.I., Molis, M.R., Zouridakis, G., and Papanicolaou, A.C. (1998). MEG correlates of categorical perception of a voice onset time continuum in humans. *Cognitive Brain Research* 7, 215-219.

Sinex, D.G. & McDonald, L.P. (1988). Average discharge rate representation of voice onset time in the chinchilla auditory nerve. *Journal of the Acoustical Society of America* 83, 1817-1827.

Sinex, D.G. & McDonald, L.P. (1989). Synchronized discharge rate representation of voice onset time in the chinchilla auditory nerve. *Journal of the Acoustical Society of America* 85, 1995-2004.

Steinschneider, M., Fishman, Y.I., and Arezzo, J.C. (2003). Representation of the voice onset time (VOT) speech parameter in population responses within primary auditory cortex of the awake monkey. *Journal of the Acoustical Society of America* 114, 307-321.

Steinschneider, M., Schroeder, C.E., Arezzo, J.C., and Vaughan, H.G. (1994). Speech-evoked activity in primary auditory cortex: Effects of voice onset time. *Electroencephalography and Clinical Neurophysiology* 92, 30-43.

Steinschneider, M., Schroeder, C.E., Arezzo, J.C., and Vaughan, H.G. (1995). Physiologic correlates of the voice onset time boundary in primary cortex (A1) of the awake monkey: Temporal response patterns. *Brain & Language* 48, 326-340.

Steinschneider, M., Volkov, I.O., Fishman, Y.I., Oya, H., Arezzo, J.C, and Howard, M.A. (2005). Intracortical responses in human and monkey primary auditory cortex support a temporal processing mechanism for encoding of the voice onset time phonetic parameter. *Cerebral Cortex* 15, 170-186.

Steinschneider, M., Volkov, I.O., Noh, M.D., Garell, P.C., and Howard, M.A. (1999). Temporal encoding of the voice onset time phonetic parameter by field potentials recorded directly from human auditory cortex. *Journal of Neurophysiology* 82, 2346-2357.

Stevens, K.N. & Klatt, D.H. (1974). Role of formant transitions in the voiced-voiceless distinction for stops. *Journal of the Acoustical Society of America* 55, 653-659.

Summerfield, Q. & Haggard, M. (1974). Perceptual processing of multiple cues and contexts: Effects of following vowel on stop consonant voicing. *Journal of Phonetics* 2, 279-295.

Summerfield, Q. & Haggard, M. (1977). On the dissociation of spectral and temporal cues to the voicing distinction in initial stop consonants. *Journal of the Acoustical Society of America* 62, 435-448.

Trébuchon-Da Fonseca, A., Giraud, K., Badier, J.M., Chauvel, P., and Liégeois-Chauvel C. (2005). Hemispheric lateralization of voice onset time (VOT) comparison between depth and scalp EEG recordings. *NeuroImage* 27, 1-14.

Tremblay, K.L. & Kraus, N. (2002). Auditory training induces asymmetrical changes in cortical neural activity. *Journal of Speech Language and Hearing Research* 45, 564-572.

Tremblay, K.L., Piskosz, M., and Souza, P. (2003). Effects of age and age-related hearing loss on the neural representation of speech cues. *Clinical Neurophysiology* 114, 1332-1343.

Werker, J.F. & Logan, J.S. (1985). Cross-language evidence for three factors in speech perception, *Perception & Psychophysics* 37, 35-44.

Werker, J.F. & Tees, R.C. (1984). Cross-language speech perception: Evidence for perceptual reorganization during the first year of life. *Infant Behavior and Development* 7, 49-63.

Williams, L. (1977). The voicing contrast in Spanish. *Journal of Phonetics* 5, 169-184.

Yeni-Komshian, G.H., Caramazza, A., and Preston, M.S. (1977). A study of voicing in Lebanese Arabic. *Journal of Phonetics* 5, 35-48.

2

Direct brain-feedback and prosody processing

GRZEGORZ DOGIL
GIUSEPPINA ROTA

Abstract: Imaging tools developed during the last decades have allowed researchers to gain insights into brain function. Real-time functional Magnetic Resonance Imaging (rtfMRI) is a new imaging technique that provides information in real-time on the level of activation recorded in brain regions of interest. rtfMRI can be employed to elicit and/or facilitate desired behavioural effects by directly self-regulating the activation of their neuronal substrates.

In this paper, we discuss the relevance of this method for the exploration of the cortical circuits responsible for language processing, and the effects of their modulation through neurofeedback.

A study that investigated the regulation of the right inferior frontal gyrus by means of rtfMRI is presented, and behavioural effects on the processing of prosodic features discussed.

1. INTRODUCTION

The advent of neuroimaging techniques has allowed researchers to gain insights into how the brain functions and processes language. The first cognitive models on language processing emerged from studies on brain-lesioned patients investigated post-mortem. Functional neuro-imaging techniques allow for a non-invasive exploration of the structures and functions of the human brain in vivo.

Newly developed, real-time functional Magnetic Resonance Imaging (rtfMRI) allows for immediate feedback on regional metabolic changes that are imposed by active mental processes. By means of rtfMRI, participants can learn to evoke mental states that trigger a desired level of activation in circumscribed brain areas. As the efficacy of the cognitive strategies adopted is mirrored in real-time, subjects are led through a process of operant learning, and achieve volitional control over the level in activation of brain regions of interest. By allowing control over fluctuations of regional brain activity, rtfMRI allows for a closer examination of the link between behavioural performances and their neuronal substrates, and can help refining our understanding of the cortical circuits involved in a wide range of cognitive processes. Moreover, it enables the elicitation of specific behavioural effects by directly regulating their neuronal bases.

Extensive work on brain-computer interfaces (BCIs) has demonstrated that neurophysiologic brain signals can be voluntarily manipulated and used to control external devices (for a review see Birbaumer et al., 2006). Operant conditioning of electrical brain activity has been investigated since in the late 60's. Pioneering studies by Barry Sterman and colleagues (1972) showed that enhancement of sensorimotor activity in animals has an inhibitory effect on epileptic seizures. These observations led to biofeedback-based methods for the treatment of epilepsy in humans (Kotchoubey et al., 1999; Daum et al., 1993). Nowadays, biofeedback of electrical brain activity is used in a number of clinical applications, such as for the treatment of the attention deficit/ hyperactivity disorder in children (Strehl et al., 2006; Lubar et al., 1995).

Numerous studies have targeted the modulation of electrical brain activity, and so far, only little research has addressed the regulation of the blood oxygen level dependent (BOLD) signal, detectable trough fMRI.

This paper is structured in two parts. After exemplifying the relevance of rtfMRI by reviewing the major findings for sensory and emotional modulation, we address its application to the processing of language, and present a study that investigated the self-regulation of the right inferior frontal gyrus (IFG).

2. SENSORY AND EMOTIONAL MODULATION

The first studies that introduced the concept of operant control of brain activity by means of fMRI-neurofeedback date back to 2002. Yoo and Jolesz (2002) first tested the feasibility of an fMRI-system for biofeedback. The researchers focused on the left somatosensory and motor areas. They presented volunteers with statistical maps of their brain activations originating in real-time from those ROIs. Over time, the participants learned to recruit a higher amount of hand-muscle groups in order to activate larger cortical areas. Yoo and Jolesz emphasized the potential utility of their fMRI-system by pointing out that it could be employed to guide subjects to voluntarily influence variations of their own brain activity, and expand or reduce them at will.

Weiskopf and colleagues (2004) trained subjects to control the BOLD responses in the supplementary motor area (SMA) and parahippocampal place area (PPA). The two target areas were chosen for their well-known functions, being respectively engaged in motor behaviour and processing of visual scenes. Behavioural performances in a name-recalling paradigm were measured. The authors reported successful differential control over SMA and PPA activations, thus suggesting that differential regulation of brain sites is achievable. A modification of performances based on the self-regulation engaged was also described.

DeCharmes and colleagues (2004) studied self-regulation of the somatomotor cortex. Before undergoing feedback-training, volunteers repeatedly performed finger movements and were engaged in trials of movement imagination. Over three sessions of feedback, the subjects used the cognitive strategies previously trained to expand the activation in the ROI. A control group was trained with pseudo-feedback, which was not related to the task. Only the experimental group achieved effective cortical control, and exhibited self-regulation also during a post-training session, which was run in the absence of direct feedback.

Yoo and colleagues (2004) implemented an fMRI-based system that allowed navigation through a 2D maze by means of thought processes alone. The BOLD responses in four ROIs were detected and translated in real-time into operational commands for moving a cursor and navigating through a 2D-maze. Mental calculation was employed to up-regulate the medial frontal gyrus and the anterior cingulate cortex (ACC), and served to generate the command "up". Mental speech generation served to regulate the activation-level in the superior temporal gyrus and to move down. Right and left hand motor imagery was used for exerting activation in respectively the right and left primary and secondary somatosensory areas and to move right and left. All the subjects could monitor in real-time their navigation through the maze and managed to reach the exit of it.

Emotional regulation through neurofeedback is a new area of investigation, which has been addressed by few studies so far. Posse and colleagues (2003) measured BOLD responses in the amygdala in a block design where trials of self-induced sadness and neutral mood were alternated with baseline trials of rest. At the end of each trial, the researchers provided the participants of the experiment with verbal feedback by informing them about the BOLD changes registered for "sad" and "neutral" conditions. At the end of the training, all volunteers had gained control over the level of activation in the amygdala by relying on mood induction strategies. Interestingly, self-mood individual ratings correlated with the level of activity detected in the amygdala.

Weiskopf and colleagues (2003) tested the feasibility of a self-implemented rtfMRI system to acquire control over the BOLD signal elicited from the dorsal "cognitive" (ACcd) division and the rostral, "affective" (ACad) division (Bush et al., 2000) of ACC. A subject was trained to increase the level of activation recorded from the ACcd while decreasing the level of activation in the ACad and vice versa. Since these brain regions appear to serve distinct functions (Bush et al., 2000), the experimenters argued that such training could be employed to further explore the role of these areas. The signal acquired from the ROIs was transformed into visual feedback and used as an operant conditioning aid to guide the individual learning process. Behavioural effects of the self-induced regulation, i.e. emotional valence and arousal, were also studied.

DeCharms and colleagues (2005) investigated the effects of fMRI-neurofeedback training on sensitivity to thermal pain. A number of imaging studies have suggested the involvement of the rostral part of ACC (rACC) in the processing of painful stimulation (Apkarian et al., 2005; Ploner & Schnitzler, 2004; Buchel et al., 2002). DeCharms and colleagues investigated whether self-modulation of rACC activation would influence pain perception in healthy subjects and in patients affected by chronic pain. Both healthy volunteers and patients underwent cycles of feedback training where their task consisted in increasing and decreasing rACC's activation. A painful thermal stimulation of identical intensity was applied during each activation block, and subjects were asked to rate intensity and unpleasantness of the painful sensation. After a two-days training, both healthy volunteers and patients were able to voluntarily increase and decrease activation in the ROI. At the beginning of the training no significant difference in intensity and unpleasantness was noted by the subjects. As an effect of the learning process, a significantly diminished perception of pain was associated with decreased activation in rACC. DeCharms and colleagues argued that ultimately this technique could lead to the development of a form of imaging therapy that could allow patients who suffer from chronic pain to alleviate their symptoms by undergoing a number of feedback sessions and learning to shut down rACC responsiveness to painful stimulation. The therapeutic perspective sketched by these researchers seems very promising, although further research needs to be conducted in order to confirm its applicability.

In a recent study, Caria and colleagues (2007) addressed the regulation of right anterior insular activity by means of rtfMRI. The insula is involved in a wide range of emotional and motivational processes, and is thought to be a key interface between affect and cognition (Wager et al., 2004). All participants were able to enhance activation in this ROI along three sessions of training. To control for training non-specific effects, two control groups were recruited. Both of them failed to show the pattern of activation exhibited by the experimental group. The authors pointed out the potential utility of this technique as a co-adjuvant tool in the treatment of anxiety disorders, for which a hyperactivity of the insula has been described (Stein et al., 2007; Simmons et al., 2006).

3. LANGUAGE PROCESSING

The topic whether rtfMRI can be employed to modulate the language cortical network and whether specific behavioural effects can be triggered by such a modulation had recently been addressed by our group (Rota et al., to appear). Neuroimaging tools have allowed the mapping of a wide range of aspects of speech processing (Dogil et al., 2003a; Demonet et al., 2005). However, the role played by the right hemisphere in language processing is still a matter of controversy.

A number of clinical studies have described neuronal plasticity processes, and functional reorganization that follows impairments of the left temporal-frontal networks, and pointed out that contralateral areas can carry out residual functioning by taking over functions of left-sided brain structures (Fernandez et al., 2004; Chapman et al., 2003; Thulborn et al., 1999; Weiller et al., 1995).

Musso and co-workers (1999) used Positron Emission Tomography (PET) to investigate short-term cortical changes correlated to recovery from Wernicke's aphasia. The recruitment of contralateral brain sites was described as key factor for the restoration of lost speech abilities.

Winhuisen and colleagues (2005) investigated the role of the right IFG for language processing in post-stroke aphasic patients, and utilized repetitive Transcranial Magnetic Stimulation (rTMS) to selectively suppress activation in the left and right IFG while they carried out a speech task. By analyzing the patients' responses to both conditions, the authors concluded that, for some of the post-stroke aphasics examined, right IFG activation was essential to carry out residual language functions. An involvement of the right hemisphere for the processing of prosody had been reported by neurolinguistic and neuroimaging literature.

Prosody is the most characteristic trait of spoken language. Prosodic features, unlike other linguistic textual-features, are often produced without conscious intention and are open to forms of interpretation which rely on emotional or non-cognitive processes. At the same time, prosodic organization of human communication is highly correlated with the semantic, syntactic, morphological and segmental packaging in speech production. Such diversity of functions is expected to be represented by very complex neural systems. However, all these functions are implemented by three simple phonetic parameters: duration, intensity and pitch. The straightforward phonetics of prosody could be expressed by an equally simple neural correlate.

The scope of prosodic functions and cues in language processing has led to multiple hypotheses concerning the neurolinguistic and neuro-

anatomical basis of prosody. At least four hypotheses have been particularly influential (Baum & Pell, 1999).
The *right hemisphere hypothesis* states that all aspects of prosody are independently processed by the right hemisphere and integrated with the linguistic information (which is processed by the left hemisphere) via interhemispheric connections of the corpus callosum (Blumstein & Cooper, 1974).
The *functional lateralization hypothesis* assumes that there is a continuum from linguistic to affective functions of prosody and that processing shifts from the left hemisphere, which is involved with the linguistically-based tasks, to the right hemisphere, which supports affectively-based tasks (Dapratto et al., 1999).
Clinical (Gandour et al., 2001) and neuroimaging evidence (Meyer, 2000) corroborating this hypothesis points out that linguistic prosody should possibly be further subdivided into phrase vs. syllable level prosody. The left hemisphere seems to be dominant for short frames (syllables) and the right hemisphere for long frames (intonational phrases).
The *subcortical processing hypothesis* claims that prosodic functions are highly dependent on subcortical processes and are not lateralized to one or the other hemisphere. According to this hypothesis, prosody is a basic, pre-linguistic channel of communication, which is neuronally the same for their human and animal ancestors (Cancelliere & Kertesz, 1990).
The *acoustic cues hypothesis* contends that duration, pitch (and possibly intensity) may be supported by highly specific and independently lateralized neural components (van Lancker & Sidtis, 1992).
All four hypotheses find support in the clinical observation of prosodically impaired subjects. There are methodological problems with the interpretations of data from patients if they are used in isolation. Such data may reflect neural reorganization or the development of compensatory strategies. Apart from that, the process of clinical observation is very complex in itself, and it can be hardly empirically traced and fractionalised into relevant cognitive components. Furthermore, modern cognitive theories question the assumption of a simple correspondence between multivariate linguistic systems (like prosody) and highly complex neural systems (like whole brain hemispheres).

In our research we assume a fractionalised and elaborated model of prosody generation (Dogil, 2003a) and test its individual components with experiments designed to reveal the functions of the active, healthy brain. The main interest in the experiment described below concerns the role of prosodic function ("intonational meaning") and the influence of the size of address frames in prosody generation.

3.1. METHODS

3.1.1. SUBJECTS AND MATERIALS

The study recruited ten healthy native German subjects (five females, five males, mean age 26.2 years, range 21-32 years). All participants were right-handed as determined by standardized inventory, and none of them had a history of neurological disorders. Informed consent had been obtained from each subject. Subjects were paid for the participation in the experiment.

The experiment was designed in accordance with the cognitive subtraction paradigm. This paradigm requires a pair of tasks which are similar except for the presence ('activation') or absence ('control') of the one cognitive process that is examined. Under activation conditions, subjects were asked to produce a sentence-like sequence consisting of five syllables [dadadadada] with various pitch-accent types and locations (the FOCUS condition), with various boundary tone types (the MODUS condition), and with various kinds of emotional state marking (the AFFECT condition). As a control condition (MONO condition) for the statistical analysis they were asked to produce the sequences [dadadadada, didididIdi, dodododo do, dudududu du] in a monotonous voice (with a syllable frequency of ca. 5 Hz). Reactions were stimulated visually.

We used reiterant syllables in order to reduce the influence of the syntactic, semantic, morphological and segmental factors on prosody generation. The aspects of prosody that were controlled in this experiment were in accordance with the model of prosody generation, correlated only with different address frames (syllables, feet, intonational phrases) and parameter settings (duration, intensity and pitch).

3.1.2. PROCEDURE AND IMAGING

Subjects lay supine in the MR scanner (1.5 Tesla whole body scanner, Siemens Vision), the heads being secured by means of foam rubber in order to minimize movement artifacts. The stimuli were presented visually every 15 s for a period of three seconds. The pauses between the stimuli were 12 s long. Subjects produced the recognized item immediately after stimulus presentation. Every 60 s there was a paradigm change, initiated by an acoustic instruction. Each stimulus was presented eight times. In four out of these presentations the 'prosodic' reaction was required. In the other four cases the subjects rendered the item in a monotonous manner. 28 parallel axial slices (thickness = 4 mm, gap = 1 mm) were acquired across the complete brain volume by means of a multislice echoplanar imaging sequence T2*EPI (TE = 39 ms, TR = 3 s, α = 90°, FOV = 192 mm, 64^2 matrix). Imaging data was processed using SPM 99 (Wellcome Institute of Cognitive Neuroscience, London). Functional images were movement corrected and coregistered with anatomical images. Spatial normalization procedures were performed. The normalized fMRI data were spatially smoothed (Gaussian filter, 6 mm FWHM). Conditions of interest were investigated by means of paired *t* tests. The activation threshold was set at $p < 0.05$ (corrected).

3.1.3. RESULTS

We observed a rather similar activation pattern for each condition compared to rest. Significant foci of activation were located in the motor cortex extending to premotor areas (MC), in the supplementary motor cortex (SMA), in the cerebellum (CER), and in occipital regions (OCC). These findings reflect the involvement of speech motor control (MC, SMA, CER) and processing of the visual stimuli (OCC).
In the direct contrasts between the prosodic conditions and their respective control condition these 'speech' networks disappeared. This indicates that all tasks were comparable concerning the required motor, visual and other paralinguistic components. As intended, the only difference between activation and control conditions was the prosody processing part – active in the former and absent in the latter. The

subtraction FOCUS-MONO revealed a pattern of activation exclusively lateralized to the left hemisphere. Foci of activation were located in the anterior part of the superior temporal gyrus (STG, BA 22) and in the IFG (BA 47). Additional clusters of activation were found in the left MC and in the anterior cingulum. The contrast MODUS-MONO revealed a focal spot of activation located also in the left IFG (BA 47). Subtracting MONO from AFFECT we observed focal activation exclusively in the right IFG (BA 47/11).

3.1.4. DISCUSSION - PROSODY PROCESSING IN THE INFERIOR FRONTAL GYRUS

The results show that both cortical hemispheres subserve processing prosody during speech production. This is clear evidence against a view that the right hemisphere is dominant for all types of prosodic computation. Furthermore, our findings do not confirm a crucial role of subcortical structures in prosody processing since we did not observe any significant activation in that part of the brain. However, our results are consistent with the functional lateralization hypothesis. Generating linguistically controlled prosodic features on the syllable level (FOCUS) as well as on the phrase level (MODUS) revealed activation patterns exclusively in the left hemisphere, while generating different emotional expressions revealed right hemisphere activation.

Considering the exact localization of the activated foci, our production data show interesting similarities with recent fMRI studies on prosody perception. In another experiment by our group, Wildgruber et al., (2000: 341) compared the identification of prosodically expressed emotions (happiness, anger, fear, sadness, disgust) with a non-prosodic, phonological control task (identification of the vowel following the first [a] in a sentence). Subtraction of the control task from the emotive identification task elicited activation in the right STG and bilateral activation in the IFG, with the right hemisphere showing overall greater activation in terms of BOLD magnitude and spatial extent.

In a different experiment, Wildgruber et al., (2001: 627) compared the perception of affective prosody (rating of emotional expressiveness of a sentence) with the perception of linguistic FOCUS (rating of appropriateness of question-answer pairs with respect to accent placement, i.e. a classical focus test). Activation patterns of both tasks again involved the IFG (BA 47/11). The linguistic task (focus identification) revealed additional activation in the left BA 44/45 (classical "Broca's area").

Focal activation in the orbito-basal frontal cortex during perceptual prosody processing was also shown by Meyer (2000) in a series of fMRI studies using low-pass filtered speech, which preserves the prosodic 'intonational' features and obliterates the segmental cues for speech. Analogous activations were found by Dapratto and colleagues (1999) in a prosody perception study which used meaningful sentences in a selective attention paradigm. Loevenbruck et al., (2005) found significant activation of the left IFG (BA 45 and/or 47) in an fMRI experiment on the production of deixis, involving both syntactic and prosodic deixis (i.e. focus).

These findings point to a crucial role of the deep frontal operculum (BA 47 and 11) of the IFG in the processing of the basic phonetic-phonological aspects of prosody. Besides adding evidence to the correlation between the function of prosody processing and the neuroanatomical region of the IFG, our results show interesting similarities between speech production and perception: both modi recruit identical anatomical structures when certain functions are executed. Based on the referenced studies and on our own data we can assume that the setting and interpretation of basic prosodic parameters is one such function. Only when these basic parameters have to be integrated with higher linguistic or paralinguistic information, other areas become additionally activated. In particular, integrating prosodic and linguistic focus activated the classical Broca's area, while generation and identification of emotions based on prosodic information activated the right IFG.

For illustrative purposes we provide an fMRI time-course representation of one subject's brain processing emotional prosody. The subject was passively listening to German sentences with different (i.e. happy, sad, angry, neutral) emotional intonations. As you can see in Figure 1, there is activation in the subject's brain prevailing for almost 15 seconds following the presentation of the sentences. The area that appears to stand out for the longest time is the IFG.

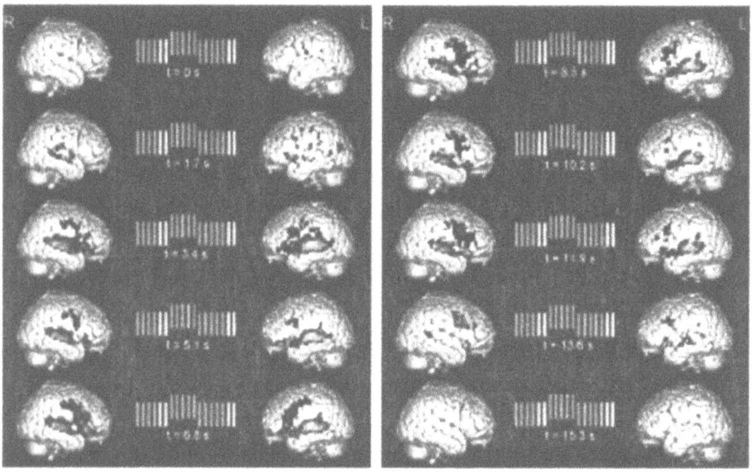

Figure 1: Processing of emotional sentences (with permission from Wildgruber et al., 2002). Brain activation is displayed in 1.7 seconds steps from left upper to lower images and continued from the right upper to the lower images.

Motivated by the discoveries of clinical neuroplasticity studies, and by neuroimaging findings on the role of the right IFG for prosody processing, we employed fMRI-neurofeedback to investigate whether healthy persons can learn to self-regulate the BOLD response in this brain area. A linguistic task and a control attentional task were employed to test short-term effects of right IFG up-regulation upon prosodic and attentive processing. The behavioural tasks required identifying emotional prosody and detecting rare visual stimuli.

3.2. REGULATION OF RIGHT IFG ACTIVITY THROUGH rtfMRI

3.2.1. MATERIALS AND METHODS

Twelve German native speakers (males, right handed, 24-30 years, mean age = 27, SD = 2.6), right handed according to the Edinburgh Handedness Inventory (Oldfield, 1971), were recruited for this study. Seven of them were trained to acquire control over the activation of the right IFG by means of rtfMRI feedback. The remaining five were recruited as control subjects. Control subjects received the same training as the experimental group, but sham-feedback only was used to guide their learning process to self-regulation.

The fMRI-neurofeedback system employed was based on a 3 Tesla whole body scanner with standard 8-channel head coil (TIM Trio, Siemens, Erlangen, Germany) in combination with the Turbo Brain Voyager software (Brain Innovation, Maastricht, The Netherlands; Goebel, 2001) and in house written scripts running on Matlab 6.5 (The Math Works, Natick, MA, USA). Figure 2 schematically illustrates the experimental set-up and data flow of the rtfMRI system implemented in the present study. Subjects' head was fixed within the head coil by means of foam rubbers in order to minimize movement. Echo-planar images (EPIs) sensitive to the BOLD response were acquired using an echo-planar imaging sequence (EPI, 16 axial slices; TR = 1.5 s, 64 x 64 matrix size, voxel size = 3.3 x 3.3 x 5 mm^3, slice gap = 1 mm, effective echo time TE = 30 ms, flip angle = 70°, bandwidth = 1.954 kHz/pixel, slice thickness = 5 mm). The first ten volumes of each session were excluded from statistical analysis to take into account T1 equilibration effects. The pars triangularis of the right IFG was chosen as the target ROI (ROI_{target}) for the experimental group, and was individually selected by means of a functional localizer run. The ROI_{target} was selected as a square region (6x6 voxels, ~ 20x20 mm) centred on the area of activation. The mean location across subjects in MNI coordinates for the centre of the selected ROI_{target} was x = 51, y = 18, z = 6.

A large reference slice ($ROI_{control}$) was used as a control area in order to account for global changes of activity, and cancel out effects due to task-unspecific activation. During training, mean differential BOLD response

[(ROI_{target} – $ROI_{control}$) $_{activation\ blocks}$ - (ROI_{target} – $ROI_{control}$) $_{baseline\ blocks}$] was transformed into the visual feedback of varying graduations of a thermometer (see Figure 2) and presented on-line to the subjects by means of video projection. As the time interval between the acquisition of new fMRI data and the presentation of its feedback was sufficiently short (about 1.5 s), subjects could monitor on-line the efficacy of their self-regulation.

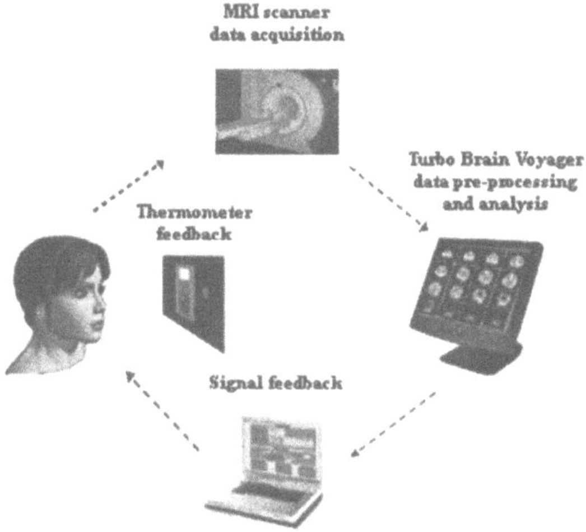

Figure 2: Experimental set-up and data flow. Raw data were collected from the scanner console, and preprocessed in real-time using the Turbo Brain Voyager software, which was running on a separate personal computer. ROI signal time-course was converted into visual feedback and displayed to the subjects with a delay of 1.5 s from image acquisition. A block design with six activation blocks (50 s each) separated by baseline blocks (50 s each) was adopted for training. During activation blocks, the subjects had to increase the level of activation recorded from the right IFG (BA 45). During baseline blocks, subjects were instructed to relax. For both types of blocks, experimental subjects received real-time visual feedback of the differential activation of the ROI_{target} (BOLD detected in the ROI_{target} minus BOLD detected in the $ROI_{control}$). Control subjects received sham feedback information. The symbols "↑" and "+" were presented on the left side of the thermometer to signal the beginning of each activation or baseline block, respectively. The whole training consisted of 4 BOLD-feedback sessions (length of each session = 8.5 minutes).

At the end of each training session, subjects were verbally asked to report the cognitive strategies adopted for both activation and baseline blocks. Subjects were provided with written information explaining the methodology of fMRI-neurofeedback, with examples of cognitive strategies. They were instructed to monitor on-line changes of the visual feedback, and learn to acquire control over the signal, increasing the level of activation displayed by the thermometer during the activation blocks. For the experimental group, achieving this goal implied finding suitable mental strategies that could reliably increase the level of activation in the right pars triangularis.

Offline data analysis was carried out using SPM2 (Wellcome Trust Centre for Neuroimaging, Queens Square, London, UK) within the framework of the General Linear Model (GLM; Friston et al., 1995). Brain Voyager QX 1.9 (Brain Innovation, Maastricht, The Netherlands) was used for ROI analysis. Pre-processing comprised motion correction, and normalization of the EPIs using the templates provided by the Montreal Neurological Institute (MNI templates, Collins et al., 1994) as implemented in SPM2. The normalized functional images were smoothed with a Gaussian kernel with a full width at half maximum (FWHM) of 12 mm. First level fixed-effects analyses were computed for every subject. Hemodynamic response amplitudes were estimated using standard regressors, constructed by convolving a boxcar function representing the block duration, with a canonical hemodynamic response function using standard SPM2 parameters. Covariates derived from motion parameters were included in the GLM (Friston, 1996) to suppress potential motor artifacts. With respect to the ROI_{target} self-regulation, learning effects were investigated by testing whether the BOLD signal increased in this brain site across sessions. The whole experiment consisted of three types of sessions: one localizer session proceeding each first training session, four training sessions, and two behavioural test sessions. Attentional skills and subjective emotional states were measured with the "d2 Test" (Brickenkamp, 1994) and the "Positive and Negative Affect Schedule" (PANAS, Watson et al., 1988).

3.2.2. BEHAVIOURAL TASKS

Stimuli belonging to two behavioural tasks were divided into two balanced sets and performed immediately before and after the whole training. At the end of the training-phase, subjects were instructed to focus on the same cognitive strategies previously successfully adopted, and to continuously up-regulate the right IFG while carrying out the two tasks. No feedback on brain self-regulation was provided to the subject in this phase.
Identification of emotional prosody was used to test short-term training effect on prosodic processing. This task consisted of four sets of German sentences belonging to the Tübingen Affect Battery (Breitenstein, 1996), describing happy, sad, angry or neutral scenarios, for a total of 16 samples. Each sentence was read by a professional actress with sad, happy, angry and neutral emotional intonations, producing a total of 64 samples. The strings lasted 2 s and were randomly presented. The participants listened to a sentence at once and were instructed to identify its emotional intonation in the shortest time possible, within a 4 s limit. Prosody judgments were performed by button pressing (i.e. selecting from a four-button device the key corresponding to the intended emotional intonation). A fixed inter-trial interval of 12 seconds was chosen. At the end of the session, subjects were debriefed, and their ability to reliably hear and understand the auditory presented stimuli was confirmed.
Accuracy of attentional processing was evaluated by means of a reaction-times visual task. The letters (N = 200) "x" (one-third the stimuli), "k" (one third of the stimuli) and "y" (one third of the stimuli) were randomly presented for 400 ms and subjects were required to press a button in the shortest time possible when the letter "k" appeared. For each task, levels of accuracy were measured as behavioural dependent variable. Stimulus presentation and collection of responses were carried out using the E-prime 1.1 software (Schneider et al., 2002). Statistical analysis of the behavioural data was carried out by means of the statistical package SPSS 14.0 (SPSS Inc., Chicago, IL, USA).

3.2.3. RESULTS AND DISCUSSION

In the present study, we tested the hypothesis that humans can learn to volitionally increase the BOLD-responses locally recorded in the pars triangularis of the right IFG. In all experimental subjects the level of activation restricted to the right BA 45 increased across training sessions. This result indicates a progressive learning effect, and suggests that real-time fMRI-biofeedback is an effective tool for non-invasively manipulating localized brain activity.

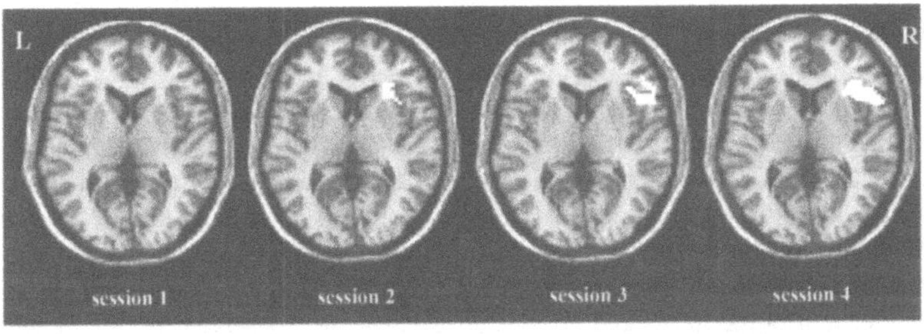

Figure 3: Experimental group: learning process across sessions of rtfMRI-training. Increased differential activation (calculated for up-regulation blocks versus rest) in the ROI_{target} across sessions was observed for the experimental group [repeated measures ANOVA, $F(3,18) = 6.379$, $P = 0.004$], but not for the control group [repeated measures ANOVA, $F(3,12) = 0.216$, $P = 0.883$]. Random effects analysis on the experimental group showed an increased level of activation for the ROI_{target} from session 1 ($N = 7$, no activation observed, $P < 0.03$, uncorrected) to session 4 ($N = 7$, $t = 2.87$, $P < 0.03$, uncorrected). Progressive increase of the level of activation in the right BA 45 (MNI = 51, 18, 6) across training sessions suggests a learning effect ($r = 0.98$; $N = 4$ sessions, $P = 0.01$ one-tailed; linear regression).

The comparison of performances in the two tasks pre and post-training suggests that the up-regulation of BA 45 correlates to a specific improvement in detecting and identifying emotional prosodic intonations. This effect was not observed for the control group.

For both groups, no significant differences in performance were measured for attentional processing. An overview of the results is illustrated by Figure 4.

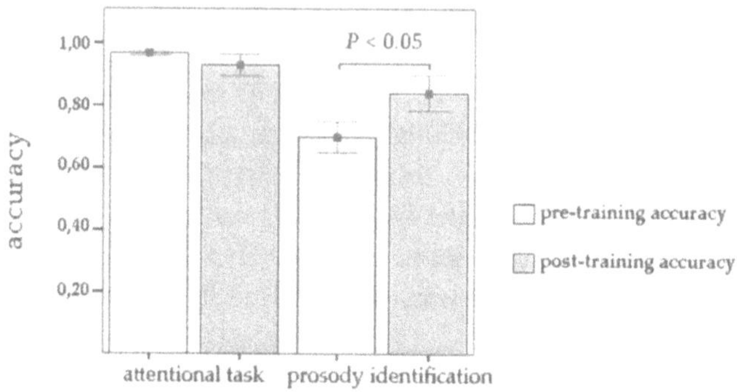

Figure 4: Experimental group: accuracy levels pre- and post-training. Experimental subjects identified 70 ± 13 % (mean ± SD) of the affective prosodic stimuli before training, and 84 ± 15 % (mean ± SD) after it. Statistical analysis showed a significant difference between the two sets of scores (two-sided Wilcoxon signed-rank test, P = 0.017). The subjects correctly responded to 96 ± 0.02 % (mean ± SD) of the attentional stimuli before the training and to 93 ± 0.09 % (mean ± SD) of to the stimuli after the training. Statistical analysis revealed no significant difference between the two levels of accuracy for the attentional task (two-sided Wilcoxon signed-rank test, P = 0.25). For the control group, no significant improvement was observed for any of these tasks.

So far, the role played by the right hemisphere, and specifically by the right BA 45, with respect to language processing has been only marginally explored, and final conclusions about hemispheric specialisations and their role for processing of distinct linguistic components of speech are far from being drawn.

Real-time fMRI feedback offers the unique and challenging possibility of exploring the role of the right hemisphere for language processing. Our findings suggest that the right IFG plays an important function in mediating the understanding of a speaker's emotional states when vehiculated by prosody.

At the onset of this section, we suggested that diverging conceptualisations exist with respect to the lateralization of prosodic processing in the brain. Coexistence of multiple phonetic cues (such as duration and pitch) and disparate functions (affective, linguistic, etc.) for the speech signal, makes it arduous to isolate the neuronal substrate of speech prosody, and might be the source for contradictory evidence about its brain mapping.

A widely supported conceptualisation highlights the dominant engagement of the right hemisphere in assessing emotional prosody regardless of valence or processing mode (Wildgruber et al., 2005; Dogil, 2003b; § 3.1.4 of this study).

In a carefully designed experiment, Gandour and colleagues, (2003) dissociated the neural circuits responsible for processing of emotional and linguistic components of prosodic speech. The researchers took advantage of the fact that in Chinese, both intonation (whether statement or question) and emotional cues can be signalled through prosody. Consistently with previous findings, Gandour and colleagues reported the exclusive recruitment of prefrontal regions (including the IFG) of the right hemisphere during the processing of emotional prosody.

Consistently with these observations, clinical studies have suggested that individuals affected by right hemisphere lesions show "a more pervasive insensitivity to emotive features of prosodic stimuli," (Pell, 2006), and a reduced decoding capacity for emotional aspects of prosody (Pell, 2007).

The findings of our experiment support this evidence and are consistent with a number of studies that indicate the involvement of the right IFG in processing of prosodic features for auditorily presented stimuli (Friederici & Alter, 2004; Kotz et al., 2003). This result indicates that the left and right hemispheres are characterized by functionally distinct specializations, and suggests that the cortical network underlying language processing can be separately modulated.

Following these lines, BOLD-biofeedback training could potentially be used to stimulate and strengthen linguistic abilities connected to emotional processing. The possibility of facilitating the processing of emotional speech appears of particular interest for a number of clinical applications, since neurofeedback aids could be employed as coadjutant therapy to normalize activation in hypo-functioning cortical networks such as for the unipolar disorder (Takami et al., 2007).

Not only clinical applications appear to be very promising. rtfMRI-neurofeedback could also be employed to potentate linguistic skills and facilitate second-language acquisition. Once brain networks responsible for second-language pronunciation are clearly identified, neurofeedback

tools could presumably be employed to train such centers in order to elicit improved linguistic performances.
To what extent neurofeedback-training can be used to stimulate and/or strengthen a wide range of cognitive skills is a topic of enormous interest that definitely will be addressed by future research.

REFERENCES

Apkarian, A.V., Bushnell, M.C., Treede, R.D. and Zubieta, J.K. (2005). Human brain mechanisms of pain perception and regulation in health and disease. *European Journal of Pain* 9, 463-484.

Baum, S. & Pell, M. (1999). The neural bases of prosody. *Aphasiology* 13, 581-608.

Birbaumer, N., Weber, C., Neuper, C., Buch, E., Haapen, K., Cohen, L. (2006). Physiological regulation of thinking: brain-computer interface (BCI) research. *Progress in Brain Research* 159, 369-391.

Blumstein, S. & Cooper, W.E. (1974). Hemispheric processing of intonation contours. *Cortex* 10, 146-158.

Breitenstein, C., Daum, I., Ackermann, H., Lütgehetmann, R., Müller, E. (1996). Erfassung der Emotionswahrnehmung bei zentralnervösen Läsionen und Erkrankungen: Psychometrische Gütekriterien der "Tübinger Affekt Batterie". *Neurologie & Rehabilitation* 2, 93-101.

Brickenkamp, R. (1994). Aufmerksamkeits- Belastungstest d2. Göttingen, Hogrefe.

Buchel, C., Bornhovd, K., Quante, M., Glauche, V., Bromm, B., Weiller, C. (2002). Dissociable neural responses related to pain intensity, stimulus intensity, and stimulus awareness within the anterior cingulate cortex: a parametric single-trial laser functional magnetic resonance imaging study. *Journal of Neuroscience* 22, 970-276.

Bush, G., Luu, P., and Posner, M.I. (2000). Cognitive and emotional influences in anterior cingulate cortex. *Trends in Cognitive Sciences* 4, 215-222.

Cancelliere, A.E., Kertesz, A. (1990). Lesion localization in acquired deficits of emotional expression and comprehension. *Brain and Cognition* 13, 133-147.

Caria, A., Veit, R., Sitaram, R., Lotze, M., Weiskopf, N., Grodd, W., and Birbaumer, N. (2007). Regulation of anterior insular cortex activity using real-time fMRI. *NeuroImage* 15, 1238-1246.

Chapman, SB., Max, J.E., Gamino, J.F., McGlothlin, J.H., and Cliff, S.N. (2003). Discourse plasticity in children after stroke: age at injury and lesion effects. *Pediatric Neurology* 29, 34-41.

Collins, D.L., Neelin, P., Peters, T.M., Evans, A.C. (1994). Automatic 3D intersubject registration of MR volumetric data in standardized Talairach space. *Journal of Computer Assisted Tomography* 18, 192-205.

Dapratto, M., Hariri, A., Bialik, M., and Bookheimer, S. (1999). Cortical correlates of affective vs linguistic prosody: an fMRI study. *NeuroImage* 9, 1054.

deCharms, R.C., Maeda, F., Glover, G.H., Ludlow, D., Pauly, J.M., Soneji, D., Gabrieli, JD., and Mackey, S.C. (2005), Control over brain activation and pain learned by using real-time functional MRI. *Proceedings of the National Academy of Sciences USA* 102, 18626-18631.

deCharms, R.C., Christoff, K., Glover, G.H., Pauly, J.M., Whitfield, S., and Gabrieli, J.D. (2004). Learned regulation of spatially localized brain activation using real-time fMRI. *NeuroImage* 21, 436-443.

Demonet, J.F., Thierry, G., and Cardebat, D. (2005). Renewal of the neu-rophysiology of language: Functional neuroimaging. *Physiological Reviews* 85, 49-95.

Daum, I., Rockstroh, B., Birbaumer, N., Elbert, T., Canavan, A., and Lutzenberger, W. (1993). Behavioural treatment of slow cortical potentials in intractable epilepsy: neuropsychological predictors of outcome. *Journal of Neurology, Neurosurgery, and Psychiatry* 56, 94-97.

Dogil, G., Ackermann, H., Mayer, J., Riecker, A., and Wildgruber, D. (2003a). Das Sprechnetzwerk im menschlichen Gehirn: Evidenz aus der funktionalen Kernspintomographie und aus der Klinik, In H. Müller, and G. Rickheit, (eds.). *Neurokognition der Sprache*, Tübingen: Narr.

Dogil, G. (2003b). Understanding Prosody. In: G. Rickheit, T. Herrmann, W. Deutsch, (eds.), *Psycholinguistics: An International Handbook*. Mouton de Gruyter, Berlin, 544-566.

Fernandez, B., Cardebat, D., Demonet, J.F., Joseph, P.A., Mazaux, J.M., Barat, M., and Allard, M. (2004). Functional MRI follow-up study of language processes in healthy subjects and during recovery in a case of aphasia. *Stroke* 35, 2171-2176.

Friederici, A.D. & Alter, K. (2004). Lateralization of auditory language functions: a dynamic dual pathway model. *Brain and Language* 89, 267-276.

Friston, K.J., Williams, S., Howard, R., Frackowiak, R.S., and Turner, R. (1996). Movement-related effects in fMRI time-series. *Magnetic Resonance Medicine* 35, 346-355.

Friston, K.J., Holmes, A., Worsley, K.J., Pline, J.P., Frith, C.D., and Frackowiak, R.S. (1995). Statistical parametric map in functional imaging: a general linear approach. *Human Brain Mapping* 2, 189-210.

Gandour, J., Wong, D., Dzemidzic, M., Lowe, M., Tong, Y., and Li, X. (2003). A cross-linguistic fMRI study of perception of intonation and emotion in Chinese. *Human Brain Mapping* 18, 149-57.

Gandour, J., Ponglorpisit, S., Khunadorn, F., Dechongkit, S., Boongirt, P., Boonklam, R., and Potisuk, S. (2001). Lexical tones in Thai after unilateral brain damage. *Brain and Language* 43, 275-307.

Loevenbruck, H., Baciu, M., Segebarth, Ch., and Abry, Ch. (2005). The left inferior frontal gyrus under focus: an fMRI study of the production of deixis via syntactic extraction and prosodic focus. *Journal of Neurolinguistics* 18, 237-258.

Lubar, J.F., Swartwood, M.O., Swartwood, J.N., and O'Donnell, P.H. (1995). Evaluation of the effectiveness of EEG neurofeedback training for ADHD in a clinical setting as measured by changes in TOVA scores, behavioral ratings, and WISC-R performance. *Applied Psychophysiology and Biofeedback* 20, 83-99.

Kotchoubey, B., Strehl, U., Holzapfel, S., Blankenhorn, V., Fröscher, W., and Birbaumer, N. (1999). Negative potential shifts and the prediction of the outcome of neurofeedback therapy in epilepsy. *Clinical Neurophysiology* 110, 683-686.

Kotz, S.A., Meyer, M., Alter, K., Besson, M., von Cramon, D.Y., and Friederici, A.D. (2003). On the lateralization of emotional prosody: an event-related functional MR investigation. *Brain and Language* 86, 366-376.

Meyer, M. (2000). *Ereignisbezogene hämodynamische Korrelate der Verarbeitung von grammatischer und prosodischer Information*. University of Leipzig (Germany): Doctoral Thesis.

Musso, M., Weiller, C., Kiebel, S., Müller, S.P., Bülau, P., and Rijntjes, M. (1999). Training-induced brain plasticity in aphasia. *Brain* 122, 1781-1790.

Oldfield, R.C. (1971). The assessment and analysis of handedness: The Edinburgh Inventory. *Neuropsychologia* 9, 97-113.

Pell, M.D. (2007). Reduced sensitivity to prosodic attitudes in adults with focal right hemisphere brain damage. *Brain and Language* 101, 64-79.

Pell, M.D. (2006). Cerebral mechanisms for understanding emotional prosody in speech. *Brain and Language* 96, 221-234.

Ploner, M. & Schnitzler, A. (2004). Cortical representation of pain. *Nervenarzt* 75, 962-969.

Posse, S., Fitzgerald, D., Gao, K., Habel, U., Rosenberg, D., Moore, G.J., and Schneider, F. (2003). Real-time fMRI of temporolimbic regions detects amygdale activation during single-trial self-induces sadness. *NeuroImage* 18, 760-768.

Rota, G., Sitaram, R., Veit, R., Erb, M., Weiskopf, N., Dogil, G., and Birbaumer, N. (2008). Self-regulation of regional cortical activity using real-time fMRI: the right inferior frontal gyrus and linguistic processing. *Human Brain Mapping, to appear.*

Schneider, W., Eschman, A., and Zuccolotto, A. (2002). *E-Prime User's Guide.* Pittsburgh: Psychology Software Tools Inc.

Simmons, A., Strigo, I., Matthews, S.C., Paulus, M.P., and Stein, M.B. (2006), Anticipation of aversive visual stimuli is associated with increased insula activation in anxiety-prone subjects. *Biological Psychiatry* 60, 402-409.

Stein, M.B., Simmons, A., Feinstein, J.S., and Paulus, M.P. (2007). Increased amygdala and insula activation during emotion processing in anxietyprone subjects. *American Journal of Psychiatry* 164, 318-327.

Sterman, M.B. & Friar, L. (1972). Suppression of seizures in an epileptic following sensorimotor EEG feedback training. *Electroencephalography and Clinical Neurophysiology* 33, 89-95.

Strehl, U., Leins, U., Goth, G., Klinger, C., Hinterberger, T., and Birbaumer, N. (2006). Self-regulation of slow cortical potentials - a new treatment for children with ADHD. *Pediatrics* 118, 1530 - 1540.

Takami, H., Okamoto, Y., Yamashita, H., Okada, G., and Yamawaki, S. (2007). Attenuated Anterior Cingulate Activation During a Verbal Fluency Task in Elderly Patients With a History of Multiple-Episode Depression. *The American Journal of Geriatric Psychiatry: Official Journal of the American Association for Geriatric Psychiatry* 15, 594-603.

Thulborn, K.R., Carpenter, P.A., and Just, M.A. (1999). Plasticity of language-related brain function during recovery from stroke. *Stroke* 30, 749-754.

Van Lancker, D. & Sidtis, J. (1992). The identification of affective-prosodic stimuli by left- and right-hemisphere-damaged subjects: All errors are not created equal. *Journal of Speech and Hearing Research* 35, 963-970.

Wager, T.D. & Feldman Barrett, L. (2004). From affect to control: functional specialization of the insula in motivation and regulation. *Published online at PsycExtra.*

Watson, D., Clark, L.A., and Tellegen, A. (1988). Development and validation of brief measures of positive and negative affect: the PANAS scales. *Journal of Personality and Social Psychology* 54, 1063-1070.

Weiller, C., Isensee, C., Rijntjes, M., Huber, W., Muller, S., Bier, D., Dutschka, K., Woods R.P., Noth J., and Diener, H.C. (1995). Recovery from Wernicke's aphasia: a positron emission tomographic study. *Annals of Neurology* 37, 723-732.

Weiskopf, N., Scharnowski, F., Veit, R., Goebel, R., Birbaumer, N., and Mathiak, K. (2004). Self-regulation of local brain activity using real-time functional magnetic resonance imaging (fMRI). *Journal of Physiology* 98, 357-373.

Weiskopf, N., Veit, R., Erb, M., Mathiak, K., Grodd, W., Goebel, R., and Birbaumer, N. (2003). Physiological self-regulation of regional brain activity using real-time functional magnetic resonance imaging (fMRI) methodology and exemplary data. *NeuroImage* 19, 577-586.

Wildgruber, D., Riecker, A., Hertrich, I., Erb, M., Grodd, W., Ethofer, T., and Ackermann, H. (2005). Identification of emotional intonation evaluated by fMRI. *NeuroImage* 24, 1233-1241.

Wildgruber, D., Pihan, H., Ackermann, H., Erb, M., and Grodd, W. (2002). Dynamic brain activation during processing of emotional intonation: influence of acoustic parameters, emotional valence, and sex. *NeuroImage* 15, 856-869.

Wildgruber, D., Hertrich, I., Ackermann, H., Riecker, A., and Grodd, W. (2001). Processing of linguistic and affective aspects of speech intonation evaluated by fMRI. *NeuroImage* 13, 627.

Wildgruber, D., Ackermann, H., Klein, M., Riecker, A., and Grodd, W. (2000). Brain activation during identification of affective speech melody: influence of emotional valence and sex. *NeuroImage* 11, 341.

Winhuisen, L., Thiel, A., Schumacher, B., Kessler, J., Rudolf, J., Haupt, W.F., and Heiss, W.D. (2005). Role of the contralateral inferior frontal gyrus in recovery of language function in poststroke aphasia: a combined repetitive transcranial magnetic stimulation and positron emission tomography study. *Stroke* 36, 1759-1763.

Yoo, S.S., Fairneny, T., Chen, N.K., Choo, S.E., Panych, L.P., Park, H.W., Lee, S.Y., and Jolesz, F.A. (2004). Brain-computer interface using fMRI: spatial navigation by thoughts. *Neuroreport* 15, 1591-1595.

Yoo, S.S. & Jolesz, F.A. (2002). Functional MRI for neurofeedback: feasibility study on hand motor task. *Neuroreport* 13, 1377-1381.

3

Phonetotopy within a neurocomputational model of speech production and speech acquisition

BERND J. KRÖGER
JIM KANNAMPUZHA
ANJA LOWIT
CHRISTIANE NEUSCHAEFER-RUBE

Abstract: A neurocomputational model of speech production is introduced in this paper. The model comprises neural maps and mappings, i.e. structure and knowledge. The structure is postulated on the basis of neurophysiological and neuropsychological facts while the knowledge is acquired during training or learning phases. The structure of the model and the training phases are described in detail in this paper. The training phases can be attributed to prelinguistic and early linguistic phases of speech acquisition. A phonetic neural map is postulated to be a central part of this model. After prelinguistic and early language-specific training phases this phonetic map exhibits an ordering of phonetic states with respect to phonetic features like the vocalic dimensions 'high-low' and 'front-back' or the consonantal place of articulation ('labial', 'apical', and 'dorsal'). This feature is labelled as *phonetotopy* in our approach.

1. INTRODUCTION

Neurologically based computational models of speech production and speech acquisition are rare. Only few approaches exist that focus on learning to produce speech and especially on learning to produce *articulatory speech movements* during speech acquisition (cf. Bailly, 1997; Guenther, 1994; 1995; 2006; and Guenther et al., 2006). These approaches complement

more linguistically oriented neural- or cognitive-based computational models of speech production which focus mainly on semantic, syntactic, and lexical processes of generating the phonological description of a word or an utterance (e.g. Levelt et al., 1999; Dell et al., 1999). These latter approaches describe *linguistic processes* but not their *concrete phonetic or sensorimotor implementation*. The organization of the neurocomputational model introduced here is based on general neurophysiological and neuropsychological principles of movement control and speech production (Kröger et al., 2008). The organization of the model (i.e. its structure) and the knowledge incorporated in the model, which results from neural learning, is described in detail in this paper.
In parallel to *tonotopy*, i.e. the fact that cells within the primary auditory cortex which are sensitive to different pitches are ordered with respect to pitch (cf. Kandel et al., 2000, p. 609), and in parallel to *somatotopy*, i.e. the fact that cells within the primary somatosensory cortex which are sensitive to somatosensory signals from different parts of the body are ordered with respect to the anatomical location of these body parts (cf. Kandel et al., 2000, p. 460), here the concept of *phonetotopy* is introduced. Our learning results using this neurocomputational production model indicate that phonetic states like sensory or motor representations of vowels are ordered with respect to phonetic dimensions like low-high and front-back and they indicate that sensory and motor states of consonantal closing gestures are ordered with respect to the place of articulation.
The structure of the model and the computer-implementation of neural maps and mappings are described in section 2. Five training experiments for silent articulation, for proto-vocalic and vocalic, and for proto-consonantal and consonantal articulation are described in sections 3 to 7. The overall results are discussed in section 8.

2. THE STRUCTURE OF THE MODEL

The organization of our neurocomputational model (Figure 1) is based on general neurophysiological and neuropsychological knowledge (Kröger et al., 2008). A main feature of the model is its subdivision into feedforward and feedback control (cf. Guenther et al., 2006; and Guenther 2006).

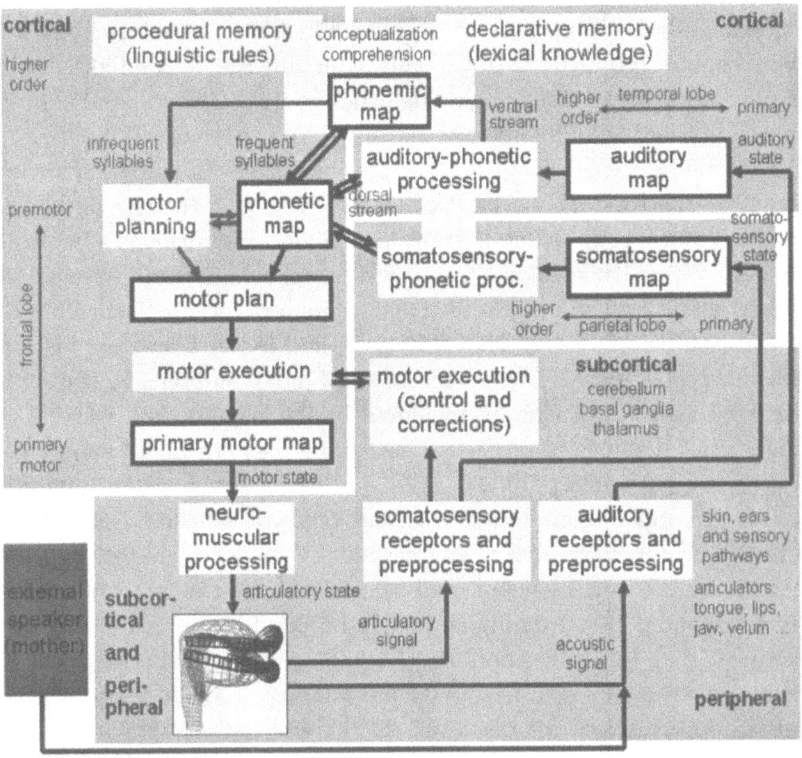

Figure 1: The neural model of speech production. Boxes with a black outline: neural maps; other boxes: neural processing units comprising neural maps and mappings not specified in detail. Arrows between neural maps indicate neural mappings or associations; arrows towards or from processing units indicate projections. The associations of the phonemic map, sensory maps, and motor plan map via the phonetic map are bidirectional, leading to a co-activation of phonemic, sensory, and motor states. In addition a bilateral connection occurs between the phonetic map and the motor planning module as well as between the cortical and the subcortical motor execution modules. Cortical, subcortical, and peripheral regions are separated. Additionally the cortical regions are separated with respect to the frontal, temporal, and parietal lobes. Modules given in grey letters and grey lines: conceptual modules, mappings and projections which are not yet been implemented.

On the *linguistic level* phonemic word forms are selected from the mental lexicon. They pass linguistic rule modules including the syllabification module (Levelt, 1992; Levelt et al., 1999; Indefrey & Levelt, 2004) and subsequently build up a chain of phonemic items (syllables) ready for sensorimotor production. This linguistic module can be subdivided into a procedural and a declarative linguistic module (Ullman, 2001) but is conceptual and not implemented in the current version of our model.
Sensorimotor *feedforward control* in our model starts with a chain of syllables specified on the level of the *phonemic map* (Kröger, Birkholz, Kannampuzha et al., 2007). If the syllable under production is a frequent syllable within the speaker's language – i.e. an already well-practised or "overlearned" syllable – the phonemic state leads to a co-activation of the appropriate auditory, somatosensory, and motor plan state via the *phonetic map*. The prelearned associations of motor and sensory states for frequent syllables or sounds are stored by the synaptic link weights of the phonemic-phonetic, phonetic-sensory and phonetic-motor mappings. Phonetic maps arise and are trained during speech acquisition for different types of sounds and different types of syllables. Sounds are ordered within these maps with respect to phonetic features like the vocalic features low-high and front-back or the consonantal feature place of articulation. This ordering is directly reflected by the neurons of the phonetic map (see our experimental results given below). The phonetic map is a self-organizing map (SOM; see Kohonen, 2001) representing the associations between the phonemic, motor, and sensory representations for all types of sounds and for all frequent syllables within the target language. Thus the phonetic map links the *phonemic map* with the *motor plan map* and with the *sensory maps (auditory and somatosensory map)*. From the viewpoint of self-organization, the phonetic map is a part of the mapping between phonemic, motor, and sensory maps. This SOM is not introduced in the approach of Guenther (2006) and Guenther et al., (2006), but in our opinion it is advantageous to introduce this neural map explicitly in a sensorimotor model of speech production since its neurons can be interpreted as *hyper-* or *supramodal state neurons* connecting the phonemic, motor and sensory states of a speech item. We hypothesize that this level is an explicit level of speech-relevant mirror neurons (cf. Fadiga et al., 2002; Fadiga and Craighero, 2004; Rizzolatti and Craighero,

2004). All maps and mappings described thus far form the mental syllabary as postulated by Levelt and Wheeldon (1994).

Infrequent syllables are not processed by the mental syllabary but by a separate motor planning module, generating the motor plan of a syllable on the basis of subsyllabic units (e.g. the sound chain; cf. Levelt and Wheeldon, 1994; Levelt et al., 1999; Varley and Whiteside, 2001). This motor planning module is linked with the phonetic map since it profits from the phonetic knowledge on the production of frequent syllables stored within the phonetic map. The motor planning unit for infrequent syllables is conceptual but not implemented in the current version of the model.

While feedforward control as described above is the main control mechanism within normal (adult) speech production and is implemented in our model for frequent syllables, online *feedback control* for supervising the ongoing flow of speech production (cf. Guenther et al., 2006) is also just conceptualised and not yet implemented in our model. However, the *feedback control* paths as given in Figure 1 are activated during the training procedures of speech acquisition in the current version of the model. Feedback control starts with the auditory and somatosensory processing of the articulatory and acoustic signals produced by the speaker's vocal tract (Figure 1). Lower level somatosensory signals (i.e. proprioceptive articulator-related joint-coordinate parameters or articulatory parameters in Kröger et al., 2006b) are directly projected to and processed by the motor execution modules (Figure 1; cf. Shadmehr and Mussa-Ivaldi, 1994; Tremblay et al., 2003; Nasir and Ostry, 2006). Higher level somatosensory and auditory information (i.e. proprioceptive tract-variable related and tactile parameters, Kröger et al., 2006b) is projected to the auditory-phonetic and somatosensory-phonetic processing module via the auditory and somatosensory map and can be compared there with the stored sensory state of a speech item (speech sound, syllable or word). In the case of differences between stored and current perceptual states for a speech item, an error signal can be generated (cf. Guenther et al., 2006).

A further feature of this model is the separation of a higher and a lower level of motor representations, i.e. the separation of a *motor plan level* and a *primary motor level* (cf. the organization of movement control in action theory, Fadiga and Craighero, 2004). In contrast, Guenther et al., (2006) directly connect phonemic, sensory and motor representations without a separation of different levels of motor control. In our approach the motor plan level is introduced in parallel to the sensory and phonemic levels. Motor plans as well as phonemic and sensory representations of syllables are processed as a whole in our approach.

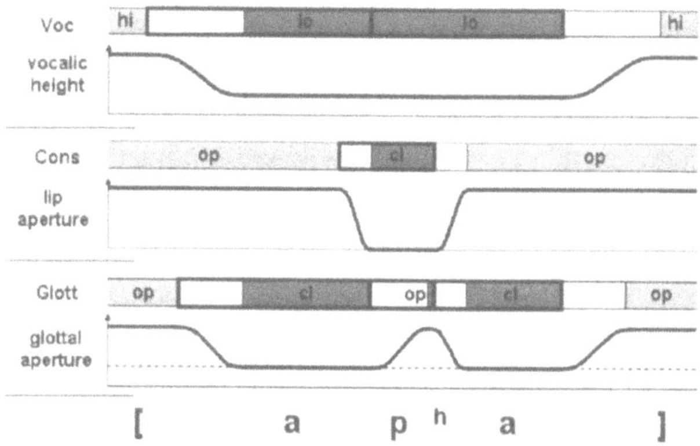

Figure 2: Temporal coordination of speech gestures for [apʰa]. Time intervals of gestural activation are marked by bold-framed boxes: two vocalic [a]-forming gestures (lo for low) on the vocalic row, one labial closing gesture (cl) on the consonantal row, and two glottal closing (cl) and three glottal opening (op) gestures on the glottal row. The time interval of gestural activation can be subdivided into transition or movement portion (white) and target portion (dark grey). Movement transitions of vocal organs are given for tongue height, for lip aperture and for glottal aperture below the tier of activation intervals for each gesture. Low and high positions of the tongue are indicated by the naming of the appropriate gesture (lo and hi). In addition target time intervals of all "neutral gestures" are indicated by light grey boxes. Neutral gestures are always activated if no other specific gesture occurs on the vocalic, consonantal or glottal row. Neutral gestures represent the pre- or post-speech articulation, i.e. high tongue position, no consonantal closure and glottal opening for breathing. For simplification, velopharyngeal gestures are omitted in this figure; for a more complete description of our gestural concept, see Kröger and Birkholz (2007).

The *motor plan* of a syllable comprises a score of executable articulatory actions. These are goal-directed speech gestures describing higher level motor features such as "produce a vocal tract closure using lips for [b]", "produce a glottal opening for [p]", or "produce a velopharyngeal opening for [m]" as well as their temporal coordination. The motor plan of the speech item [apa] is given in Figure 2.

One labial closing gesture and one glottal opening gesture for the production of [p], two coordinated gestures for tongue, lower jaw, and lips for producing the [a]-articulation, and two glottal closing gestures for producing phonation have to be coordinated in time on the motor plan level. Subsequently, motor execution leads to a concrete specification of each gesture on the level of the *primary motor map*. For example, a labial closing gesture involves coordinated movement of at least three articulators, i.e. the lower jaw and the lower and the upper lips, and each of these articulators is controlled by an ensemble of different motor units. Thus the concrete realization of a gesture is not specified on the higher motor plan level but spelled out during motor execution. Concepts for speech gesture coordination are suggested by different authors (cf. Ito et al., 2004; Sanguineti et al., 1997; Saltzman, 1979; Saltzman and Munhall, 1989; Saltzman and Byrd, 2000).

One-layer feedforward networks (Figure 3) are currently used for modelling the motor plan to primary motor mapping, and *self-organizing networks* are used in the case of the phonemic to sensory and phonetic to motor mapping (Figure 4), where the phonetic map represents the self-organizing map (SOM, i.e. the central map of the self-organizing network; cf. Kröger, Birkholz, Kannampuzha et al., 2007; Kröger, Birkholz, Neuschaefer-Rube, 2007).

Furthermore our model is capable of processing acoustic signals of external speakers (Figure 1). This information is processed via the same auditory signal processing pathway as is used for feedback control during training. An external auditory signal is also able to activate states of the phonetic map via the dorsal stream of the auditory pathway (cf. Hickok and Poeppel, 2007) and can co-activate pre-stored sound or syllable information of the auditory, phonetic, and phonemic parts of the mental syllabary (Figure 1). The ventral stream of the auditory pathway (cf. Hickok and Poeppel, 2007), which directly activates lexical items (e.g. words), is conceptualised but not implemented in the current version of the model.

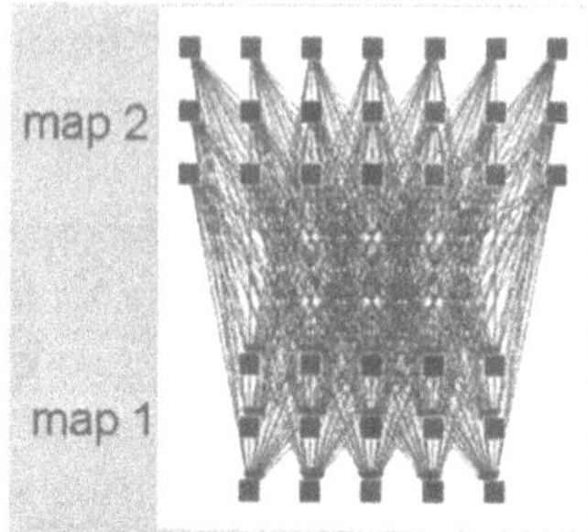

Figure 3: Example of a one-layer feedforward network (cf. Zell 2003). Grey lines indicate the heap of neural connections between two maps (motor plan and primary motor maps). The two heaps of squares indicate neuron collectives (i.e. neural maps). Black squares indicate activated neurons. The neural activation pattern of each neural map determines a distinct motor plan state (map 2) or primary motor state (map 1).

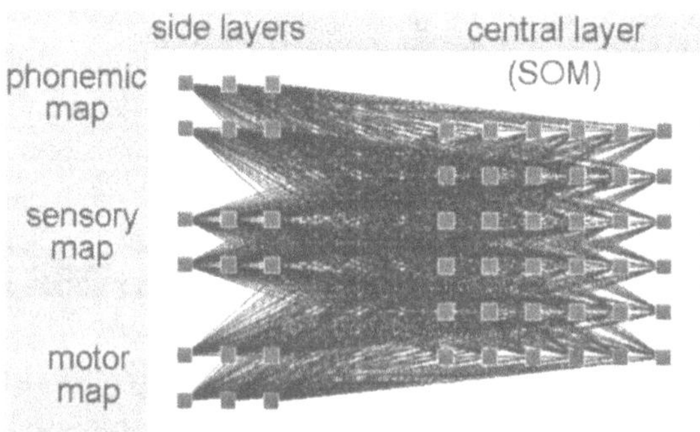

Figure 4: Example of a self-organizing network (cf. Kohonen, 2001). The heaps of grey squares indicate neuron collectives (i.e. neural maps). Black lines indicate the neural connections between side layers (i.e. neural maps for input and output representations) and the central layer (i.e. self-organizing map, SOM; the phonetic map in our model). The central layer (SOM) and all neural connections represent the self-organizing network.

The validity of the training results for our neurophonetic model, i.e. the quality of the neural mappings, strongly depends on the quality of the acoustic and articulatory signals generated by the included *vocal tract model*. These signals are the basis for calculating somatosensory and auditory feedback information and are needed for training the neural networks of the model during the speech acquisition phases. Our vocal tract model comprises a highly elaborate three-dimensional articulatory model (Birkholz, 2005; Birkholz et al., 2006; Birkholz and Kröger, 2006; 2007) and a highly elaborate articulatory-acoustic model (Birkholz and Jackel, 2004; Birkholz, 2005; Birkholz et al., 2007) capable of producing all speech-relevant vocal tract states (vocalic openings, critical closures for fricatives, complete closures, velopharyngeal coupling, etc.). The articulatory model generates vocal tract geometries for each time point on the basis of the lower level motor commands (articulatory commands; primary motor level). A vocal tract area function is calculated on the basis of the resulting geometrical information, which stipulates the acoustically relevant information of the vocal tract cavities (pharyngeal, mouth, and nasal cavity). The acoustic speech signal is then calculated using a multi-tube approximation of the vocal tract by applying the transmission line circuit approach (Birkholz and Jackel, 2004; Birkholz, 2005; Birkholz et al., 2007).

The gross or broad anatomical location of each map and mapping considered within this model can be assigned with respect to brain imaging literature (Figure 1; cf. Huang et al., 2001; Blank et al., 2002; Hillis et al., 2004; Guenther et al., 2006; Sörös et al., 2006). It is important that most of these maps, mappings, and modules are located *bilaterally* since they model the general phonetic sensorimotor processes of speech production. Lateralization occurs mainly for the *higher level language processing units* (Blank et al., 2002; Indefrey and Levelt, 2004; Liebenthal et al., 2005; Rimol et al., 2005).

In order to validate the functional aspects of the model, a number of experiments were performed to test whether it could simulate normal speech acquisition observed in infants. Central to this approach are the neural link weights of the mappings, i.e. the strength of the synaptic connection of neurons of two associated neural maps, which arise during the learning or training phase of the model (Guenther et al., 2006; Kröger et al., 2006b; Kröger, Birkholz & Neuschaefer-Rube, 2007).

Normal *speech acquisition* is divided in our model into three stages, i.e. (i) silent articulations, (ii) proto-vocalic and proto-consonantal articulation, and (iii) language-specific training of vowels and consonants (Kröger et al., 2006b). Whilst the first two phases are part of the *prelinguistic speech acquisition phase* (also called *babbling phase*), the third phase is part of *language-specific learning or training* (also called *imitation phase*; cf. Oller et al., 1999). The proto-vocalic training phase defined in our model is comparable to the phonation stage defined by Oller et al. (1999). The proto-consonantal training phase of the model can be associated mainly with the primitive articulation stage and in part with the expansion and the canonical stage defined by Oller et al. (1999). During babbling the toddler tries to collect "sensorimotor experience" from playing with his/her own speech apparatus and thus produces all kinds of possible speech (as well as non-speech) motor events and perceives the resulting sensory consequences. This contrasts with the language-specific stage, where the toddler learns to imitate external speech from carers (mother, father, etc.). Each stage or phase in the learning process depends at least in part on the previous phase, i.e. information acquired at an early stage is further modified and built on at the next stage.

All three model training phases defined above have been processed in our approach so far. Table 1 outlines how the training phases were attributed to mappings of our model trained during these phases. Both vowels and consonants were used in this training.

Table 1: The assignment of training phases defined within the neurophonetic model with the mappings trained during these phases. Mappings are indicated in Figure 1 by arrows.

Training phase	*Mappings trained during each training phase*
silent articulations (prelinguistic babbling)	motor plan → primary motor
proto-vocalic or proto-consonantal articulation (prelinguistic babbling)	phonetic → motor plan → primary motor somatosensory ←→ phonetic, auditory ←→ phonetic
language-specific training: vocalic and consonantal (development of the mental syllabary by imitation of external speech)	phonetic → motor plan → primary motor somatosensory ←→ phonetic, auditory ←→ phonetic phonemic ←→ phonetic

The following four sections describe the experimental set-up and the results of the training phases for the acquisition and the later production of vowels and consonants within VC-syllables using the neurocomputational model.

3. EXPERIMENT I: SILENT ARTICULATION TRAINING

3.1. METHOD

The training phase for *silent articulation* is based on a training set consisting of 4608 items of lower level and related higher level motor states (i.e. primary motor and motor plan states). The 4608 items cover the whole range of static articulatory states which can be produced by the vocal tract model (cf. Kröger et al., 2006a; 2006c). Within this training phase the mapping of higher level to lower level motor parameters, i.e. motor plan to primary motor mapping (see Figure 1), is learned or trained. This mapping is also known as the spatial-to-joint coordinate mapping (cf. Saltzman and Munhall, 1989).

3.2. RESULTS

Training this static part of the motor plan to primary motor mapping was successful using a one-layer feedforward network (Figure 3) and using standard training algorithms (Zell, 2003). Within a one-layer feedforward network all neurons representing the higher level spatial motor parameters are connected with all neurons representing the lower level joint motor parameters (Figure 3; a detailed discussion of neural representations for motor parameters is given in Kröger et al., submitted). Approximately 100,000 training steps were needed to obtain acceptable training results, i.e. to obtain a mean error for predicting a lower level motor state by higher level parameters below 10%. The prediction error was measured using a test set of 1152 test items which also cover the whole range of articulatory states but use combinations of parameter values different from those used in the training set. An example of training results is given in Figure 5 for the production of three types of vocal tract closures, a labial, an apical, and a dorsal closure. Vocal tract closure is controlled here by higher level motor parameters. The closures were stable, even with strong distortions on the level of the primary motor parameters, i.e. by fixing of the lower jaw in a very high or very low position. This result is a typical illustration of motor equivalence (for the concept of motor equivalence in speech, see Perkell et al., 1993; Guenther 1995).

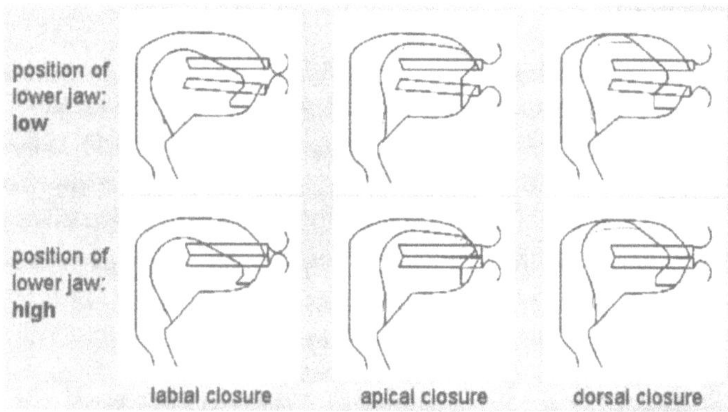

Figure 5: Mediosagittal contours generated by our three-dimensional vocal tract model for the production of a labial, an apical, and a dorsal closure defined by higher level motor parameters (the light grey lines indicate lateral articulator contours). Higher level motor parameters are constant for each column defining the labial, apical, or dorsal closure. The jaw parameter is fixed by lower level motor parameters as low or high (see both rows). It can be seen that the production of these three closures is stable despite the distortion introduced by different jaw positions.

4. EXPERIMENT II: PROTO-VOCALIC ARTICULATION TRAINING

4.1. METHOD

The training of *proto-vocalic articulation* is based on a training set comprising 1078 items, i.e. proto-vocalic higher level motor states, which cover the entire vowel space bordered by a high-front [i]-like, a high-back [u]-like and a low [a]-like articulation (Figure 6a, and see Kröger et al., 2006a and 2006b). For this training set the primary motor parameters are constrained with respect to an articulatory variation in two vocalic motor plan parameter dimensions: high-low and front-back. This set of training items is used for training the sensory to motor mapping via the phonetic map (Figure 1). The main goal of this training phase is to predict proto-vocalic higher level motor states from sensory states.

4.2. RESULTS

Training was successful using a self-organizing neural network or self-organizing map (SOM) comprising 15x15 neurons and using standard training algorithms (Kohonen, 2001). The 15x15 neurons represent the central SOM within this mapping (see Figure 4) and this SOM represents the vocalic part of the phonetic map (Figure 1). Preliminary experiments indicated that the size of the SOM can be varied between 10x10 and 20x20 without changing the results substantially. In order to keep the computational time practicable (below one hour for a complete training phase), a 15x15-sized SOM was chosen. Approximately 500,000 training steps were necessary to obtain good training results, i.e. a mean error below 2% for predicting a proto-vocalic motor state from a sensory state. The prediction error was measured using a test set of 270 test items which also cover the same range of vocalic states as defined by the training set, which use different proto-vocalic parameter values with respect to the training items. The synaptic link weights for the neural connections between self-organizing phonetic map and auditory map are displayed by the intersection points (i.e. net nodes) of the grid network in Figure 6b. Each intersection point within the grid network (Figure 6b) represents one neuron of the SOM and its link weights with the auditory map. The grid network itself displays the neighbourhood relations of these neurons.

Firstly a comparison of Figure 6a and Figure 6b indicates that the grid network for proto-vowels (Figure 6b) not only unfolds in a regular way but also covers the whole (stimulus) range of the vowel space (Figure 6a).

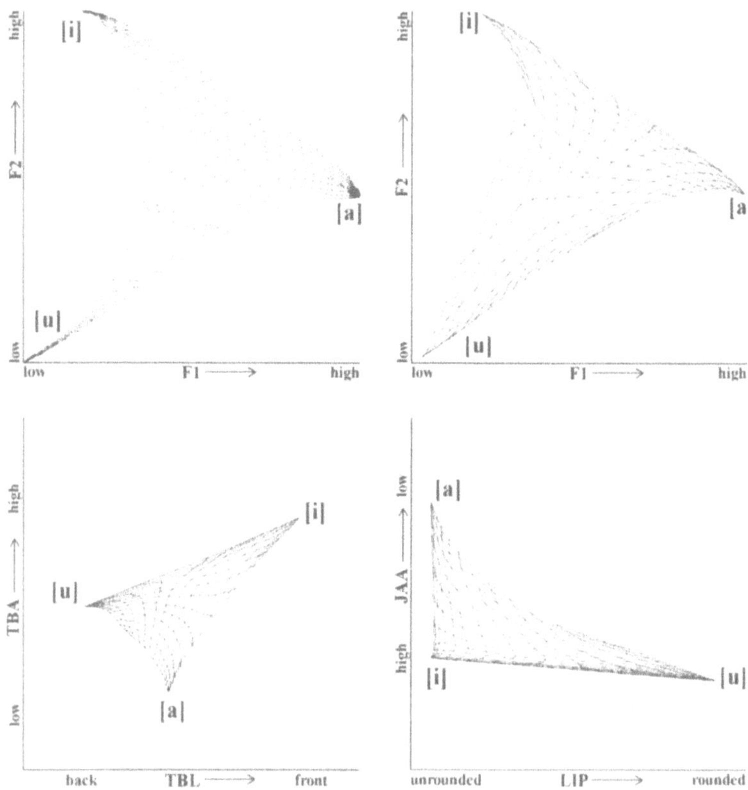

Figure 6: (a) Top, left : Distribution of the proto-vocalic training items in the auditory domain (bark-scaled F1 and F2 values). (b) Top, right: Typical training result for the self-organizing map displayed as a grid network. The nodes of the grid network represent the auditory F1-F2-link weights of the self-organizing map after proto-vocalic training. Data and training results are displayed in the acoustic-auditory F1-F2-plane (F3-link weights were also trained but are not displayed here). Both formant frequency axes are bark scaled. (c) Bottom, left: Training result for the same SOM for the motor parameter link weights tongue body horizontal location (TBL) and tongue body angle (TBA). (d) Bottom, right: Training result for the same SOM for the motor parameter link weights lip protrusion (LIP) and lower jaw angle (JAA).

Secondly the regular unfolding grid network (Figure 6b, 6c, and 6d) indicates that the differences of synaptic link weight values of neighbouring SOM neurons (represented by the distance of the neurons within the grid network) are small, i.e. link weight values from neuron to neuron vary continuously with respect to the neural ordering within the SOM. Thirdly this continuous variation of link weight values displayed in Figure 6b for the auditory link weights and in Figure 6c and Figure 6d for the motor plan link weights indicates in addition an ordering of proto-vocalic phonetic states within the grid network. Since the motor parameter dimensions of tongue body parameters (tongue body horizontal location, TBL, and tongue body angle, TBA) and the motor parameter dimensions of lip and lower jaw parameters (lip protrusion, LIP, and jaw angle, JAA) as well as the auditory (bark-scaled) F1-F2-dimensions can also be interpreted as vocalic low-high and front-back dimensions, it appears that proto-vocalic states represented by the net nodes of the grid network are ordered with respect to these dimensions. Thus the SOM displayed in Figure 6b, 6c, and 6d for the auditory and the motor plan dimensions is capable of organizing or arranging vowel states in an ordered and phonetic manner with respect to the vocalic attributes high-low and front-back. This feature of our neurocomputational network is called *phonetotopic ordering* of vocalic states or just *phonetotopy*. This SOM and its link weight distribution displayed in Figure 6b, 6c, and 6d form the *vocalic part of the phonetic map*.

5. EXPERIMENT III: LANGUAGE-SPECIFIC VOCALIC ARTICULATION TRAINING

5.1. METHOD

After proto-vocalic training the model is capable of learning vocalic phoneme realizations by using a *language-specific vocalic training set*. The aim of this phase is to train the model to produce correct phoneme realizations, i.e. to activate correct motor and sensory representations for each phonemic state. This training is based here on a training set representing a five-phoneme vowel system (/i/, /e/, /a/, /o/, and /u/) comprising 100 realizations of each phoneme. The distribution of these 500 phoneme realizations (training items) over the acoustic-auditory F1-F2 vowel space is shown in Figure 7a. The 100 realizations per phoneme form a "phoneme realization region" within the vowel space. They are generated by random spreading or scattering with respect to a Gaussian density distribution. The training is done after proto-vocalic training and leads to a further adjustment of the link weights of the phonetic-sensory and phonetic-motor mappings. In addition, however, the phonetic-phonemic mapping is trained at this point (Figure 1). The link weight values of the phonetic-phonemic mapping are initially zero during proto-vocalic training since that training does not by definition include a phonemic labelling of the stimuli. Thus during the proto-vocalic acquisition phase only those synaptic link weights within the SOM are trained which connect the vocalic phonetic map with the sensory and motor maps. However, during language-specific vocalic training the synaptic link weights connecting the SOM with the phonemic map (Figure 1 and Figure 4) are also adjusted.

5.2. RESULTS

Using standard training SOM algorithms, approximately 5,000 training steps were necessary to obtain a mean error below 1% for predicting a motor state from a sensory state at the language-specific stage for the 5-vowel system. This training leads to a shift of neural net nodes within the sensory and motor link-weight dimensions. These net nodes then concentrate in the phoneme regions of the vowel space in all motor and sensory dimensions (see Figure 7b, 7c, and 7d). Each phoneme realization region is thus represented by a heap of neighbouring net nodes within the grid network.

Since the language-specific training also comprises training of the phonetic-phonemic mapping (Figure 1) in addition to the synaptic link weights for the phonetic-motor and phonetic-sensory mappings, the synaptic link weights of the phonetic-phonemic mapping (i.e. the phonemic link weights for the SOM neurons) are adjusted and can also be displayed (Figure 8). In Figure 8 the link weight distribution is not displayed using a *grid network display* but a *neuron box display*.

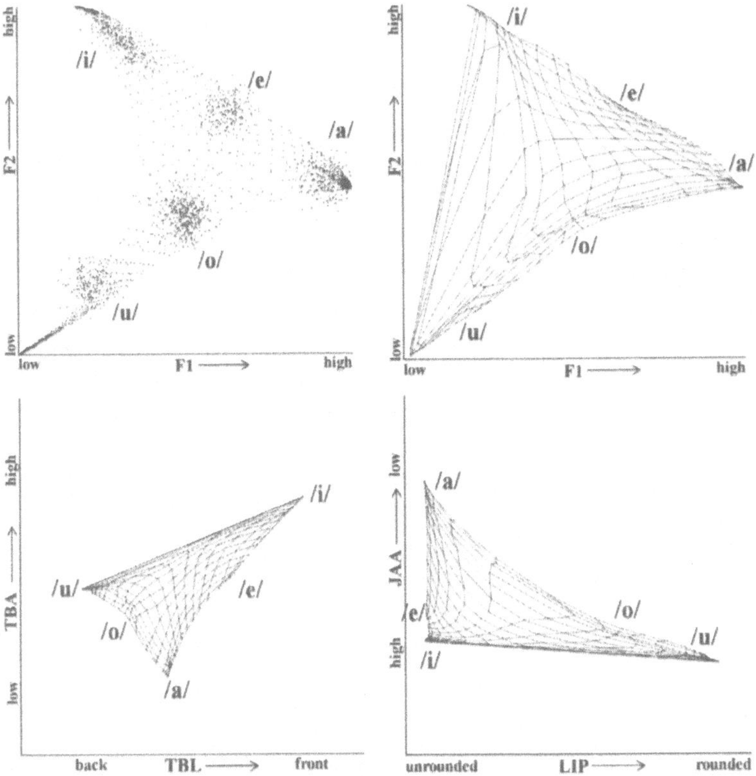

Figure 7: (a) Top, left: The distribution of 1078 proto-vocalic training items of the proto-vocalic training set (light grey dots) is overlaid by 500 language-specific training items (dark grey dots) representing a typical five-vowel phonemic system. (b) Top, right: Training results for the phonetic-auditory mapping of the self-organizing map displayed as a grid network. Both formant frequency axes are bark scaled. (c) Bottom, left: Training result for the same SOM for the motor parameter link weights tongue body horizontal location (TBL) and tongue body angle (TBA). (d) Bottom, right: Training result for the same SOM for the motor parameter link weights lip protrusion (LIP) and lower jaw angle (JAA).

Here (Figure 8) the neurons of the 15x15 SOM (i.e. vocalic part of the phonetic map) are displayed as boxes and the link weights (in this case the phonemic link weights) are displayed by a bar chart. The distribution of these phonemic link weights clearly indicates that bundles of neighbouring neurons within the phonetic map are strongly connected with one neuron of the phonemic map, i.e. that bundles of neighbouring neurons represent realizations of a definite phoneme on the level of the phonetic map. Furthermore the phonetotopic ordering of vowel states within the phonetic map is apparent. It should be noted that this phonetotopic ordering of phoneme realizations only appears when language-specific training is done in parallel or even after proto-vocalic training. Phonetotopic ordering always occurs in these cases, but the distribution of the phonetic vocalic dimensions low-high and front-back differs from training to training because of the random distribution of initial link weight values (see Figure 9). If proto-vocalic training is omitted, our training results indicate no phonetotopic ordering (Figure 10).

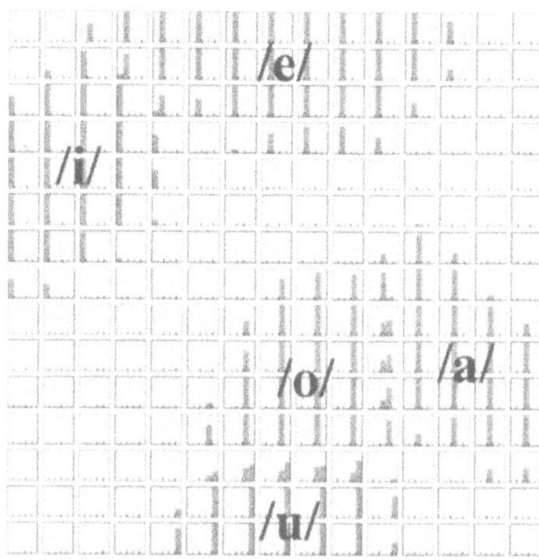

Figure 8: Training results for the phonemic-phonetic mapping of the self-organizing map given in the neuron box display. Each grey box represents one neuron of the SOM (as do the nodes in the grid network display in Figure 8). The five bars within each box represent the phonemic link weights of the SOM after language-specific vocalic training. Bars from left to right represent link weight values for /i/, /e/, /a/, /o/, and /u/. This bar plot indicates that some neurons can be clearly associated with distinct vowel phonemes while other neurons exhibit no association with any vowel phoneme.

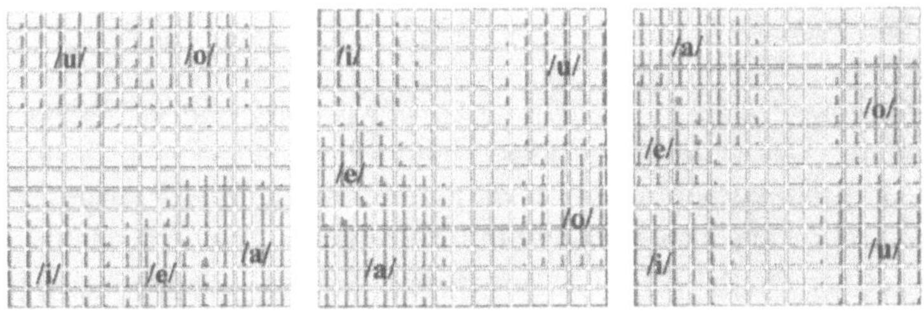

Figure 9: Training results for the phonemic-phonetic mapping of the self-organizing map given in the neuron box display for three other instances (training procedures). Each grey box represents one neuron of the SOM (cf. Figure 8). In all three cases a phonetotopic ordering occurs (as occurs in Figure 8), but the ordering differs with respect to the x- and y-axes of the neural map.

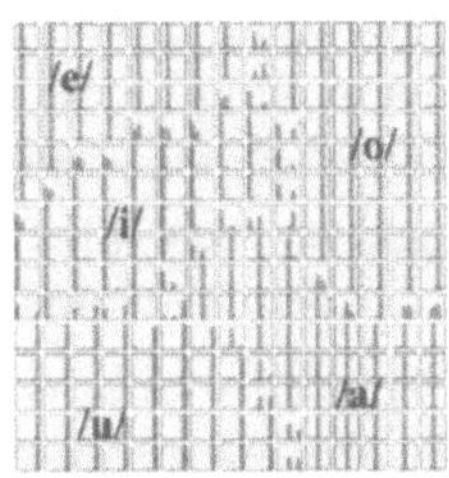

Figure 10: Training results for the phonemic-phonetic mapping of the self-organizing map given in the neuron box display for a further instance of the model (cf. Figure 8 and Figure 9). Not babbling training, but imitation training was executed and no phonetotopic ordering occurred.

6. EXPERIMENT IV: PROTO-CONSONANTAL ARTICULATION TRAINING

Up to this point, only steady state motor events, i.e. vowels, had been trained. As a next step, the model underwent prelinguistic and linguistic training phases for consonants, more specifically for labial, apical and dorsal full closing gestures.

6.1. METHOD

The training of *proto-consonantal articulation* is based on a training set comprising 225 closing gestures. The training items start from 25 different proto-vocalic states, covering the whole vowel space. Each proto-vocalic state is combined with nine different closing positions, i.e. three positions for labial, apical, and dorsal closures. In natural babbling, the exact closing position for a vocal tract organ (lips, tongue tip, tongue body) is in part determined by the vocalic starting position of this articulator (henceforth "natural closing position"). This is reflected in this training set by the association of rounded vowels with rounded labial closures, unrounded vowels with unrounded labial closures, back vowels with a slightly more back velar dorsal closure and front vowels with a slightly more front velar closure. In addition, a forward- or backward-shift from these natural closing positions was implemented in the training set in order to have a training set comprising all physiologically possible consonantal closure positions. This results in three closing positions (front, mid, and back) for each of the three articulatory gestures (labial, apical, and dorsal), i.e. it results in nine different closing positions per proto-vocalic starting position.

The *motor plan representation* of each proto-consonantal closing gesture comprises the following motor plan parameters: (i) The parameters 'front-back' and 'high-low' define the proto-vocalic state; (ii) the parameter 'gesture-executing vocal organ' (lips, tongue tip, or tongue body), and (iii) a label for the 'exact proto-consonantal place of articulation' (front, mid, or back) define the closing gesture. The exact movement of the gesture-executing vocal tract organ on the level of the primary motor map is defined by calculating the distance between the current and target position of the closure-producing vocal tract organ and then by specifying a movement velocity which is proportional to this distance.

The *auditory representation* of each proto-consonantal closing gesture comprises the first three (bark-scaled) formant transitions of the closing gesture starting from the proto-vocalic state and ending at the beginning of vocal tract closure (Figure 11). Formant values were extracted at 5 equidistant time points covering the entire transition interval. In addition, somatosensory information are added to the training items (i) representing the tactile pattern (contact pattern) of the tongue tip or tongue body with the hard and soft palate during vocal tract closure and (ii) representing the proprioceptive state of tongue and lips for the initial proto-vowel and for the final proto-consonantal closure.

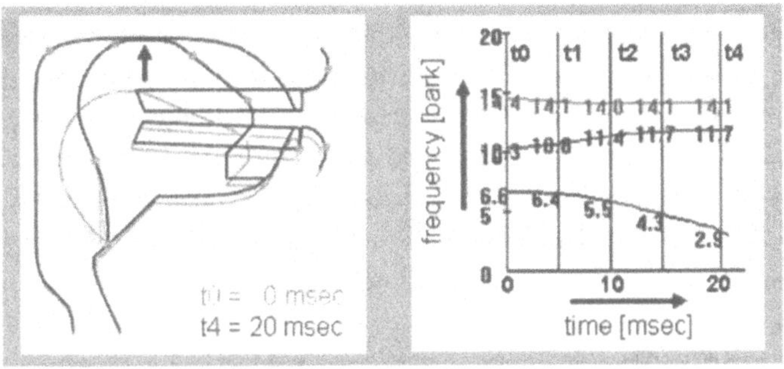

Figure 11: Auditory state (right side) for a dorsal closing gesture (left).

6.2. RESULTS

The aim of the *proto-consonantal training phase* is to predict the higher level motor representation of closing gestures from the auditory representation, i.e. from the formant transitions. Training was successful using a 10x10 self-organizing map (voiced plosive VC part of the phonetic map) for training the phonetic-sensory and phonetic-motor mappings (simulations using 15x15 maps led to similar results; 20x20 maps have not been tested yet). Standard training algorithms were used (Kohonen, 2001). Approximately 150,000 training steps were sufficient to obtain good training results, i.e. a mean error below 5% for predicting all motor plan parameters of a proto-consonantal closing gesture from its auditory state (i.e. its formant transition). The prediction of just the gesture-executing vocal tract organ (lips, tongue tip or tongue body) leads to a prediction error of lower than 1%. The prediction errors were measured using a test set of 198 test items which cover the whole range of proto-vocalic states and proto-consonantal closures as defined by the training set (Figure 6a). Different motor plan parameter values were used here in comparison to the training set items. The synaptic link weights after training are given in a neuron box display for the neurons of the SOM (Figure 12). This SOM represents the *VC-proto-consonantal part* of the phonetic map. The first three bars indicate the motor link weight values for identifying the gesture-executing vocal tract organ (labial, apical, or dorsal). The map shows a clear separation of three regions for labial, apical, and dorsal closures indicating that these three types of closing gestures can be clearly separated by our production model on the level of this SOM (Figure 12b). It should be emphasized that the formant transitions displayed within each box in Figure 12a do *not* show training *data* but training *results*. They display the auditory *link weight values* of this SOM. Thus this display delivers *100 typical formant transitions*, learned from all combinations of proto-vocalic starting positions and closure positions given in the training set. This is the *formant-transition knowledge for closure gestures* gained from the proto-consonantal training. In addition, on the basis of this 10x10 system of formant transitions, a clear auditory separation of labial, apical, and dorsal closing gestures is given. This means that the network is capable of predicting motor plan representations for closing gestures or at least the closure-performing articulator and thus the place of articulation on the basis of these 100 auditory states.

The SOM displayed in Figure 12 indicates not only an ordering of phonetic states with respect to the type of closing gesture (labial, apical, and dorsal; Fig 12b) but also with respect to the proto-vocalic starting position (Figure 12c). Distinct SOM regions can not only be detected for the closure-forming vocal tract organ but also for the proto-vocalic starting position, at least for the front-high and back-high feature combinations (Figure 12c) across different types of closing gestures (labial, apical, and dorsal). This illustrates *phonetotopy* for the type of closing gesture. Strict phonetotopy cannot occur here in the sense that a strict ordering occurs for the proto-vocalic starting positions of the gestures with respect to the phonetic dimensions 'front-back' and 'high-low', as it is impossible from a topological viewpoint to order all closing gesture states with respect to three phonetic dimensions (i.e. consonantal closing position 'labial-apical-dorsal' and two vocalic dimensions 'front-back' and 'high-low'), since it is a physiological fact that cortical neural maps are two-dimensional.

It must be emphasized that proto-consonantal training can start in parallel with proto-vocalic training. A finalization of proto-vocalic training is not needed for starting the proto-consonantal training.

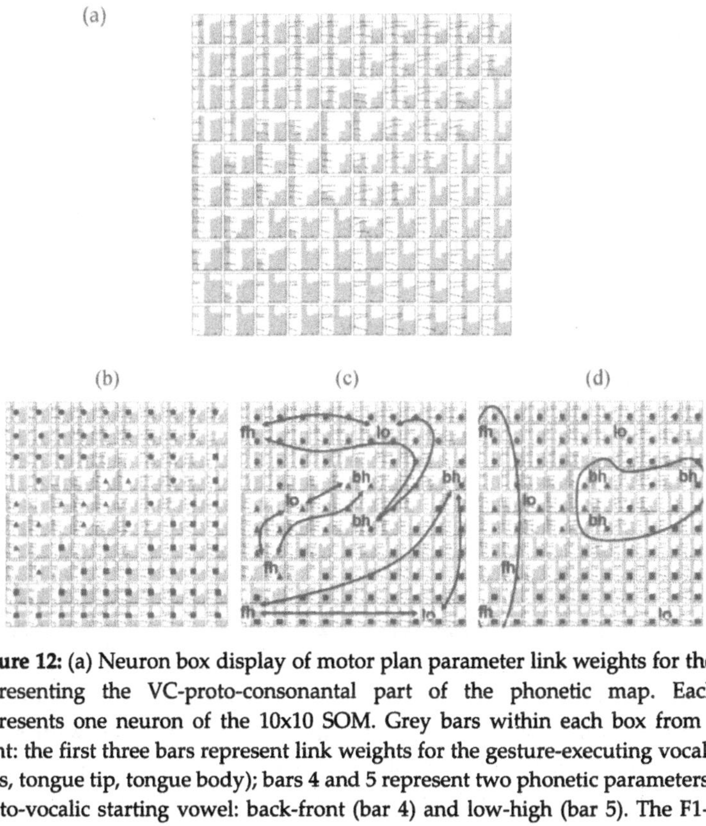

Figure 12: (a) Neuron box display of motor plan parameter link weights for the SOM representing the VC-proto-consonantal part of the phonetic map. Each box represents one neuron of the 10x10 SOM. Grey bars within each box from left to right: the first three bars represent link weights for the gesture-executing vocal organ (lips, tongue tip, tongue body); bars 4 and 5 represent two phonetic parameters of the proto-vocalic starting vowel: back-front (bar 4) and low-high (bar 5). The F1-F2-F3-formant trajectories (lines) represent the auditory link weights. (b) Same SOM as in Figure 10; in addition gesture-executing vocal organs are marked if the link weight value is above 98% for this organ: labial (triangle), apical (dot), dorsal (square). (c) Same SOM; in addition feature combinations for the proto-vocalic starting position are marked: front-high or [i]-like (fh), back-high or [u]-like (bh), and low or [a]-like (lo); also transitions from front-high to back-high and from front-high or back-high to low are marked by arrows for each gesture-executing vocal tract organ. (d) Same SOM; in addition connected regions can be found for front-high ([i]-like) and back-high ([u]-like) feature combinations for the proto-vocalic starting positions across labial-apical-dorsal boundaries.

7. EXPERIMENT V: LANGUAGE-SPECIFIC CONSONANTAL ARTICULATION TRAINING

7.1. METHOD

After proto-consonantal training a typical *language-specific consonantal phoneme system* is trained using a VC-syllable training set, i.e. the *VC voiced plosive training set*. This training set comprises all combinations of 50 vowel phoneme realizations (10 realizations per vowel /i/, /e/, /a/, /o/, /u/ were chosen from the language-specific vocalic training set) and three consonantal closures (labial, apical, and dorsal) using the natural closing position (see section 6.1). Thus the training set comprises 150 items. Similar to the process described in the training experiments for vowels, training items are now in addition labelled as /Vb/, /Vd/, or /Vg/ (V = vowel phoneme label).

7.2. RESULTS

Training was successful using a 10x10 SOM. In comparison with the proto-consonantal SOM, now in addition the phonemic-phonetic mapping was trained. 100 training cycles (approximately 5,000 training steps) were sufficient to obtain good training results, i.e. to predict the phonemic state (/b/, /d/, or /g/) from an auditory state with a prediction error below 1% for all VC-combinations. The resulting map of phonetic-sensory and phonetic-motor link weights is nearly identical with those trained earlier during the proto-consonantal training. In addition phonemic link weights for /b/, /d/, and /g/ were trained now, leading to a distribution similar to the motor link weight distribution for the gesture-executing vocal tract organ (lips, tongue tip, tongue body). Thus in the case of proto-consonantal and language-specific consonantal training, the fact of three discrete closure-forming articulators (lips, tongue tip, and tongue body) already anticipates the phonemic separation in the case of a three-plosive phoneme system /b/, /d/, and /g/ during the proto-consonantal (prelinguistic) training phase.

It must be emphasized that language-specific consonantal training can also start in parallel with language-specific vocalic training as well as in parallel with proto-vocalic and proto-consonantal training. A finalization of proto-vocalic and vocalic training as well as a finalization of proto-consonantal training is not needed to start the language-specific consonantal or syllabic training.

8. MAIN RESULTS AND DISCUSSION

A neurocomputational model of speech production is introduced which defines the structure of neural maps and mappings. Training or learning phases are described for acquiring sensorimotor, phonetic and phonemic knowledge for the mappings which build up this model.

In the structural part the model differentiates feedforward and feedback control (cf. Guenther, 2006). In the case of feedforward control, motor plans and sensory states of sounds, syllables or words are activated from phonological (i.e. linguistic) descriptions of these speech items via a phonetic map. The phonetic map introduced in our approach exhibits bilateral mappings with phonemic, sensory, and motor maps and can be interpreted as a computer-implemented spell-out of the mental syllabary (cf. Levelt and Wheeldon, 1994). In the case of feedback control, already learned and stored sensory states of speech items can be compared with auditory signal states currently produced by the model (or speaker). The neural feedback pathway is active during all training phases described above but cannot be activated in the current implementation of our model as an online control system during speech production.

The phonetic map introduced in our approach results from the fact that the neural mapping of sensory, motor plan, and phonemic states is implemented as a self-organizing map (SOM; Kohonen, 2001). This SOM is the central part of the sensory-motor-phonemic mapping. The cells within the SOM representing these connections can be labelled as *hyper-* or *supramodal* since they comprise direct neural connections towards all sensory maps and towards the motor plan map. The SOM in addition can be labelled as *phonetic* since it comprises the whole range of phonetic realizations of a phonemic item. Different SOMs were trained for different phonemic items (e.g. V and VC in this paper). Our training results indicate that the ordering of phonetic states within these SOMs reflects phonetic dimensions like the vocalic dimensions 'high-low' and 'front-back' or classes of plosives like 'labial', 'apical', and 'dorsal' plosives. This ordering is called *phonetotopic ordering* and has recently been verified by brain imaging experiments for vowels (Obleser et al., 2006). Furthermore, regarding the phonetic map, i.e. the vocalic and consonantal phonetic submaps trained during this study, it has been found that the neurons within the phonetic submaps exhibit an ordering of phonetic states with respect to phonetic features like high-low and front-back in the case of the vocalic submap or high-low, front-back and consonantal place of articulation (labial, apical, dorsal) in the case of VC-syllables. The same results gained for VC-syllables can also be reproduced for CV-syllables (not shown in this paper).

Speech items like syllables are processed as a whole in this model. The motor plan and its sensory consequences are stored for each frequent syllable *as a whole pattern* by the phonetic to sensory and by the phonetic to motor mappings. Thus the temporal succession of a motor and its appropriate sensory states is represented as one chunk on the level of the sensory and motor maps including the time succession for this speech item. Therefore time occurs implicitly in our model. As a result this model in its current implementation does not process temporal aspects of speech production in the same way or in such a detailed way as is done in the Guenther et al. (2006) approach.

Moreover in contrast to the gestural control approach introduced by Browman and Goldstein (1992), which is a mainly articulatory-based and not acoustically or perceptually based concept, the goals of gestures are coded within a hypermodal phonetic domain in our approach. For example, targets of speech gestures, which are defined on the level of the motor plan in our approach (and which are defined in parallel within the tract-variable space in the Browman and Goldstein approach), have in addition closely related sensory (i.e. auditory and somatosensory) correlates in our approach. This results from the bidirectional mappings of motor plan and sensory states (Figure 1). Thus gestural targets are coded in parallel in motor plan and sensory domains in our approach.

In order to gather speech knowledge, the mappings are trained in five basic training or learning phases. These phases are described in detail in this paper (i.e. silent articulation training, proto-vocalic and vocalic articulation training, proto-consonantal and consonantal articulation training). Silent articulation training results in the ability to accomplish a certain local or overall vocal tube geometry (i.e. formation of a certain consonantal closure or near-closure or formation of a certain vocalic tube geometry) using different relative articulatory positioning patterns (e.g. accomplishment of a certain vocal tube geometry using different articulatory positions of the lower jaw). Proto-vocalic and proto-consonantal articulation training are prelinguistic phases and lead to the gathering of general (language-independent) phonetic knowledge. These training phases result in the ability to predict proto-speech (or speech-like) articulation from sensory, mainly auditory speech-like patterns. This prelinguistic sensorimotor babbling training is the basis for language-specific imitation training. In the case of imitation training, vocalic and consonantal articulation training are language-specific and are exemplified in this paper for (i) a five-vowel phoneme system (/i/, /e/, /a/, /o/, and /u/) and (ii) for VC-syllables with a phoneme system of three voiced plosives (/b/, /d/, and /g/). The vocalic phoneme realizations form realization clouds within the articulatory and acoustic vowel space as is illustrated above (Figure 7).

It may be a shortcoming of our study that the (external) acoustic phoneme realization clouds for imitation training are generated in an artificial way representing a "hypothetical" 5-phoneme vowel system, but preliminary tests which vary the location and the degree of overlap of the phoneme realization clouds indicate that the resulting self-organizing phonetic map is stable with respect to the features mentioned in this paper, e.g. the feature of phonetotopy.

It may be a further limitation of our model that the babbling training sets are associated with random production of motor events, although this is an oversimplification (cf. McNeilage et al., 1997; McNeilage et al., 2000). Better training sets should be found, but currently there exist no complete phonetic data sets of toddlers' productions during the first year of life.

As a result of the phonetotopic ordering of phonetic states within the phonetic SOM for *all* motor and sensory dimensions, this SOM network is capable of predicting motor and somatosensory states for each speech item directly from the auditory state (auditory information). However, in addition the network is also capable of predicting, for example, sensory (auditory and/or somatosensory) states from motor states with comparable accuracy. This *multidirectionality* – i.e. multidirectional prediction of motor and sensory states for a speech item via the phonetic map – is represented by the bidirectional arrow bundles in Figure 1. Furthermore this multidirectionality means *co-activation* of motor or sensory states: If a specific state within one map in the side layer of the self-organizing network (motor, auditory, or somatosensory) is initially stimulated, a co-activation of all other side-layer maps immediately occurs via the central layer (phonetic map).

Thus assuming the proposed structure or organization of this neurocomputational model as introduced here – which is based on existing neurophysiological and neuropsychological knowledge – our simulation experiments for acquiring prelinguistic and basic linguistic or language-dependent knowledge lead to three main results: (i) The model is capable of predicting effects like ordering of vocalic and consonantal states with respect to phonetic features, which is labelled as phonetotopy. (ii) The model is capable of predicting motor states from auditory states after prelinguistic babbling training, here exemplified for proto-vocalic and proto-consonantal articulation training. This ability is the basis for imitation training. (iii) During language-specific imitation training the model is capable of learning sets of sound or syllable realizations for each phonemic representation (here exemplified for V and VC with C = voiced plosives). These sets of sound or syllable realizations are clustered within the phonetic map.

Future work has to be done in order to train other sound types (nasals, fricatives, approximants, etc.) and other and even more complex syllable types (like CV, CVC, CCV, CCVC, etc.). This would lead to an exemplification of the mapping between the phonetic map and the motor planning module (Figure 1) and would lead to the concretisation of language-specific timing rules for speech gestures. Furthermore, corrective processes due to feedback signals occurring during the sensorimotor process of speech production (cf. Guenther et al., 2006) should be implemented in our approach immediately.

ACKNOWLEDGEMENTS

This work has been supported in part by the German Research Council DFG research grant No. KR 1439/13-1. I deeply thank the editors of this book and all people who gave fruitful comments on this paper and who contributed in correcting this manuscript.

REFERENCES

Bailly, G. (1997). Learning to speak: sensory-motor control of speech movements. *Speech Communication* 22, 251-267.

Birkholz, P. (2005). *3D articulatory speech synthesis*. University of Rostock: Unpublished PhD thesis. [In German: 3D-Artikulatorische Sprachsynthese].

Birkholz, P. & Jackel, D. (2004). Influence of temporal discretization schemes on formant frequencies and bandwidths in time domain simulations of the vocal tract system. *Proceedings of the International Conference on Speech and Language Processing (Interspeech 2004)*, Jeju, Korea, 1125-1128.

Birkholz, P. & Kröger, B.J. (2006) Vocal tract model adaptation using magnetic resonance imaging. *Proceedings of the 7th International Seminar on Speech Production*, Ubatuba, Brazil, 493-500.

Birkholz, P. & Kröger, B.J. (2007). Simulation of vocal tract growth for articulatory speech synthesis. *Proceedings of the 16th International Congress of Phonetic Sciences*, Saarbrücken, Germany, 377-380.

Birkholz, P., Jackel, D., and Kröger, B.J. (2006). Construction and control of a three-dimensional vocal tract model. *Proceedings of the International Conference on Acoustics, Speech, and Signal Processing (ICASSP 2006)*, Toulouse, France, 873-876.

Birkholz, P., Jackel, D., and Kröger, B.J. (2007). Simulation of losses due to turbulence in the time-varying vocal system. *IEEE Transactions on Audio, Speech, and Language Processing* 15, 1218-1225.

Blank, S.C., Scott, S.K., Murphy, K., Warburton, E., and Wise, R.J.S. (2002). Speech production: Wernike, Broca and beyond. *Brain* 125, 1829-1838.

Browman, C.P., Goldstein, L. (1992). Articulatory phonology: An overview. *Phonetica* 49, 155-180.

Dell, G.S., Chang, F., and Griffin, Z.M. (1999). Connectionist models of language production: lexical access and grammatical encoding. *Cognitive Science* 23, 517-541.

Fadiga, L., Craighero, L., Buccino, G., and Rizzolatti, G. (2002). Speech listening specifically modulates the excitability of tongue muscles: a TMS study. *European Journal of Neuroscience* 15, 399-402.

Fadiga, L. & Craighero, L. (2004). Electrophysiology of action representation. *Journal of Clinical Neurophysiology* 21, 157-168.

Guenther, F.H. (1994). A neural network model of speech acquisition and motor equivalent speech production. *Biological Cybernetics* 72, 43-53.

Guenther, F.H. (1995). Speech sound acquisition, coarticulation, and rate effects in a neural model of speech production. *Psychological Review* 102, 594-621.

Guenther, F.H. (2006). Cortical interaction underlying the production of speech sounds. *Journal of Communication Disorders* 39, 350-365.

Guenther, F.H., Ghosh, S.S., and Tourville, J.A. (2006). Neural modeling and imaging of the cortical interactions underlying syllable production. *Brain and Language* 96, 280-301.

Hickok, G. & Poeppel, D. (2007). Towards a functional neuroanatomy of speech perception. *Trends in Cognitive Sciences* 4, 131-138.

Hillis, A.E., Work, M., Barker, P.B., Jacobs, M.A., Breese, E.L., and Maurer, K. (2004). Re-examing the brain regions crucial for orchestrating speech articulation. *Brain* 127, 1479-1487.

Huang, J., Carr, T.H., and Cao, Y. (2001). Comparing cortical activations for silent and overt speech using event-related fMRI. *Human Brain Mapping* 15, 39-53.

Indefrey, P. & Levelt, W.J.M. (2004). The spatial and temporal signatures of word production components. *Cognition* 92, 101-144.

Ito, T., Gomi, H., and Honda, M. (2004) Dynamical simulation of speech cooperative articulation by muskle linkages. *Biological Cybernetics* 91, 275-282.

Kandel, E.R., Schwartz, J.H., and Jessell, T.M. (2000). *Principles of Neural Science*. New York: MacGraw-Hill.

Kohonen, T. (2001). *Self-organizing maps*. Berlin: Springer.

Kröger, B.J., Birkholz, P. (2007). A gesture-based concept for speech movement control in articulatory speech synthesis. In: A. Esposito, M. Faundez-Zanuy, E. Keller, and M. Marinaro (eds.) *Verbal and Nonverbal Communication Behaviours*, 174-189, Berlin: Springer.

Kröger, B.J., Birkholz, P., Kannampuzha, J., and Neuschaefer-Rube, C. (2006a). Modeling sensory-to-motor mappings using neural nets and a 3D articulatory speech synthesizer. *Proceedings of the 9th International Conference on Spoken Language Processing (Interspeech 2006 – ICSLP)*, Pittsburgh, USA, 565-568.

Kröger, B.J., Birkholz, P., Kannampuzha, J., and Neuschaefer-Rube, C. (2006b). Learning to associate speech-like sensory and motor states during babbling. *Proceedings of the 7th International Seminar on Speech Production (ISSP 2006)*, Ubatuba, Brazil, 67-74.

Kröger, B.J., Birkholz, P., Kannampuzha, J., and Neuschaefer-Rube, C. (2006c). Spatial-to-joint mapping in a neural model of speech production. *DAGA-Proceedings of the 32th Annual Meeting of the German Acoustical Society*, Braunschweig, Germany, 561-562. (for download see also http://www.speechtrainer.eu)

Kröger, B.J., Birkholz, P., Kannampuzha, J., and Neuschaefer-Rube, C. (2007). Multi-directional mappings and the concept of a mental syllabary in a neural model of speech production. *DAGA-Proceedings of the 33th Annual Meeting of the German Acoustical Society*, Stuttgart, Germany), 91-92. (for download see also http://www.speechtrainer.eu)

Kröger, B.J., Birkholz, P., and Neuschaefer-Rube, C. (2007). Modeling developmental aspects of sensorimotor control os speech production. *Laryngo-Rhino-Otologie* 86, 365-370. [In German: Ein neuronales Modell zur sensomotorischen Entwicklung des Sprechens]

Kröger, B.J., Schnitker, R., and Lowit, A. (2008). The organization of a neurocomputational control model for articulatory speech synthesis. In: A. Esposito, N. Bourbakis, N. Avouris, and I. Hatzilygeroudis (eds.) *Verbal and Nonverbal Features of Human-Human and Human-Machine Interaction*, Berlin: Springer, 126-141.

Kröger, B.J., Birkholz, P., and Lowit, A. (submitted). Phonemic, sensory, and motor representations in a neural model of speech production.

Levelt, W.J.M. (1992). Accessing words in speech production: stages, processes and representations. *Cognition* 42, 1-22.

Levelt, W.J.M. & Wheeldon, L. (1994). Do speakers have access to a mental syllabary? *Cognition* 50, 239-269.

Levelt, W.J.M., Roelofs, A., and Meyer, A. (1999). A theory of lexical access in speech production. *Behavioral and Brain Sciences* 22, 1-75.

Liebenthal, E., Binder, J.R., Spitzer, S.M., Possing, E.T., and Medler, D.A. (2005). Neural substrates of phonemic perception. *Cerebral Cortex* 15, 1621-1631.

McNeilage, P.F., Davis, B.L., and Matyear, C.L. (1997). Babbling and first words: phonetic similarities and differences. *Speech Communication* 22, 269-277

McNeilage, P.F., Davis, B.L., Kinney, A., and Matyear, C.L. (2000). A motor core of speech: a comparison of serial organization patterns in infants and languages. *Child Development* 71, 153-163.

Nasir, S.M. & Ostry, D.J. (2006) Somatosensory precision in speech production. *Current Biology* 16, 1918-1923.

Obleser, J., Boecker, H., Drzezga, A., Haslinger, B., Hennenlotter, A., Roettinger, M., Eulitz, C., and Rauschecker, J.P. (2006). Vowel sound extraction in anterior superior temporal cortex. *Human Brain Mapping* 27, 562-571.

Oller, D.K., Eilers, R.E., Neal, A.R., and Schwartz, H.K. (1999). Precursors to speech in infancy: the prediction of speech and language disorders. *Journal of Communication Disorders* 32, 223-245.

Perkell, J.S., Matthies, M.L., Svirsky, M.A., and Jordan, M.I. (1993). Trading relations between tongue-body raising and lip rounding in production of the vowel /u/: a pilot "motor equivalence" study. *Journal of the Acoustical Society of America* 93, 2948-2961.

Rimol, L.M., Specht, K., Weis, S., Savoy, R., and Hugdahl, K. (2005). Processing of sub-syllabic speech units in the posterior temporal lobe: an fMRI study. *Neuroimage* 26, 1059-1067.

Rizzolatti, G. & Craighero, L. (2004). The mirror neuron system. *Annual Review of Neuroscience* 27,169-192.

Saltzman, E. (1979). Levels of sensorimotor representation. *Journal of Mathematical Psychology* 20, 91-163.

Saltzman, E. & Byrd, D. (2000). Task-dynamics of gestural timing: Phase windows and multifrequency rhythms. *Human Movement Science* 19, 499-526.

Saltzman, E. & Munhall, K.G. (1989). A dynamic approach to gestural patterning in speech production. *Ecological Psychology* 1, 333-382.

Sanguineti, V., Laboissiere, R., and Payan, Y. (1997). A control model of human tongue movements in speech. *Biological Cybernetics* 77, 11-22.

Shadmehr, R., Mussa-Ivaldi, A. (1994). Adaptive representation of dynamics during learning of a motor task. *Journal of Neuroscience* 14, 3208-3224.

Sörös, P., Sokoloff, L.G., Bose, A., McIntosh, A.R., Graham, S.J., and Stuss, D.T. (2006). Clustered functional MRI of ouvert speech production. *NeuroImage* 32, 376-387.

Tremblay, S., Shiller, D.M., and Ostry, D.J. (2003). Somatosensory basis of speech production. *Nature* 423, 866-869.

Ullman, M.T. (2001). A neurocognitive perspective on language: the declarative / procedural model. *Nature Reviews Neuroscience* 2, 717-726.

Varley, R. & Whiteside, S. (2001). What is the underlying impairment in acquired apraxia of speech. *Aphasiology* 15, 39-49.

Zell, A. (2003). *Simulation neuronaler Netze*. München: Oldenbourg.

4

Some aspects of language plasticity in epileptic patients as assessed by functional MRI

MONICA BACIU
EMILIE COUSIN

Abstract: We explored the cerebral reorganisation (plasticity) of language in adult patients with temporal lobe epilepsy. This fMRI study aimed at assessing patterns of cerebral language reorganisation according to several factors of interest such as a) hippocampal sclerosis (associated or not) and b) age of seizure onset (early or late). Seven right-handed control volunteers and seven preoperative adult epileptic patients performed a rhyme (language condition) and a visual (control condition) detection task with visually presented words and unreadable characters, respectively. All patients were left hemisphere dominant for language as determined by classical methods (SEEG, video-EEG). fMRI analyses yielded the following preliminary results:

1. Patients compared to healthy subjects showed a lower degree of hemispheric lateralization with supplementary involvement of the right hemisphere. 2. The degree of hemispheric specialisation varies according to the investigated region. 3. Patients with early seizures show signs of temporal and parietal reorganization more frequently than patients with late onset of seizures. 4. Patients with early seizures tend to exhibit intra-hemispheric frontal reorganisation. 5. Epilepsy-associated hippocampal sclerosis facilitates the inter-hemispheric shift of temporal activation. Our results appear to indicate the presence of atypical lateralization of language in epileptic patients. The pattern of cerebral reorganization can be different according to extrinsic variables (i.e. age of seizure onset).

1. INTRODUCTION

The term "focal epilepsy" classically refers to seizures generated by a specific brain region, the epileptogenic zone (Lüders et al., 2006; Rosenow and Lüders, 2001). The majority of focal epilepsies in adults are temporal lobe epilepsies (TLE) (Engel, 2001; Thomas and Genton, 1992). Unlike healthy subjects, patients with chronic temporal epileptogenic zone exhibit reorganized temporal language networks (Breier et al., 2005; Hertz-Pannier et al., 2002; Pataraia et al., 2005; Pataraia et al., 2004). Inasmuch as the left hemisphere is involved in language (Billingsley et al., 2001; Gitelman et al., 2005; Seghier et al., 2004), atypical representation (bilateral hemispheric representation or right hemispheric dominance) may occur in the subjacent cerebral regions (Adcock et al., 2003; Demonet et al., 2005). When the epileptogenic zone is located within the predominant hemisphere for language, two types of cerebral reorganisation are generally observed: a) intra-hemispheric, i.e., the non-affected cerebral regions from the hemisphere containing the epileptogenic zone take over language functions, e.g. the language function of the temporal region may "shift" within the frontal region of the same hemisphere in cases where the epileptogenic zone is located in the temporal lobe (Bell et al., 2002; Brazdil et al., 2003; Kadis et al., 2007; Pataraia et al., 2005; Pataraia et al., 2004), and b) inter-hemispheric, i.e. the homologue cerebral regions in the non-predominant hemisphere for language become involved in language (Breier et al., 2005; Helmstaedter et al., 2006; Hertz-Pannier et al., 2002; Pataraia et al., 2005; Pataraia et al., 2004; Thivard et al., 2005). The type of reorganisation is determined by several factors of interest such as the age of seizure onset (Berl et al., 2005; Demonet et al., 2005; Goldmann and Golby 2005; Hertz-Pannier et al., 2002; Liegeois et al., 2004; Thivard et al., 2005), the language region (temporo-parietal or frontal) being investigated (Hertz-Pannier et al., 2002; Kurthen et al., 1992; Liegeois et al., 2004; Thivard et al., 2005) or epilepsy-associated hippocampal sclerosis (Janszky et al., 2006; Knecht 2004; Weber et al., 2006) that can be observed in case of temporal epilepsy.

The age of seizure onset has often been investigated in this regard (Bell et al., 2002; Brazdil et al., 2003; Muller et al., 1999a; Pataraia et al., 2004). Seizures that occur before the age of six (Goldmann and Golby 2005;

Yuan et al., 2006) and originate in the left predominant hemisphere can induce either inter-hemispheric (bilateral or right hemispheric) (Liegeois et al., 2004; Muller et al., 1999a; Muller et al., 1999b; Voets et al., 2006) or intra-hemispheric (Bell et al., 2002; Pataraia et al., 2004) reorganisation of language. The right shift of language tends to be stronger and involves more numerous language regions in patients with early seizures, as compared to patients with late lesion onset, i.e. after the age of six (Muller et al., 1999a). The fact that intra-hemispheric reorganisation occurs indicates that language operations depend on regions that are not originally dedicated to these operations. The incidence of intra-hemispheric reorganisation is significantly higher if seizures start early in life (Bell et al., 2002; Pataraia et al., 2004).

Epileptics with associated hippocampal sclerosis are more likely to exhibit atypical reorganisation of language than non-sclerotic patients (Janszky et al., 2003; Knecht, 2004; Liegeois et al., 2004; Maccotta et al., 2007; Weber et al., 2006). It has been suggested that hippocampal pathology influences the type (intra- and inter-hemispheric) of language reorganisation (Knecht, 2004). For instance, some fMRI studies have shown that patients with left hippocampal sclerosis exhibit a high level of involvement of the right medial temporal lobe during semantic language tasks (Weber et al., 2006; Richardson et al., 2003). Epileptics with hippocampal sclerosis show evidence of supplementary ipsilateral recruitment of non-temporal areas such as frontal regions (Maccotta et al., 2007). The aforementioned studies suggest that inter-hemispheric temporal as well as intra-hemispheric reorganisation of language occurs when the hippocampal sclerosis is involved.

The pattern of language plasticity also varies according to which language region is being investigated. According to Thivard et al. (2005), the inter-hemispheric shift of language from the left to the right hemisphere is more likely to occur for temporal than for frontal regions in patients with TLE. Moreover, these authors found that lateralization indices calculated for regions of interest rather than for the hemisphere as a whole, exhibit a greater degree of bilateral activation when the temporal region is taken into account for the LI calculation, and much less frontal region activation. These findings are consistent with other results (Billingsley et al., 2001) indicating that there is a larger inter-hemispheric shift of activation for temporal than for frontal regions, and

suggest that language plasticity should be investigated at the regional rather than global hemispheric level.
The aim of the present fMRI study was to determine whether language is reorganized in epileptic patients with focal temporal lobe epilepsy differently than in healthy participants.
Toward this end, we investigated the following: a) regional (frontal, temporal, parietal) language reorganisation; and b) the effect of the age of seizure onset and the associated hippocampal sclerosis. All subjects performed a rhyme detection task. Inasmuch as this task induces robust lateralized activation in the predominant hemisphere for language (Baciu et al., 2001; Baciu, Watson et al., 2005; Billingsley et al., 2001; Cousin et al., 2006; Lurito et al., 2000; Seghier et al., 2004), and particularly in the left peri-sylvian (frontal, temporal, parietal) regions (Baciu, Juphard et al., 2005; Pugh et al., 1996) that are essential for language (Ojemann et al., 1989), it allowed for the detection of language reorganisation at both the global hemispheric and regional levels.
Our investigations were based on the following working hypotheses:
1. At the hemispheric level, the difference between left and right hemisphere activity will be greater in healthy participants than in epileptic patients owing to significant involvement of the right hemisphere.
2. At the regional level, the reorganisation will involve the temporo-parietal regions to a significantly greater extent than the frontal regions, owing to the fact that the epileptogenic zone is temporal.
3. The TLE associated with hippocampal sclerosis will induce a higher degree of atypical temporal lateralization than TLE without hippocampal sclerosis.

2. MATERIAL AND METHODS

2.1. PARTICIPANTS

Seven healthy right-handed (Oldfield, 1971), native French speaker volunteers (3 women and 4 men, mean age 28.28) with no history of neurological disorders, and seven preoperative adult patients (see Table 1 for demographic data) with medically intractable temporal lobe epilepsy (TLE).

Table 1: Shows demographic data for the epileptic patients examined in this study. For each of them the following information is mentioned: Age; Sex; Handedness (R = right-handed, L = left-handed), VIQ (verbal IQ assessed by Mill Hill Part B or WAIS III), age of seizures onset, VEEG (video-EEG monitoring showing the clinical features and the EEG during seizures or intercritical), SEEG (stereo-EEG). Location of the EZ (epileptogenic zone), HD= hemispheric predominance assessed by VEEG, SEEG, fMRI (all patients had LH= left hemispheric predominance), Associated hippocampal sclerosis (L = left, R = right). In all patients the neurological examination was normal and MRI excluded tumours or scars. The epileptogenic zone in all patients was dysplasia.

Patient	Age, Sex	Handed-ness	VIQ	Age at seizures onset (y)	VEEG	SEEG	EZ location	HD VEEG	HD SEEG	HD fMRI	Hippocampal sclerosis
1.	14, m	R	105	12	Clinical features and EEG spikes	Yes	L temporal (VEEG, SEEG)	-	LH	LH	-
2.	15, m	R	Not avail.	12	Intercritical EEG spikes	Yes	L temporal (VEEG, SEEG)	LH	LH	LH	-
3.	39, f	L	95	14	Clinical features and EEG spikes	Yes	R temporal (VEEG, SEEG)	LH	LH	LH	R
4.	17, f	L	Not avail.	3	Clinical features	Yes	L temporal (VEEG, SEEG)	-	LH	LH	-
5.	17, f	R	85	5	EEG spikes	Yes	L temporal (VEEG, SEEG)	LH	LH	LH	L
6.	43, m	L	100	1	Clinical features and EEG spikes	No	L temporal (VEEG)	LH	-	LH	L
7.	34, f	R	Not avail.	5	EEG spikes	No	L temporal (VEEG)	LH	-	LH	L

6/7 had left TLE, 4/7 had ipsilateral hippocampal sclerosis, 4/7 had early seizures (prior to age six, mean age 3.5) and 3/7 had late seizures (after age six, mean age 12.3). The 4/7 right-handed and 3/7 left-handed patients were considered as a single group for the statistical analyses. Each patient included in the study was diagnosed in the neurology department and the type of seizures was determined based on clinical features, video-EEG and stereo-EEG. None of the patients underwent surgery during the study. The temporal location of the epileptogenic zone was determined using VEEG and SEEG (5/2 patients). All patients had "functional" epileptogenic zones, i.e. no tumours or scars were detected via MRI, although some had hippocampal sclerosis. In all patients the left hemisphere was predominant for language (as determined by VEEG and SEEG and confirmed by fMRI examination, see Table 1). This study was reviewed by the relevant ethics committee and all participants gave their informed consent.

2.2. STIMULI

The stimuli consisted of word pairs displayed at the centre of the screen, written either in a readable (Times New Roman) or unreadable (Karalyn Patterson) font. A total of 58 pairs of readable and 58 pairs of unreadable word pairs were presented per scan. The stimuli were generated using Psyscope V.1.1 software (Carnegie Mellon Department of Psychology) on a Macintosh computer (Power Macintosh 9600) and were transmitted in the scanner by means of a video projector (Eiki LC 6000), a projection screen situated behind the scanner, and a mirror centred above the patient's eyes. The duration of each stimulus (one pair of readable and unreadable words) was 3 seconds.

2.3. TASKS

Patients and control subjects were instructed to decide whether the two words rhymed (rhyme detection task, task epoch). With respect to "words" in unreadable font, patients and controls were instructed to decide if the "words" contained at least one character which overshot the others (visual detection task, "control epoch"). The responses were given by using two response keys pressed with the index finger for "yes" and with the middle finger for "no."

2.4. PARADIGM AND MR ACQUISITION

A "block" paradigm was used during the fMRI examination, consisting of five periods, each composed of a "control" and a "task" epoch. Each epoch lasted 48 seconds. Each patient underwent a single fMRI scan. Before entering into the magnet, the subjects were positioned in front of a computer screen, and carefully instructed and trained to execute the tasks by using stimuli which were different from those used during the experiment.

Functional MR imaging was performed on a 1.5 Tesla MR imager (Philips NT) equipped with echo-planar (EPI) acquisition. Twenty five adjacent, axial slices (thickness 5 mm each) were imaged sequentially. The imaging volume was oriented parallel to the bicommissural (AC-PC) plane. It was measured sixteen times during each epoch. Positioning of the image planes was performed on scout images acquired in the sagittal plane. An EPI MR Pulse sequence was used. The major MR acquisition parameters of this sequence were: TR = 3000 ms, TE = 45 ms, flip angle = 90°, acquisition time per slice = 37 ms, field-of-view = 256x256 mm^2, imaging matrix = 64x64, reconstruction matrix = 128x128. Subsequent to the functional scan, a high resolution 3D anatomical MR scan was obtained from the volume examined functionally.

2.5. DATA PROCESSING

Data analysis was performed by using the SPM2 software (Friston et al., 1995) and based on the general linear model (boxcar function convolved with the hemodynamic response). The MR images were spatially pre-processed as follows. First, motion correction was applied and all images were realigned by means of a rigid body transformation with respect to the first acquired image. Subsequently, all images (patients and controls) were normalized, first the anatomical and then, the functional volumes.

In order to avoid left-right morphological asymmetries that could bias the inter-hemispheric comparison, a symmetrical template was built by averaging the standard MNI template and its mirror with respect to the mid-sagittal plane. This average template was then used for a normalization of all participants, including patients as they did not have anatomical brain deformation, confirmed by MRI. To conform to the underlying assumption in SPM that the data are normally distributed, the functional images were spatially smoothed by an 8-mm FWHM (Full Width at Half Maximum) Gaussian kernel. Time-series for each voxel were high-pass filtered (1/128 Hz cutoff) to remove low-frequency noise and signal drift.

The general linear model was then used to generate parameter estimates of activity at each voxel, for each condition, and each participant. Statistical parametric maps were generated from linear contrasts between the HRF parameter estimates for the two experimental conditions. At the individual level, we assessed the whole network of cerebral areas involved for each contrast (*rhyme vs control, control vs rhyme*). Subsequently, we performed in healthy participants a random-effect group analysis on the contrast images from individual analyses (Friston et al., 1998) using one-sample t tests. Clusters of activated voxels were then identified as significant at a voxel level of $p < 0.001$, $T > 4.50$, extended threshold of 15 voxels. The group analysis allowed identifying language regions significantly more activated within one hemisphere with respect to the other one. The brain regions were reported according to the stereotaxic atlas of Talairach and Tournoux (Talairach and Tournoux, 1988) and the activation's peak (x, y, z co-ordinates) of regions of interest (ROI) were identified. The considered ROIs were the regions classically activated by previous studies for this task for healthy participants (Baciu, Juphard et al., 2005; Baciu et al., 2001; Demonet et al., 1992; Lurito et al., 2000; Seghier et al., 2004). They were the inferior frontal gyrus (IFG, BA 44, 45), the inferior and middle temporal regions (IMTG, BA 37, 21) and the inferior parietal lobule (IPL, BA 39, 40). Subsequently, the peak of activation was used for drawing ROI in each participant (healthy controls and patients) by using the Marsbar tool (http://marsbar.sourceforge.net). Each ROI was delineated as a sphere of 20 mm radius (Liegeois et al., 2004) centred on the peak (x,y,z) and symmetrically within hemispheres (one ROI to the left and the

symmetrical to the right for each participant). Then, the parameter estimates (% of signal intensity variation for task and control conditions) were extracted from all left and right ROIs, in each participant.
The parameter estimate values for all left ROIs and all right ROIs of individual participants were submitted to a three way ANOVA analysis (by using STATISTICA 5.0 software) with *activated regions* (IFG, IMTG, IPL) and *hemispheres* (Right and Left) as within-subjects factors, and *pathological condition* (Controls and Patients) as between-subject factor. We checked first, if patients were significantly differently lateralized than healthy subjects. If significant difference in lateralization between the groups had been detected, we subsequently tested for each ROI if the factors of interest (age of seizure onset and associated hippocampal sclerosis) influenced plasticity. Their influence was checked for the intra- and inter-hemispheric reorganisation of language. The parameter estimates for each left and homologue right ROI were correlated with the two variables (age of onset and associated hippocampal sclerosis). Because of the small sample size, a non-parametric procedure was used (Spearman correlations). The critical significance threshold of correlations was considered at $p < .05$. Significant correlations suggested that these factors may have an effect on the cerebral reorganisation of language in epileptic patients.

3. RESULTS

3.1. HEALTHY PARTICIPANTS

Activated regions (ROI) during rhyming task
Brain areas involved in 'task' (rhyme) condition relative to 'control' (visual detection) condition and in 'control' relative to 'task' condition are listed in Table 2. During rhyme, the activated regions of interest were exclusively located to the left: inferior frontal gyrus (IFG, BA 44, x y z, -40 17 25), inferior parietal lobule (supramarginal gyrus, SMG, BA 40, x y z, -44 -41 35) and infero-medial temporal gyrus (IMTG, BA 37/21, x y z, -44 -63 -7). During visual detection, the activated regions were exclusively located to the right: middle frontal gyrus (BA 9, x y z, 51 10 36) and middle occipital gyrus (BA 19, x y z, 44 -40 -15).

3.2. EPILEPTIC PATIENTS

MR signal intensity variation (parameter estimates, magnitude) in left and right ROI in individual patients

The parameter estimates were extracted from the ROI identified in healthy subjects: IFG, IPL (SMG) and IMTG. Then, these values were subsequently analysed by using ANOVA analyses. First, when all participants (Controls and Patients) and all regions (IFG, IPL, IMTG) were considered, we obtained significantly greater activation of the left ($F_{1, 12} = 5.295$, $p < .05$) than of the right hemisphere. Furthermore, ANOVA revealed an interaction (Figure 1) between hemispheres and pathological condition ($F_{1, 12} = 7.60$, $p < .01$) with greater inter-hemispheric difference (i.e. left hemispheric dominance) for healthy than for epileptic patients. This result suggests that the right hemisphere is significantly more involved in patients than in controls, although patients keep left hemispheric predominance.

Table 2: Cerebral activated regions obtained for "Task" versus "Control" (T > C) and for "Control" versus "Task" (C > T). The statistical significance threshold for individual voxels was set at p<0.001 uncorrected (random-effect analysis). The Talairach peak coordinates (x, y, z) are indicated for each cluster. Abbreviations: H = Hemisphere; R = right hemisphere; L = left hemisphere; BA = Brodmann area; k = number of voxels in the cluster; T = Rhyme task; C = Control task.

Contrast	Cerebral activated regions	H	BA	k	x	y	z	T
T vs C	*Frontal cortex*							
	Inferior frontal gyrus	L	44	133	-40	17	25	10.75
	Superior frontal gyrus	R	11	22	32	-63	-24	5.79
	Parietal cortex							
	Inferior parietal lobule (supramarginal gyrus)	L	40	114	-44	-41	35	8.52
	Temporal cortex							
	Inferomedial temporal gyrus	L	21/37	41	-44	-63	-7	5.95
	Cerebellum	L	-	46	-16	-90	-6	6.77
C vs T	*Frontal cortex*							
	Middle frontal gyrus	R	9	22	51	10	36	5.65
	Occipital cortex							
	Middle occipital gyrus	R	19	55	44	-40	-15	7.27
	Cerebellum	L	-	46	-16	-90	-6	6.77

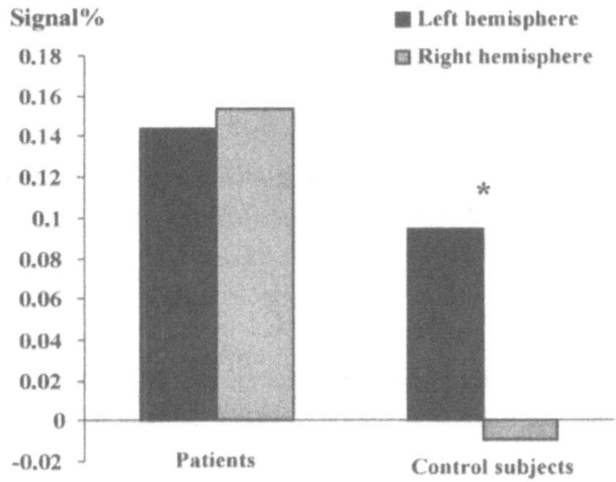

Figure 1: Significant interaction between hemisphere (Left and Right) and pathological condition (Control and Patient). The y-axis shows the degree of hemispheric lateralization (magnitude difference between conditions in left and right ROI for patients and controls (x-axis). It shows significantly a left-right difference for controls in comparison to patients.

The effect of seizure onset and hippocampal sclerosis on plasticity

This effect was assessed for each individual left ROI and right ROI by performing correlations between the parameter estimates extracted from these regions and the two variables (age of seizure onset and associated hippocampal sclerosis). In the following section we describe each specific 'plastic' region.

Inferomedial temporal gyrus (IMTG, BA 37/21)

We obtained significant correlations between the parameter estimates extracted from the left IMTG and the age of seizure onset ($r_s = .83$, $p<.01$), as well as between the parameters estimates extracted from the right IMTG and the age of seizure onset ($r_s = .89$, $p<.006$). This result suggests that seizures starting early in life induce more bilateral activation of the IMTG. Interestingly, we also obtained significant correlation between the parameter estimates extracted from the right IMTG and the associated left hippocampal sclerosis ($r_s = .77$, $p<.05$). This result suggests that patients with associated hippocampal sclerosis are more likely to involve their homologue lMTG during language processing.

Inferior parietal lobule (IPL, SMG, BA 40)

Significant correlation was obtained between the parameter estimates extracted from the right IPL and the age of seizure onset ($r_s = .89$, $p<.006$). This result suggests that early age of seizure onset could induce supplementary activation of the right homologue parietal region in patients.

No significant correlation has been obtained between the parameter estimates extracted from this region and the presence/absence of hippocampal sclerosis.

Inferior frontal gyrus (IFG, BA 44)

The correlation between the parameter estimates extracted from the left IFG and the age of seizure onset failed to reach significance ($r_s = .71$, $p=.06$) suggesting only a tendency of the intra-hemispheric reorganisation for this region when seizures start early in life.

No significant correlation was observed between the parameter estimates extracted from the IFG and the presence/absence of hippocampal sclerosis.

We remind the reader that the random analysis has been used for defining ROI. It means that inter-subject variability has been taken into account. Thus, significant group activation for a given region means that each participant presented significant activation within that region.

As an example, the following figure (Figure 2) shows in each participant (healthy and patient) the activation of one region of interest, the temporal region.

Our patient population was not homogeneous with respect to the handedness: 4/7 of patients were right-handed and 3/7 were left-handed. This sample was too small for splitting patients in right and left-handed. Although the right and the left handedness were confounded because we did not explore the relationship between handedness and cerebral reorganisation, we checked the possible effect of this factor. To this purpose, Spearman correlations between handedness and left and right homologues ROI have been calculated. No significant effect was obtained ($.43<r_s<.14$, $.33<p<.75$) suggesting that the handedness did not significantly affect the cerebral reorganisation in our sample.

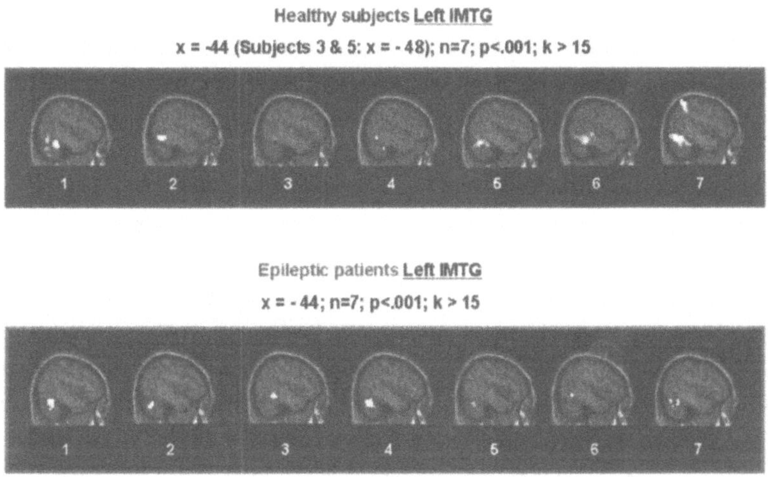

Figure 2: Significant activation of temporal region in each participant.

4. DISCUSSION

The present fMRI study investigated the influence of two variables (age of seizure onset and associated hippocampal sclerosis) on cerebral reorganisation of language in seven adult epileptic patients relative to seven healthy subjects during a rhyme detection task. We first identified language ROI based on a random-effect group analysis for delineating the left and symmetrical right ROI of individual patients. We then extracted the parameter estimates from each ROI (magnitude or percentage of MR signal variation) for each condition ('task' and 'control') and incorporated these values into ANOVAs with a view to detect significant differences between patients and controls in these ROI. For the patient group, we additionally estimated (using Spearman correlations) the effect of the two variables (age of seizure onset and hippocampal sclerosis) on the reorganisation of language.

Regions of interest during rhyme detection

This task presupposes predominant grapho-phonemic conversion (phonological analysis) of words in order to detect rhyming, as well as, automatic semantic analysis on presentation of a word (Baciu et al., 2001; Seghier et al., 2004). Hence this task was used in the present study for the purpose of assessing regions that are related to the phonological and semantic dimensions of language. The task mainly induced the activation of left hemisphere regions, in line with the results from previous studies (Binder et al., 1997; Binder et al., 1996; Demonet et al., 1992; Lurito et al., 2000; Price, 2000). We obtained a) left frontal activation (BA 44, x y z, -40 17 25), which is responsible for output phonological processes (Demonet et al., 1992), planning and execution of language (i.e. articulation) and post-lexical processing (Gitelman et al., 2005), b) left temporal activation (BA 37/21, x y z, -44 -63 -7), which is related to semantic associations (Billingsley et al., 2001; Gitelman et al., 2005; Lurito et al., 2000; Schaefer et al., 2006); and c) left parietal activation (BA 40, x y z, -44 -41 35), which is related to short term storage of phonological items (Gitelman et al., 2005). Visual detection (i.e. the control condition) induced very limited activation within the right hemisphere, related to visual attentional processes (Corbetta et al., 1998).

Hemispheric lateralization of language in patients relative to control subjects

Our results suggest that left hemispheric lateralization for language is significantly less prevalent in epileptic patients than in healthy individuals, who classically are strongly left lateralized (Baciu, Juphard et al., 2005; Fiez, 2001; Seghier et al., 2004). The reduced left hemisphere predominance in epileptics suggests that they exhibit a tendency toward bilateralization with supplementary involvement of the right hemisphere (Adcock et al., 2003; Springer et al., 1999). Other research has revealed differences between the degree or pattern of hemispheric specialisation in patients (Brazdil et al., 2005; Pataraia et al., 2005; Pataraia et al., 2004; Thivard et al., 2005; Yuan et al., 2006) relative to healthy subjects. However, the assessment of left-right hemispheric differences in these studies was not statistically robust, since lateralization index calculations were used for most parts. This method is known to be threshold-dependent, and the results engendered by it vary according to the number of voxels activated in the hemispheres under investigation

(Baciu, Juphard et al., 2005; Liegeois et al., 2002). In the present study, the use of robust statistical analyses of MR signal intensity variation (parameter estimates) extracted from ROIs generated robust evidence, indicating that the lateralization patterns in patients and controls differ.

The effect of seizure onset and associated hippocampal sclerosis on language reorganisation

It has been found (Lehericy et al., 2002; Ries et al., 2004; Thivard et al., 2005) that language reorganisation is best investigated at the regional rather than the hemispheric level since a) reorganisation patterns vary according to region, b) reorganisation is more prevalent in temporal than in frontal regions, c) reorganisation patterns are affected by a number of factors, the following two of which were investigated in the present study:

1. Age of seizure onset

Cerebral plasticity is affected by the age of seizure onset (Brazdil et al., 2003; Hertz-Pannier et al., 2002; Liegeois et al., 2004; Thivard et al., 2005). Although it is difficult to distinguish between neuropathological changes and normal language development (Yuan et al., 2006), it is widely accepted that age is the primary factor for predicting recovery, and that the prognosis is far better for children with seizure onset prior to age six. In such patients, the presence of language plasticity is indicated by a) supplementary involvement of the homologue hemisphere and a reduction in the degree of specialisation (Brazdil et al., 2003; Demonet et al., 2005; Helmstaedter et al., 2006; Liegeois et al., 2004; Muller et al., 1999a; Pataraia et al., 2005; Thivard et al., 2005; Voets et al., 2006; Yuan et al., 2006), and b) intra-hemispheric reorganisation of cerebral networks (Bell et al., 2002; Lazar et al., 1997; Pataraia et al., 2004). In other words, regions not originally involved in a specific language operation become involved following reorganisation. In the present study, the age of seizure onset was significantly correlated with the activity of each ROI that was investigated. We shall now describe the plasticity mechanism in each of the relevant regions.

Frontal region: Our results indicate only a tendency toward intra-hemispheric reorganisation of frontal activation in healthy subjects, thus suggesting that early seizures induce greater activation and involvement of frontal regions than late-onset seizures. This hypothesis (and our results) are supported by other research (Hertz-Pannier et al., 2002) indicating that language reorganisation occurs in pre-existing bilateral networks that are only detectable postoperatively. This pattern, which is also referred to as the *translocation of language function* (Lazar et al., 1997), is thought to result from frontal region hyperactivity with probably taking into account the function of other language regions, such as the posterior (temporo-parietal) ipsilateral areas (Lehericy et al., 2002). This pattern may also indicate that the presence of pathology in temporal regions reduces their involvement in language tasks (Ries et al., 2004).

Parietal region: Our results indicate that inter-hemispheric reorganisation occurs in the parietal region and is correlated with the age of seizure onset, i.e. reorganisation is more likely to occur in cases of early onset. These findings are consistent with other studies of temporo-parietal reorganisation for language that treat the two regions as a single entity (Helmstaedter et al., 2006; Thivard et al., 2005) or investigate them separately (Hertz-Pannier et al., 2002).

Temporal region: We observed a significant correlation between age of seizure onset and signal intensity variation in the right and left IMTG, which suggests that early seizures induce bilateral representation of language for temporal regions. In addition, the significant correlation between the left IMTG and the age of seizure onset suggests that the injured hemisphere is still able to handle language functions (DeVos et al., 1995), inasmuch as the epileptogenic area in the majority of our patients was located in the left temporal lobe. The correlation we observed between age of onset and the right IMTG is consistent with previous studies showing similar results when the left temporal region is injured (Brazdil et al., 2003; Hertz-Pannier et al., 2002; Janszky et al., 2006; Liegeois et al., 2004; Sabbah et al., 2003; Thivard et al., 2005).

In our view, all of the aforementioned results suggest that left temporal lobe segregation occurs in early-onset TLE patients. Their functional temporal sub-regions are unable to handle certain language operations, which are taken over either by other intra-hemispheric language regions (such as the frontal region via intra-hemispheric "shift") or by homologue language regions (right temporal, via inter-hemispheric "shift"). This takeover process may induce hyperactivation in some other functional temporal sub-regions.

2. Associated hippocampal sclerosis

Hippocampal sclerosis appears to play an important role in cerebral plasticity for language, which in our study was significantly correlated with right IMTG activity. Other research has demonstrated right lateralization of temporal lobe activation in TLE with accompanying hippocampal sclerosis (Grunwald et al., 1999; Richardson et al., 2003; Schaefer et al., 2006; Weber et al., 2006). The right "shift" is regarded as a compensatory mechanism a) for verbal memory processes that is induced by the injured left hippocampal structures (medial temporal regions) and/or b) language, since hippocampal structures may be involved in the development of language lateralization (Knecht, 2004).

The handedness of our epileptic patients was not homogenous. Hand preference should be taken into account (Knecht et al., 2000; Pujol et al., 1999) in investigations of language plasticity as a linear relationship has been demonstrated between handedness and atypical dominance with increased incidence of reorganisation in strongly left-handed patients (Knecht et al., 2000; Pujol et al., 1999). Our results do not indicate a correlation between handedness and MR signal intensity values in left and right ROIs. However, this finding needs to be confirmed, since our patient sample was very small and the handedness of our controls and patients did not match up. In future studies, we plan to investigate the effect of hand preference on language reorganisation using a larger group of epileptic patients and by comparing patient data with that of appropriate and matched left- and right-handed healthy subjects.

5. CONCLUSION

Relative to healthy subjects, the focal TLE patients we investigated exhibited significantly reduced hemispheric lateralization during language task performance. The significant correlation we observed between age of seizure onset and the signal magnitude of temporo-parietal regions points to the involvement of the right hemisphere as well (Thivard et al., 2005). The presence of a relatively weak correlation between seizure onset and left frontal region magnitude suggests that intra-hemispheric reorganisation may occur in this region, but additional investigations are needed in order to obtain more robust results. The preliminary findings of the present study indicate that cerebral reorganisation can be assessed by using statistical evaluation as a function of various regions and variables. With respect to the relatively small patient sample in the present study, our results should be regarded carefully at the individual patient. However, our results suggest that neuroimaging may be a useful tool for further language plasticity research.

REFERENCES

Adcock, J.E., Wise, R.G., Oxbury, J.M., Oxbury, S.M., and Matthews, P.M. (2003). Quantitative fMRI assessment of the differences in lateralization of language-related brain activation in patients with temporal lobe epilepsy. *NeuroImage* 18(2), 423-438.

Baciu, M., Juphard, A., Cousin, E., and Le Bas, J.F.(2005). Evaluating fMRI methods for assessing hemispheric language dominance in healthy subjects. *European Journal of Radiology* 55(2), 209-218.

Baciu, M., Kahane, P., Minotti, L., Charnallet, A., David, D., Le Bas, J.F., and Segebarth, C (2001). Functional MRI assessment of the hemispheric predominance for language in epileptic patients using a simple rhyme detection task. *Epileptic Disorder* 3(3), 117-124.

Baciu, M., Watson, J.M., Maccotta, L., McDermott, K.B., Buckner, R.L., Gilliam, F.G., and Ojemann, JG. (2005). Evaluating functional MRI procedures for assessing hemispheric language dominance in neurosurgical patients. *Neuroradiology* 47(11), 835-844.

Bell, B., Hermann, B., Seidenberg, M., Davies, K., Cariski, D., Rosenbek, J., Woodard, A., Rutecki, P., and Bishop, M. (2002). Ipsilateral Reorganization of Language in Early-Onset Left Temporal Lobe Epilepsy. *Epilepsy & Behavior* 3(2), 158-164.

Berl, M.M., Balsamo, L.M., Xu, B., Moore, E.N., Weinstein, S.L., Conry, J.A., Pearl, P.L., Sachs, B.C., Grandin, C.B., Frattali, C., Ritter, F.J., Sato, S., Theodore, W.H., and Gaillard, W.D. (2005). Seizure focus affects regional language networks assessed by fMRI. *Neurology* 65(10), 1604-1611.

Billingsley, R.L., McAndrews, M.P., Crawley, A.P., and Mikulis, D.J. (2001). Functional MRI of phonological and semantic processing in temporal lobe epilepsy. *Brain* 124(6), 1218-1227.

Binder, J.R., Frost, J.A., Hammeke, T.A., Cox, R.W., Rao, S.M., and Prieto, T. (1997). Human brain language areas identified by functional magnetic resonance imaging. *Journal of Neuroscience* 17(1), 353-362.

Binder, J.R., Swanson, S.J., Hammeke, T.A., Morris, G.L., Mueller, W.M., Fischer, M., Benbadis, S., Frost, J.A., Rao, S.M., and Haughton, V.M. (1996). Determination of language dominance using functional MRI: a comparison with the Wada test. *Neurology* 46(4), 978-984.

Brazdil, M., Chlebus, P., Mikl, M., Pazourkova, M., Krupa, P., and Rektor, I. (2005). Reorganization of language-related neuronal networks in patients with left temporal lobe epilepsy - an fMRI study. *European Journal of Neurology* 12(4), 268-275.

Brazdil, M., Zakopcan, J., Kuba, R., Fanfrdlova, Z., and Rektor, I. (2003). Atypical hemispheric language dominance in left temporal lobe epilepsy as a result of the reorganization of language functions. *Epilepsy & Behavior* 4(4), 414-419.

Breier, J.I., Castillo, E.M., Simos, P.G., Billingsley-Marshall, R.L., Pataraia, E., Sarkari, S., Wheless, J.W., and Papanicolaou, A.C. (2005). Atypical language representation in patients with chronic seizure disorder and achievement deficits with magnetoencephalography. *Epilepsia* 46(4), 540-548.

Corbetta, M., Akbudak, E., Conturo, T.E., Snyder, A.Z., Ollinger, J.M., Drury, H.A., Linenweber, M.R., Petersen, S.E., Raichle, M.E., Van Essen, D.C., and Shulman, GL. (1998). A common network of functional areas for attention and eye movements. *Neuron* 21(4), 761-773.

Cousin, E., Peyrin, C., and Baciu, M. (2006). Hemispheric predominance assessment of phonology and semantics: a divided visual field experiment. *Brain and Cognition* 61(3), 298-304.

Demonet, J.F., Chollet, F., Ramsay, S., Cardebat, D., Nespoulous, J.L., Wise, R., Rascol, A., and Frackowiak, R. (1992). The anatomy of phonological and semantic processing in normal subjects. *Brain* 115 (6), 1753-1768.

Demonet, J.F., Thierry, G., and Cardebat, D. (2005). Renewal of the neurophysiology of language: functional neuroimaging. *Physiological Reviews* 85(1), 49-95.

DeVos, K.J., Wyllie, E., Geckler, C., Kotagal, P., and Comair, Y. (1995). Language dominance in patients with early childhood tumors near left hemisphere language areas. *Neurology* 45(2), 349-356.

Engel, J., Jr. (2001). Mesial temporal lobe epilepsy: what have we learned? *Neuroscientist* 7(4), 340-352.

Fiez, J.A. (2001). Neuroimaging studies of speech an overview of techniques and methodological approaches. *Journal of Communication Disorders* 34(6), 445-454.

Friston, K.J., Fletcher, P., Josephs, O., Holmes, A., Rugg, M.D., and Turner, R. (1998). Event-related fMRI: characterizing differential responses. *NeuroImage* 7(1), 30-40.

Friston, K.J., Frith, C.D., Frackowiak, R.S., and Turner, R. (1995). Characterizing dynamic brain responses with fMRI: a multivariate approach. *NeuroImage* 2(2), 166-172.

Gitelman, D.R., Nobre, A.C., Sonty, S., Parrish, T.B., and Mesulam, M.M. (2005). Language network specializations: an analysis with parallel task designs and functional magnetic resonance imaging. *NeuroImage* 26(4), 975-985.

Goldmann, R.E. & Golby, A.J. (2005). Atypical language representation in epilepsy: implications for injury-induced reorganization of brain function. *Epilepsy & Behavior* 6(4), 473-487.

Grunwald, T., Beck, H., Lehnertz, K., Blumcke, I., Pezer, N., Kutas, M., Kurthen, M., Karakas, H.M., Van Roost, D., Wiestler, O.D., and Elger, C.E. (1999). Limbic P300s in temporal lobe epilepsy with and without Ammon's horn sclerosis. *European Journal of Neuroscience* 11(6), 1899-1906.

Helmstaedter, C., Fritz, N.E., Gonzalez Perez, P.A., Elger, C.E., and Weber, B. (2006). Shift-back of right into left hemisphere language dominance after control of epileptic seizures: evidence for epilepsy driven functional cerebral organization. *Epilepsy Research* 70(2-3), 257-262.

Hertz-Pannier, L., Chiron, C., Jambaque, I., Renaux-Kieffer, V., Van de Moortele, P.F., Delalande, O,. Fohlen, M., Brunelle, F., and Le Bihan, D. (2002). Late plasticity for language in a child's non-dominant hemisphere: a pre- and post-surgery fMRI study. *Brain* 125(2), 361-372.

Janszky, J., Jokeit, H., Heinemann, D., Schulz, R., Woermann, F.G., and Ebner, A. (2003). Epileptic activity influences the speech organization in medial temporal lobe epilepsy. *Brain* 126(9), 2043-2051.

Janszky, J., Mertens, M., Janszky, I., Ebner, A., and Woermann, F.G. (2006). Left-sided interictal epileptic activity induces shift of language lateralization in temporal lobe epilepsy: an fMRI study. *Epilepsia* 47(5), 921-7.

Kadis, D.S., Iida, K., Kerr, E.N., Logan, W.J., McAndrews, M.P., Ochi, A., Otsubo, H., Rutka, J.T., Iii, O.C., Weiss, S.K., and Smith, M.L. (2007). Intrahemispheric reorganization of language in children with medically intractable epilepsy of the left hemisphere. *Journal of the International Neuropsychological Society* 13(3), 505-516.

Knecht, S. (2004). Does language lateralization depend on the hippocampus? *Brain* 127(6), 1217-1218.

Knecht, S., Drager, B., Deppe, M., Bobe, L., Lohmann, H., Floel, A., Ringelstein, E.B., and Henningsen, H. (2000). Handedness and hemispheric language dominance in healthy humans. *Brain* 123 (12), 2512-8.

Kurthen, M., Linke, D.B., Elger, C.E., and Schramm, J. (1992). Linguistic perseveration in dominant-side intracarotid amobarbital tests. *Cortex* 28(2), 209-219.

Lazar, R.M., Marshall, R.S., Pile-Spellman, J., Hacein-Bey, L., Young, W.L., Mohr, J.P., and Stein, B.M. (1997). Anterior translocation of language in patients with left cerebral arteriovenous malformation. *Neurology* 49(3), 802-8.

Lehericy, S., Biondi, A., Sourour, N., Vlaicu, M., du Montcel, S.T., Cohen, L., Vivas, E., Capelle, L., Faillot, T., Casasco, A., Le Bihan, D., and Marsault, C. (2002). Arteriovenous brain malformations: is functional MR imaging reliable for studying language reorganization in patients? Initial observations. *Radiology* 223(3), 672-682.

Liegeois, F., Connelly, A., Cross, J.H., Boyd, S.G., Gadian, D.G., Vargha-Khadem, F., and Baldeweg, T. (2004). Language reorganization in children with early-onset lesions of the left hemisphere: an fMRI study. *Brain* 127(6), 1229-1236.

Liegeois, F., Connelly, A., Salmond, C.H., Gadian, D.G., Vargha-Khadem, F., and Baldeweg, T. (2002). A direct test for lateralization of language activation using fMRI: comparison with invasive assessments in children with epilepsy. *NeuroImage* 17(4), 1861-1867.

Lüders, H.O., Najm, I., Nair, D., Widdess-Walsh, P., and Bingman, W. (2006). The epileptogenic zone: general principles. *Epileptic Disorders* 8(Supplement 2), 1-9.

Lurito, J.T., Kareken, D.A., Lowe, M.J., Chen, S.H., and Mathews, VP. (2000). Comparison of rhyming and word generation with FMRI. *Human Brain Mapping* 10(3), 99-106.

Maccotta, L., Buckner, R.L., Gilliam, F.G., and Ojemann, J.G. (2007). Changing frontal contributions to memory before and after medial temporal lobectomy. *Cerebral Cortex* 17(2), 443-456.

Muller, R.A., Behen, M.E., Rothermel, R.D., Muzik, O., Chakraborty, P.K., and Chugani, HT. (1999a). Brain organization for language in children, adolescents, and adults with left hemisphere lesion: a PET study. *Progress in Neuropsychopharmacology and Biological Psychiatry* 23(4), 657-668.

Muller, R.A., Rothermel, R.D., Behen, M.E., Muzik, O, Chakraborty, PK & Chugani, HT. (1999b). Language organization in patients with early and late left-hemisphere lesion: a PET study. *Neuropsychologia* 37(5), 545-557.

Ojemann, G., Ojemann, J., Lettich, E., and Berger, M. (1989). Cortical language localization in left, dominant hemisphere. An electrical stimulation mapping investigation in 117 patients. *Journal of Neurosurgery* 71(3), 316-326.

Oldfield, R.C. (1971). The assessment and analysis of handedness: the Edinburgh inventory. *Neuropsychologia* 9(1), 97-113.

Pataraia, E., Billingsley-Marshall, R.L., Castillo, E.M., et al. (2005). Organization of receptive language-specific cortex before and after left temporal lobectomy. *Neurology* 64(3), 481-487.

Pataraia, E., Simos, P.G., Castillo, E.M., Billingsley-Marshall, R.L., McGregor, A.L., Breier, J.I., Sarkari, S., and Papanicolaou, AC. (2004). Reorganization of language-specific cortex in patients with lesions or mesial temporal epilepsy. *Neurology* 63(10), 1825-1832.

Price, C.J. (2000). The anatomy of language: contributions from functional neuroimaging. *Journal of Anatomy* 197(3), 335-339.

Pugh, K.R., Shaywitz, B.A., Shaywitz, S.E., Constable, R.T., Skudlarski, P., Fulbright, R.K., Bronen, R.A., Shankweiler, D.P., Katz, L., Fletcher, J.M., and Gore, J.C. (1996). Cerebral organization of component processes in reading. *Brain* 119(4), 1221-1238.

Pujol, J., Deus, J., Losilla, J.M., and Capdevila, A. (1999). Cerebral lateralization of language in normal left-handed people studied by functional MRI. *Neurology* 52(5), 1038-1043.

Richardson, M.P., Strange, B.A., Duncan, J.S., and Dolan, R.J. (2003). Preserved verbal memory function in left medial temporal pathology involves reorganisation of function to right medial temporal lobe. *NeuroImage* 20(Supplement 1), 112-119.

Ries, M.L., Boop, F.A., Griebel, M.L., Zou, P., Phillips, N.S., Johnson, S.C., Williams, J.P., Helton, K.J., and Ogg, R.J. (2004). Functional MRI and Wada determination of language lateralization: a case of crossed dominance. *Epilepsia* 45(1), 85-89.

Rosenow, F. & Lüders, H. 2001. Presurgical evaluation of epilepsy. *Brain* 124(9), 1683-1700.

Sabbah, P., Chassoux, F., Leveque, C., Landre, E., Baudoin-Chial, S., Devaux, B., Mann, M., Godon-Hardy, S., Nioche, C., Ait-Ameur, A., Sarrazin, J.L., Chodkiewicz, J.P., and Cordoliani, Y.S. (2003). Functional MR imaging in assessment of language dominance in epileptic patients. *NeuroImage* 18(2), 460-467.

Schaefer, M., Heinze, H.J., and Rotte, M. (2006). Verbal memory encoding in patients with left-sided hippocampal sclerosis. *Neuroreport* 17(11), 1219-1223.

Seghier, M.L., Lazeyras, F., Pegna, A.J., Annoni, J.M., Zimine, I., Mayer, E., Michel, C.M., and Khateb, A. (2004). Variability of fMRI activation during a phonological and semantic language task in healthy subjects. *Human Brain Mapping* 23(3), 140-155.

Springer, J.A., Binder, J.R., Hammeke, T.A., Swanson, S.J., Frost, J.A., Bellgowan, P.S., Brewer, C.C., Perry, H.M., Morris, G.L., and Mueller, W.M. (1999). Language dominance in neurologically normal and epilepsy subjects: a functional MRI study. *Brain* 122(11), 2033-2046.

Talairach, J. & Tournoux, P. (1988). *Co-planar stereotaxic atlas of the human brain.3-dimensional proportional system: An approach to cerebral imaging.* New York: Thieme.

Thivard, L., Hombrouck, J., du Montcel, S.T., Delmaire, C., Cohen, L., Samson, S., Dupont, S., Chiras, J., Baulac, M., and Lehericy, S. (2005). Productive and perceptive language reorganization in temporal lobe epilepsy. *NeuroImage* 24(3), 841-851.

Thomas, P. & Genton, P. (1992). *Epilepsies*. Paris: Masson.

Voets, N.L., Adcock, J.E., Flitney, D.E., Behrens, T.E., Hart, Y., Stacey, R., Carpenter, K., and Matthews, P.M. (2006). Distinct right frontal lobe activation in language processing following left hemisphere injury. *Brain* 129(3), 754-766.

Weber, B., Wellmer, J., Reuber, M., Mormann, F., Weis, S., Urbach, H., Ruhlmann, J., Elger, C.E., and Fernandez, G. (2006). Left hippocampal pathology is associated with atypical language lateralization in patients with focal epilepsy. *Brain* 129(2), 346-351.

Yuan, W., Szaflarski, J.P., Schmithorst, V.J., Schapiro, M., Byars, A.W., Strawsburg, R.H., and Holland, S.K. (2006). fMRI shows atypical language lateralization in pediatric epilepsy patients. *Epilepsia* 47(3), 593-600.

5

Functional neuroimaging of speech production in Parkinson's disease: Towards a better understanding of dysarthria physiopathology

SERGE PINTO
GAELLE FILLATRE
ALAIN GHIO

Abstract: Dysarthria in Parkinson's disease (PD) is generally described by a monotony of pitch and loudness, reduced stress, variable rate, imprecise consonants, and a breathy and harsh voice. Among surgical treatments, only subthalamic nucleus (STN) stimulation seems able to notably improve some motor components of speech, while intelligibility decreases after surgery. Results available often confirm the lower degree of speech improvement following STN stimulation compared with the total motor state, even showing a potential exacerbation of speech production following stimulation. Thus, management of dysarthria is still challenging for the clinician, and functional brain imaging can address issues to better understand the particular physiopathology of PD dysarthria. It has been suggested that PD dysarthria is associated with an altered recruitment of the principal brain motor regions (orofacial primary motor cortex, cerebellum) and an increased involvement of premotor and prefrontal cortices (notably the supplementary motor area). This pathological pattern does not parallel the compensatory strategy developed for hand motor tasks and may explain the frequent therapeutical difficulties encountered by the clinician who has to deal with the heterogeneous responses of limb and speech movements to pharmacological and surgical therapies.

1. SPEECH IMPAIRMENT IN PARKINSON'S DISEASE

Parkinson's disease (PD) affects between one and two per cent of the world's population aged 60 and older; the mean age at which symptoms appear is about 58 years (Marsden, 1994), but patients can develop the symptoms before the age of 40. Seventy per cent of patients with PD indicate that their speech is impaired during the progression of the disease (Hartelius and Svensson, 1994; Ramig et al., 1994).

1.1. PARKINSON'S DISEASE PHYSIOPATHOLOGY

The main cerebral lesion leading to the disease is the progressive dopaminergic neurodegeneration of the nigro-striatal pathway, projecting from the substantia nigra pars compacta (SNc) to the striatum (Agid et al., 1990). Notably, this represents the origin of the inherent basal ganglia (BG) motor loop dysfunction. According to the model described by several authors (Albin et al., 1989; Alexander and Crutcher, 1990; Alexander et al., 1990; Delong, 1990), neural degenerations in PD lead to several dysfunctions of basal ganglia activity. We can point out three main aspects (Figure 1): 1) an increased activation of basal ganglia output structures, the internal pallidum (GPi) and the substantia nigra pars reticulata (SNr), 2) an increased thalamic inhibition and 3) a decreased activation of the motor cortex. Thus, the nigro-striatal denervation leads to the appearance of the motor symptoms (Lee et al., 1994) that characterize PD: akiesia, bradykinesia and hypokinesia.
Akinesia represents the slowness of movement initiation, while bradykinesia is the slowness of movement execution. The reduced amplitude movements are described as hypokinesia. These three symptoms are often subsumed under the general term akinesia; the classic PD symptomatic triad associates this symptom with hypertonia and rest tremor. Other signs of the disease (e.g. gait impairment, postural impairment, blocks and freezings, hypomimia, hypersyalorrhea, micrographia, ocular convergence impairment, hypotension, weight loss, depression, dementia etc., mainly axial signs, take part in the multimodal symptomatology of the disease. However, akinesia frequently remains the more disabling one according to the patients' complaints. A frequent

axial sign limits oral communication and is involved in the loss of quality of life and the progressive social isolation of the patient: the speech impairment, so-called dysarthria in PD.

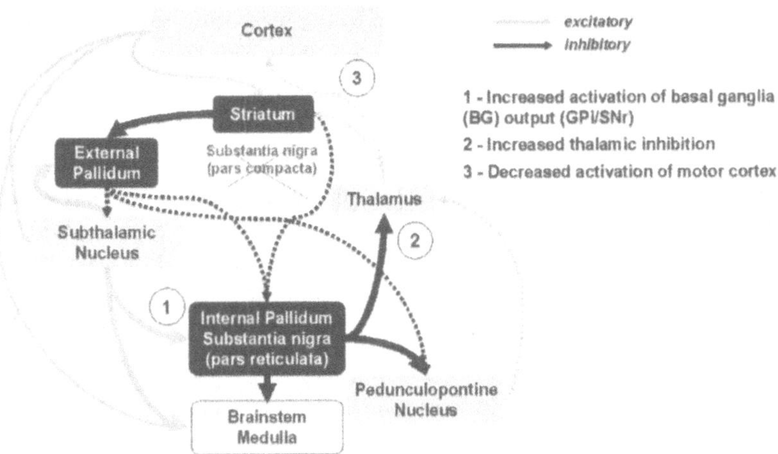

Figure 1: Functional impact of the dopaminergic degeneration in Parkinson's disease: the model (inspired by Alexander et al., 1990; Obeso et al., 2000; Kopell et al., 2006). Bold arrows refer to increased activations; dotted arrows represent decreased activations.

1.2. DYSARTHRIA IN PARKINSON'S DISEASE

"*Dysarthria is a collective name for a group of related speech disorders that are due to disturbances in muscular control of the speech mechanisms resulting from any impairment of the basic motor processes involved in the execution of speech*" (Darley et al., 1969a).

In other words, dysarthria characterizes an impairment of speech organ motor control resulting from a lesion of the peripheral or central nervous system (Darley et al., 1969a; 1969b; 1975). Dysarthria can appear at any stage of PD, and worsens in the later stages of the disease (Klawans, 1986; Mutch et al., 1986). After several years of disease progression, the classic symptom triad is usually still improved by pharmacological strategies whereas the response of dysarthria to treatment is highly variable (Klawans, 1986).

PD patients generally have a favourable response to levodopa at the beginning of treatment. This response decreases with time as dopaminergic and non-dopaminergic systems degrade. Aggravation of PD with time, concomitant with aggravation of dysarthria, suggests that the decrease in response is also linked to the increasing severity of non-dopaminergic cerebral lesions (Agid et al., 1990). This latter fact might be a reason for the partial response of dysarthric speech to levodopa therapy: some speech components tend to improve with dopatherapy while others do not; the effect of dopaminergic treatment is limited and variable among patients. In addition, motor fluctuations appear with an alternate state of severe Parkinsonism ("off" period) and a state of improved mobility ("on" period), often impaired by dyskinesias. These fluctuations can contribute to the aggravation of dysarthria (see Pinto, Ozsancäk et al., 2004 for a review).

According to the work and classification made by Darley and colleagues in the late 1960s, PD dysarthria is usually characterized by a monotony of pitch and loudness, reduced stress, variable rate, short rushes of speech, imprecise consonants and a breathy and harsh voice (Figure 2). These characteristics have been attributed to the weakness and slowness of movement (respectively referred to as hypokinesia and bradykinesia), rigidity and tremor at rest. Any or all components of speech production may be affected, including alterations of the respiratory, phonatory and articulatory systems. The observed bradykinetic and hypokinetic articulatory movements are frequently associated with a facial hypomimia. Thus, impaired neuromuscular function is the basis of dysarthria in PD.

The use of the term dysarthria to qualify speech impairment in PD could is debated. Although dysarthria is not only associated with articulatory/arthric difficulties according to the definition given by Darley and colleagues, it might be possible that there may be confusion in regard to respiratory, laryngeal and/or prosodic functions. Some authors would prefer to refer to the Parkinsonian case as dysarthrophonia (Ackermann & Ziegler, 1989; Baumgartner et al., 2001; Klostermann et al., 2008) in order to stress the laryngeal level of dysfunction among the various modalities of PD speech.

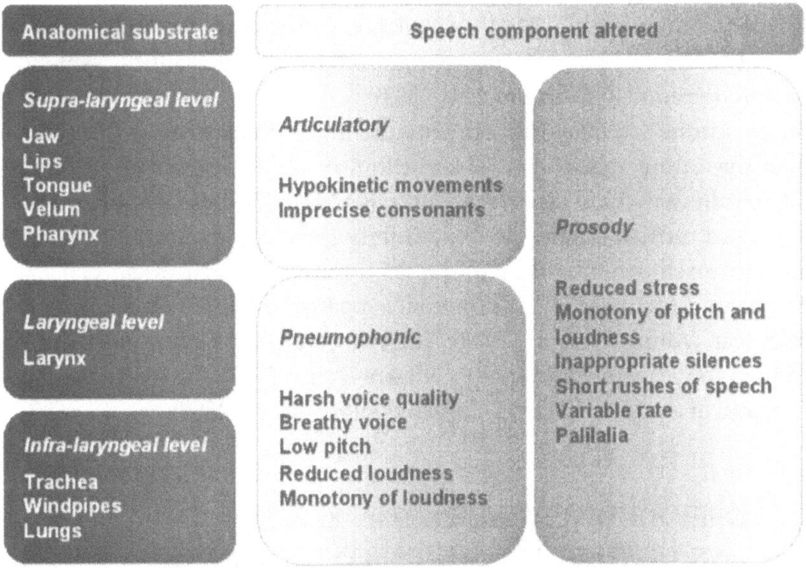

Figure 2: Anatomical substrate and related speech component alterations underlying Parkinsonian dysarthria (according to Darley et al.'s descriptions, 1969a, 1969b and 1975).

1.3. OTHER LANGUAGE DIFFICULTIES IN PARKINSON'S DISEASE

Apart from the motor aspects of the speech dysfunction in PD described above, some linguistic impairments have also been observed in PD patients. Significant deficits in verb generation (Bertella et al., 2002; Péran et al., 2003; Castner, Chenery, Silburn et al., 2007), aspects of lexical-semantic inhibitory mechanisms (Castner, Copland et al., 2007), semantic and affective priming (Castner, Chenery, Copland et al., 2007), as well as sentence comprehension (Angwin et al., 2005; 2007) and processing (Grossman et al., 2002) have been reported by various studies. All these data together suggest that high-level language difficulties can be present in PD (Berg et al., 2003), and that they may be linked with basal ganglia non-motor loop dysfunction (Castner, Chenery, Copland et al., 2007). Notably, impairment of a fronto-temporal network associated with word production has been suggested (Castner,

Chenery, Silburn et al., 2007), as well as overaction of the "right inferior frontal and left posterolateral temporal-parietal areas during sentence comprehension" (Grossman et al., 2003).

These studies address impairments of linguistic aspects in PD rather than dysarthric speech as a dysfunction of motor performance. This is the reason why these aspects are only mentioned in this chapter and not discussed further. Indeed, it would is important to combine both types of data to reach a global state-of-the-art level of research on speech and language difficulties in PD, especially regarding the effects of pharmacological (Angwin et al., 2006; Angwin et al., 2007) and deep brain stimulation (Castner, Chenery, Silburn et al., 2007; Castner, Chenery, Copland et al., 2007; Castner, Copland, Silburn et al., 2007).

2. DEEP BRAIN STIMULATION EFFECTS ON DYSARTHRIA IN PARKINSON'S DISEASE

Electrical stimulation of deep brain structures has been used since the early years of PD surgical treatment to guide ablative gesture. Since the 1990s, improved knowledge of basal ganglia functions and development of neurosurgical procedures have led to a great interest in high frequency deep brain stimulation as a treatment of choice for Parkinsonian signs.

2.1. EFFECTS OF SUBTHALAMIC NUCLEUS STIMULATION ON SPEECH IN PARKINSON'S DISEASE

The effects of thalamus and internal pallidum stimulations on speech have never been well studied; few references addressing this specific issue can be found in the literature (see Pinto, Ozsancäk et al., 2004, for a review). This has principally been attributed to the fact that positive effects of subthalamic nucleus (STN) stimulation on motor Parkinsonian symptoms have led most of the centres to consider this nucleus as the best target.

Two main groups of speech studies should then be considered: first, those involving a subjective assessment of speech intelligibility using the

speech items of the Unified Parkinson's Disease Rating Scale (UPDRS; Fahn et al., 1987) or other perceptual tools (Table 1); and second, studies involving instrumental motor speech tools for the measurement of specific speech components (Table 2). To inventory the studies that have reported data on the question, we sought articles from the "Pubmed" search engine on our subject (references are listed until April 2008) and selected the articles written in English, and published in international peer-reviewed journals. We identified the references using the following associated terms: "Parkinson, speech, stimulation", "Parkinson, dysarthria, stimulation", "Parkinson, subthalamic, stimulation", "Parkinson, speech, subthalamic stimulation", "Parkinson, stimulation, side effect", and "Deep brain stimulation, side effect". Then we classified the relevant articles according to the two main groups described above and further divided them into the following subgroups: beneficial, neutral and deleterious effects of STN stimulation on Parkinsonian speech.
Initial clinical assessments of the effect of STN stimulation by means of the UPDRS (speech item 18) report no change in or beneficial impact on PD dysarthria, although there does seem to be some beneficial effect on the limbs (Limousin et al., 1998). However, the use of the UPDRS subjective five-point scale seems to be insufficient to accurately assess speech disorders and discriminate between the observed impairments. A worsening of speech intelligibility can frequently be observed after surgery (Table 1); in some cases, when this stimulation-induced dysarthria persists, it may be necessary to adjust (that means decrease) stimulation parameters, leading to a lesser improvement in limb motor function (evaluated perceptually).
Thus, this possible improvement in speech intelligibility would tend to decrease in the long term.

Table 1: Review of the literature on the effects of STN stimulation on PD dysarthria; qualitative and perceptual assessments.

	Beneficial effect
Limousin et al., 1998	*24 patients, UPDRS*
Vingerhoets et al., 2002	*20 patients, UPDRS*
Rousseaux et al., 2004	*9 patients, UPDRS, dysarthria test*
Tabbal et al., 2007	*72 patients, UPDRS*
	No change
Bejjani et al., 2000	*10 patients, UPDRS*
Rousseaux et al., 2004	*9 patients, UPDRS, dysarthria test*
	Deleterious effect
Saint-Cyr et al., 2000	*11 patients, UPDRS, verbal fluency*
Brusa et al., 2000	*3 patients, UPDRS, verbal fluency*
Hariz et al., 2000	*Case report, qualitative rating scale*
Thobois et al., 2002	*18 patients, UPDRS*
Krack et al., 2003	*49 patients, UPDRS*
Romito et al., 2003	*33 patients, UPDRS*
Moretti et al., 2003	*Case report, neurolinguistic evaluation*
Krause et al., 2004	*27 patients, UPDRS*
Rousseaux et al., 2004	*9 patients, UPDRS, dysarthria test*
Rodriguez-Oroz et al., 2005	*49 patients, UPDRS*
Schüpbach et al., 2005	*37 patients, UPDRS*
Törnqvist et al., 2005	*10 patients, UPDRS, phoniatric assessment*
DeGaspari et al., 2006	*26 patients, UPDRS*
Ostergaard & Dunde, 2006	*22 patients, UPDRS*
Guehl et al., 2006	*44 patients, UPDRS*
Zhang et al., 2006	*46 patients, UPDRS*
Derost et al., 2007	*53 young & 34 older patients, UPDRS, quality of life questionnaire*
Kenney et al., 2007	*182 patients, medical assessments (metanalysis)*
Castelli et al., 2007	*19 patients, verbal fluency*
Klostermann et al., 2008	*19 patients, qualitative ratings*

Using instrumental assessments, articulatory and phonatory aspects of speech have been investigated individually; most of the parameters considered in these studies showed an improvement in speech with STN stimulation compared to the off-stimulation condition (Table 2). However, worsening of loudness and voice quality could also be observed, especially with inadequate stimulation parameters (Pinto et al., 2005). A common thread running through all these investigations is the question as to why STN stimulation worsens speech in some patients and not in others. The variation among the patients studied, in most of the investigations, leads to a weak level of evidence in terms of reliability and reproducibility of the results. Moreover, some articles appear more than once, in different subgroups, as they report various effects.

Table 2: Review of the literature on the effects of STN stimulation on PD dysarthria; instrumental investigations.

Beneficial effect	
Gentil, Tournier et al., 1999	*Case report, articulatory forces*
Gentil, Garcia-Ruiz et al., 1999	*10 patients, articulatory forces*
Dromey et al., 2000	*7 patients, acoustic analysis*
Gentil et al., 2001	*26 patients, acoustic analysis*
Pinto et al., 2003	*26 patients, articulatory forces*
Gentil et al., 2003	*16 patients, articulatory forces and acousic analysis*
Pinto, Thobois et al., 2004	*10 patients, articulatory forces, acoustic analysis, PET*
Pinto et al., 2005	*4 case reports, acoustic analysis*
Deleterious effect	
Santens et al., 2003	*7 patients, acoustic analysis*
Wang et al., 2003	*6 patients, acoustic analysis*
Pinto et al., 2005	*4 case reports, acoustic analysis*
Wang et al. 2006	*20 case reports, articulatory force and acoustic analysis*

2.2. CAN WE PREDICT HOW SPEECH WILL CHANGE AFTER STN STIMULATION?

Every scientific study has its own advantages and disadvantages. The selection and number of patients are frequent constraints that researchers have to deal with. Most of the studies evaluate the surgical effects on Parkinsonian signs, among which is dysarthria. However, dysarthria is never the reason why the patients are operated on; the patients are selected for displaying all inclusion and exclusion criteria needed for the surgery, and this point should obviously be mentioned when reporting the results. The severity of the disease and the dysarthria may also lead to variation in the response to treatments. In the case of STN stimulation, the fact that pre-surgery selection of patients is needed to ensure minimum risks for those patients in terms of surgical gesture also adds a bias that affects the populations studied. The period between the surgery and speech assessment is also one point that has to be mentioned.

Results are different when a single aspect of speech production is considered as compared to the intelligibility of speech in general. Each aspect of speech production is interesting on its own in terms of understanding the physiopathology of the symptom, but in terms of communication in daily live, intelligibility of speech should remain the primary measure in order to help the clinician to best adjust the treatment of the patient. As mentioned above, speech intelligibility responds poorly to STN stimulation, sometimes controlled by modulation of stimulation, while motor subcomponents of speech (lip or laryngeal movements assessed individually, etc.) may show some improvement induced by surgery.

Furthermore, medication should always be considered since the effects of STN stimulation on speech impairment depend on medication states. Although PD patients often experience a considerable reduction in dopaminergic treatment after surgery, clinicians usually consider it necessary to maintain a levodopa dose. Synergistic effects of both treatments together can thus be observed on dysarthric speech, both in terms of improvement and exacerbation of the symptom (Rousseaux et al., 2004; Pinto et al., 2005). In this context, clinicians have to address all these considerations when trying to develop the best treatment program for each patient.

The reading of these articles led us to consider the importance of the selection criteria for the patients and the adjustment of the stimulation parameters in optimizing the effects of STN stimulation on dysarthria. According to the numerous studies (particularly those reported in Tables 1 and 2) emerging from the international community interested in STN stimulation and PD speech research, the most common adverse effect observed following STN stimulation is the continuance and/or the exacerbation of dysarthric speech. Consequently, it would be important for the patients if clinicians could respond to the opening question of the present section with a consensual argumentation based on physiopathological considerations. Predictive factors still need to be identified, as well as the best location for stimulation in the STN. Fortunately, recent studies report on some issues that will be crucial to answering this important question.

3. WHY ARE THERE DISCREPANCIES BETWEEN STN STIMULATION EFFECTS ON LIMB AND SPEECH MOVEMENTS?

To answer this question, it is important to consider cerebral activations associated with motor tasks in PD. The development of neuroimaging techniques has led to a better knowledge of cerebral area dysfunctions related to various experimental tasks in PD. In particular, recent findings have revealed that dysfunctions observed during motor speech tasks do not parallel those associated with limb movements.

3.1. FUNCTIONAL NEUROIMAGING OF LIMB MOVEMENTS IN PARKINSON'S DISEASE

In recent years, functional brain imaging techniques such as positron emission tomography (PET) or functional magnetic resonance imaging (fMRI) have provided an additional approach to the investigation of the cerebral activations underlying various functions.
Functional imaging has given researchers the opportunity to assess brain activation during hand movements. The contralateral primary sensorimotor cortex involvement in hand movement has been well established (Olesen, 1971), as well as the involvement of several cortical areas such as the supplementary motor area (SMA) (Roland et al., 1980; Deiber et al., 1991; Colebatch et al., 1991; Seitz & Roland, 1992), the lateral premotor cortex (Deiber et al., 1991; Colebatch et al., 1991; Seitz & Roland, 1992), the anterior cingulate cortex (Deiber et al., 1991; Paus et al., 1993) and Brodmann's parietal area 7 (Deiber et al., 1991; Grafton et al., 1992). Remy and colleagues (1994) showed in a PET study that all-finger movement only activated the primary sensorimotor cortex and the

supplementary motor area contralateral to the movement. The middle finger movement induced a much more complex pattern: a high degree of sensorimotor cortex and SMA activation contralateral to the movement, as well as a slight ipsilateral activation of these areas (Remy et al., 1994).

During the execution of a freely chosen unilateral motor task, underactivation (i.e. a reduction in regional cerebral blood flow) was found in the SMA, dorsolateral prefrontal cortex (DLPFC) and anterior cingulate in PD patients compared to normal subjects. These cerebral areas are respectively the main output projections of the basal ganglia to the motor, associative and limbic loops (Playford et al., 1992; Jahanshahi et al., 1995). Conversely the primary motor (M1), parietal and lateral premotor cortices were normally activated. Apomorphine administration normalized the activation profile when patients turned on-medicated (Jenkins et al., 1992). More recent studies have demonstrated overactivations involving a lateral cerebello-parieto-premotor circuit rather than the impaired mesial SMA-cingulate circuit (Rascol et al., 1997; Samuel et al., 1997; Sabatini et al., 2000). Circuits showing overactivity are implicated more in externally cued motor tasks (Jahanshahi et al., 1995). These studies have also demonstrated that SMA underactivation involves anterior SMA while the caudal part is overactivated (Sabatini et al., 2000). Furthermore, the primary motor cortex, both ipsi- and contralateral to a motor task, may also be overactivated in PD even in early stages of the disease (Sabatini et al., 2000; Thobois et al., 2000). These abnormal activation patterns are obviously highly task-dependent. During an externally cued, sequential and repetitive motor task, the SMA is normally activated in PD while the M1 cortex and the cerebellum are underactivated (Turner et al., 2003). In contrast, lesser activation of the SMA is observed in PD during a task that requires more attentional and selection processes (Rowe et al., 2002).

All these data together represent the commonly accepted background that characterizes PD cerebral dysfunctions associated with (proximal) limb movements (Ceballos-Baumann, 2003): 1)a decreased activation of the motor circuitry involving the BG and reaching the SMA; 2) an increased activation of the M1 cortex (corresponding to the upper limb somatotopy); and 3) an increased activation of the cerebello-thalamo-cortical motor circuit. These two latter points suggest a compensatory recruitment of this cerebello-thalamo-cortical motor circuit in order to make up for the dysfunction of the one involving the BG. More recent studies have obtained similar results and supported this compensation hypothesis (*e.g.* Wu & Hallett, 2005; Yu et al., 2007). Studies investigating the effects of pharmacological treatments are also important in addressing some issues regarding the physiopathology of limb movements in PD: the compensatory mechanism has been confirmed off-medication, associated with a normalization of the cerebral activation profile on-medication (Haslinger et al., 2001). However, this question is still debated based on results obtained with apomorphine administration which are in opposition to these trends (Peters et al., 2003).

3.2. FUNCTIONAL NEUROIMAGING OF DYSARTHRIA IN PARKINSON'S DISEASE

In normal subjects, speech production and language processes have been widely investigated. As an example, speech articulation and vocalization have been separately investigated under different conditions using PET (Murphy et al., 1997). Regions specifically implicated in the motor component of speech were the inferior part of the primary sensorimotor cortex bilaterally, the left and right cerebellum and the right thalamus and caudate nucleus. In another PET study, the activated regions associated with articulation were the left anterior insula, lateral premotor cortex and basal ganglia (Wise et al., 1999). The authors suggested that the left anterior insula plays a major role in the planning and accuracy of speech movements. In addition, speech articulation in stroke patients specifically affected by a disorder in the motor planning of articulatory movements, apraxia of speech, was studied by magnetic resonance imaging (MRI) and computerized tomography scans (Dronkers, 1996). All the patients had brain lesions that included a discrete region of the left precentral gyrus of the insula, which suggests a role of this area in the motor planning of speech (Donnan et al., 1997).

So far, only two PET studies and one fMRI investigation are available in regard to the cerebral activations associated with Parkinsonian speech. Although important issues have been addressed, it is still difficult to come to a conclusion on the cerebral changes related to PD dysarthria.

Liotti and colleagues (Liotti et al., 2003) have studied the cerebral haemodynamic responses with respect to various speech production tasks. They showed that abnormalities of brain activation were essentially represented by an overactivation of the orofacial M1 cortex, inferior lateral premotor cortex and SMA. However, the findings concerned a small number of patients and did not include any control subjects. Another study showed that in PD, there is 1) a lack of activation in the right orofacial M1 cortex and bilateral cerebellar hemispheres (Figure 3), 2) an abnormal increase in haemodynamic response in the right superior premotor cortex and bilateral dorsolateral prefrontal cortex (DLPFC), and 3) an overactivation of the SMA (Pinto, Thobois et al., 2004).

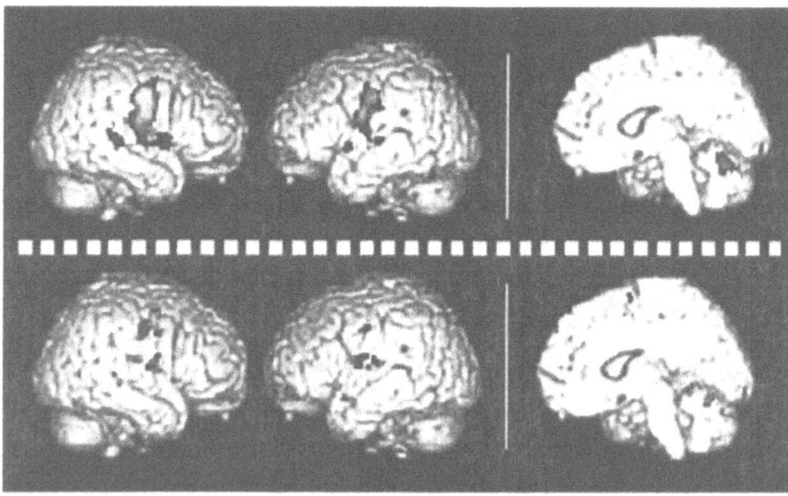

Figure 3: Cerebral activations during speech in normal subjects (top panel) and Parkinsonian patients (bottom panel). Decreased activation in the primary motor cortex and the cerebellum are observed bilaterally.

It has been suggested that Parkinsonian dysarthria is associated with an altered recruitment of the principal brain motor regions (orofacial M1 cortex, cerebellum) and an increased involvement of premotor and prefrontal cortices (DLPFC, SMA, superior premotor cortex). This would represent either a compensatory phenomenon or the inherent activation pattern underlying brain dysfunctions of PD dysarthria. In both cases, this pattern does not parallel the one associated with hand motor tasks and may explain the frequent therapeutical challenge encountered by the clinician who has to deal with the heterogeneous responses of limb and speech movements to pharmacological and surgical therapies. Evolution of the disease along time is concomitant with aggravation of dysarthria, which suggests that it is also linked to the increasing severity of cerebral non-dopaminergic lesions (Agid et al., 1990). Due to its complexity, speech production cannot be restricted to the motor basal ganglia loop: it should be emphasized that the cerebellum M1 cortex circuitry (Ackermann et al., 1998) may compensate for the lack of basal ganglia motor loop.

These data reinforce the finding that speech and hand movements differentially recruit the basal ganglia and the cerebello-thalamo-cortical motor loops. The common result of the two studies (Liotti et al., 2003; Pinto, Thobois et al., 2004) is the overactivation of the SMA, interpreted by both groups as a consequence of complex task performance. However, it is still important to consider the lack of activation in the cerebellum. The cerebellum projects its fibres massively towards the ventro-lateral nucleus of the thalamus, which is tightly connected with the motor cortex, Broca's area and the SMA (Nakano et al., 1992). Furthermore, Ackermann has pointed out the crucial role of the predominant right cerebellar projection to the left motor cortex in the control of speech (Ackermann et al., 1998). In regard to cerebellar dysfunction in dysarthric speech revealed by neuroimaging techniques, some case studies have been described (Urban et al., 1999; Okuda et al., 1999). Apart from the consistent cerebellar metabolism, other cerebral areas such as frontal, temporal and sensorimotor cortices have also displayed a reduction in rCBF. Ischaemic lesions in superior and inferior cerebellar arteries are known to be the source of appearance of dysarthric speech (Ackermann et al., 1992 ; Urban et al., 1999 ; Urban et al., 2001). A recent study carried out with stuttering patients showed a cerebellar underactivation during speech in comparison with control subjects; this lack of activation has been interpreted as a reflection of the increased voluntary control of speech in these patients who have lost speech automatisms (De Nil et al., 2001).

A more recent fMRI investigation reports data obtained in a group of 9 PD patients under medication (Rektorova et al., 2007). The speech paradigm studied was a reading task. The main result, interpreted by the authors as a compensatory phenomenon to preserve speech production in PD, was a significantly higher regional cerebral blood flow in the right primary orofacial sensorimotor cortex in PD patients as compared to controls. Interestingly, since the patients were on-medicated, the authors stress the fact that this overactivation is consistent with the two previous PET studies (Liotti et al., 2003; Pinto, Thobois et al., 2004) and may likely be associated with a "response to treatment" (Rektorova et al., 2007). Indeed, functional abnormalities in the speech-related cerebral activation profile were displayed in the patients involved in the study.

4. CONCLUSIONS

4.1. SOME PHYSIOPATHOLOGICAL HYPOTHESES FOR PARKINSONIAN DYSARTHRIA

PD dysarthria is less responsive to pharmacological and deep brain stimulation treatments than akinesia and rigidity. In addition, UPDRS perceptual evaluations (Table 1) seem to reveal a trend towards a worsening of speech. On one hand, the use of the UPDRS subjective five point scale seems to be insufficient to estimate speech disorders accurately: the major change from understandable speech to that which is difficult to understand corresponds to only one point. It appears that a more standardised dysarthria assessment procedure would certainly be more precise and relevant in order to provide a more informative profile of speech production characteristics. Some additionnal issues have been reported using more qualitative dedicated assessments (Ozsancäk et al., 2002; Rousseaux et al., 2004; see also Table 1).

On the other hand, the trend towards a worsening of speech revealed by the perceptual evaluations reflects the clinical global impression of most of the clinicians. We have already mentioned that in order to explain the differences between the effects of STN stimulation on limbs and speech organs, the brain activation profile associated with dysarthric speech would represent either a compensatory phenomenon or the inherent specific activation pattern underlying brain dysfunctions of PD dysarthria. Heterogeneity of individual motor performances according to tasks should also be taken into account when carrying out group analyses. This reality represents a methodological constraint that requires a rigorous verification of individual brain activation profiles prior to the pooling of data.

One can also consider that the observed discrepancies may be directly due to the stimulation itself. The idea can be proposed of a potential current spread towards neighbouring structures of the STN and the basal ganglia, such as the pyramidal tract. This might explain a sort of confusing message delivered to speech organ motoneurones; indeed, the pyramidal cortico-bulbar tract represents the origin of the cranial nerves which provide the innervation of the facial area. More generally, current spread to structures that should not be stimulated could occur in two ways: increasing the stimulation voltage, thus creating a larger region exposed to the current, and the inadequate localization of the stimulation. Previous observations involving such testing procedures would be in favour of this hypothesis (Pinto et al., 2005).

On the other hand, preliminary data (Pinto et al., 2006) from a larger study have showed that in control subjects, simultaneous performance of two movements by two different motor effectors, hand and speech organs, combined cerebral activations with respect to both motor functions. This combination seems difficult in PD patients, which may explain the pathophysiological mechanism of the patients' difficulties in performing simultaneous movements. This is an important issue which is still under investigation.

4.2. DYSARTHRIC SPEECH IN MOVEMENT DISORDERS AS A MODEL TO INVESTIGATE NEURAL CORRELATES OF SPEECH MOTOR AND NON-MOTOR ASPECTS

Movement disorders are often associated with motor speech impairment, which classically does not involve linguistic deficits; this is probably due to the fact that motor deficits are predominant in dysarthria. Dysarthria is considered as a motor speech disorder, and it is thus complicated to find aspects of linguistic alterations on dysarthria in the literature. However, evidence has been reported regarding verb generation deficits in non-demented PD patients (Péran et al., 2003). These findings may suggest that linguistic alteration could be part of speech impairment in PD.

Neuronal degeneration of the disease is characterized by the early loss of dopaminergic neurons emerging from the SNc, the projections of which, apart from those to the motor cortical regions, are also directed towards the frontal and orbito-frontal cortices. Thus, it is quite reasonable to imagine that the dopaminergic loss could also influence the activity of frontal language areas. This is another investigation track that has to be considered to further our understanding of dysarthria physiopathology.

REFERENCES

Ackermann, H., Vogel, M., Petersen, D. and Poremba, M. (1992). Speech deficits in ischaemic cerebellar lesions. *Journal of Neurology* 239, 223-227.

Ackermann, H., Wildgruber, D., Daum, I. and Grodd, W. (1998). Does the cerebellum contribute to cognitive aspects of speech production? A functional magnetic resonance imaging (fMRI) study in humans. *Neuroscience Letters* 247, 187-190.

Ackermann, H. & Ziegler, W. (1989). Dysarthrophonia of Parkinson syndrome. *Fortschritte der Neurologie-Psychiatrie* 57, 149-160.

Agid, Y., Graybiel, A.M., Ruberg, M., Hirsch, E., Blin, J., Dubois, B. & Javoy-Agid, F. (1990). The efficacy of levodopa treatment declines in the course of Parkinson's disease: Do nondopaminergic lesions play a role? *Advances in Neurology* 53, 83-100.

Albin, R.L., Young, A.B. and Penney, J.B. (1989). The functional anatomy of basal ganglia disorders. *Trends in Neurosciences* 12, 366-375.

Alexander, G.E. and Crutcher, M.D. (1990). Functional architecture of basal ganglia circuits: Neural substrates of parallel processing. *Trends in Neurosciences* 13, 266-271.

Alexander, G.E., Crutcher, M.D. & DeLong, M.R. (1990). Basal ganglia-thalamocortical circuits: Parallel substrates for motor, oculomotor, "prefrontal" and "limbic" functions. *Progress in Brain Research* 85, 119-146.

Angwin, A.J., Chenery, H.J., Copland, D.A., Murdoch, B.E., and Silburn, P.A. (2005). Summation of semantic priming and complex sentence comprehension in Parkinson's disease. *Brain Research. Cognitive Brain Research* 25, 78-89.

Angwin, A.J., Chenery, H.J., Copland, D.A., Murdoch, B.E. and Silburn, PA. (2007). The speed of lexical activation is altered in Parkinson's disease. *Journal of Clinical Experimental Neuropsychology* 29, 73-85.

Angwin, A.J., Copland, D.A., Chenery, H.J., Murdoch, B.E. and Silburn, PA. (2006). The influence of dopamine on semantic activation in Parkinson's disease: Evidence from a multipriming task. *Neuropsychology* 20, 299-306.

Baumgartner, C.A., Sapir, S. and Ramig, L. (2001). Voice quality changes following phonatory-respiratory effort treatment (LSVT) versus respiratory effort treatment for individuals with Parkinson disease. *Journal of Voice* 15, 105-114.

Bejjani, B.P., Gervais, D., Arnulf, I., Papadopoulos, S., Demeret, S., Bonnet, A.M., Cornu, P. and Agid, Y. (2000). Axial Parkinsonian symptoms can be improved: The role of levodopa and bilateral subthalamic stimulation. *Journal of Neurology, Neurosurgery & Psychiatry* 68, 595-600.

Berg, E., Björnram, C., Hartelius, L., Laakso, K., and Johnels, B. (2003). High-level language difficulties in Parkinson's disease. *Clinical Linguistics and Phonetics* 17, 63-80.

Bertella, L., Albani, G., Greco, E., Priano, L., Mauro, A., Marchi, S., Bulla, D., and Semenza, C. (2002). Noun verb dissociation in Parkinson's disease. *Brain and Cognition* 48, 277-280.

Brusa, L., Pierantozzi, M., Peppe, A., Attibrandi, M.G., Giacomini, P., Mazzone, P., and Stanzione, P. (2000). Deep brain stimulation attentional effects parallel those of l-dopa treatment. *Journal of Neural Transmission* 108, 1021-1027.

Castelli, L., Lanotte, M., Zibetti, M., Caglio, M., Rizzi, L., Ducati, A., Bergamasco, B., and Lopiano, L. (2007). Apathy and verbal fluency in STN-stimulated PD patients. An observational follow-up study. *Journal of Neurology* 254, 1238-1243.

Castner, J.E., Chenery, H.J., Copland, D.A., Coyne, T.J., Sinclair, F. & Silburn, P.A. (2007). Semantic and affective priming as a function of stimulation of the subthalamic nucleus in Parkinson's disease. *Brain* 130, 1395-1407.

Castner, J.E., Chenery, H.J., Silburn, P.A., Smith, E.R., Coyne, T.J., Sinclair, F., and Copland, D.A. (2007). The effects of subthalamic deep brain stimulation on noun/verb generation and selection from competing alternatives in Parkinson's disease. *Journal of Neurology, Neurosurgery, & Psychiatry,* Oct 2007; doi:10.1136/jnnp.2007.118729

Castner, J.E., Copland, D.A., Silburn, P.A., Coyne, T.J., Sinclair, F., and Chenery, H.J. (2007). Lexical-semantic inhibitory mechanisms in Parkinson's disease as a function of subthalamic stimulation. *Neuropsychologia* 45, 3167-3177.

Ceballos-Baumann, A.O. (2003). Functional imaging in Parkinson's disease: Activation studies with PET, fMRI and SPECT. *Journal of Neurology* 250, I/15-I/23.

Colebatch, J.G., Deiber, M.P., Passingham, R.E., Friston, K.J., and Frackowiak, R.J.S. (1991). Regional cerebral blood flow during voluntary arm and hand movements in human subjects. *Journal of Neurophysiology* 65, 1392-1401.

Darley, F.L., Aronson, A.E., and Brown, J.R. (1969a). Differential diagnostic patterns of dysarthria. *Journal of Speech and Hearing Research* 12, 246-269.

Darley, F.L., Aronson, A.E., and Brown, J.R. (1969b). Clusters of deviant speech dimensions in the dysarthrias. *Journal of Speech and Hearing Research* 12, 462-496.

Darley, F.L., Aronson, A.E., and Brown, J.R. (1975). *Motor speech disorders.* Philadelphia: Saunders.

DeGaspari, D., Siri, C., DiGioia, M., Antonini, A., Isella, V., Pizzolato, A., Landi, A., Vergani, F., Gaini, S.M., Appolonio, I.M., and Pezzoli, G. (2006). Clinical correlates and cognitive underpinnings of verbal fluency impairment after chronic subthalamic stimulation in Parkinson's disease. *Parkinsonism and Related Disorders* 12, 289-295.

Deiber, M.P., Passingham, R.E., Colebatch, J.G., Friston, K.J., Nixon, P.D., and Frackowiak, RJ.S. (1991). Cortical areas and the selection of movement: A study with positron emission tomography. *Experimental Brain Research* 84, 393-402.

DeLong M.R. (1990). Primate models of movement disorders of basal ganglia origin. *Trends in Neurosciences* 13, 281-285.

De Nil, L.F., Kroll, R.M., and Houle, S. (2001). Functional neuroimaging of cerebellar activation during single word reading and verb generation in stuttering and nonstuttering adults. *Neuroscience Letters* 302, 77-80.

Derost, P.P., Ouchchane, L., Morand, D., Ulla, M., Llorca, P.M., Barget, M., Debilly, B., Lemaire, J.J., and Durif, F. (2007). Is DBS-STN appropriate to treat severe Parkinson disease in an elderly population? *Neurology* 68, 1345-1355.

Donnan, G.A., Darby, D.G., and Saling, M.M. (1997). Identification of brain region for coordinating speech articulation. *Lancet* 349, 221-222.

Dromey, C., Kumar, R., Lang, A.E., and Lozano, A.M. (2000). An investigation of the effects of subthalamic nucleus stimulation on acoustic measures of voice. *Movement Disorders* 15, 1132-1138.

Dronkers, N.F. (1996). A new brain region for coordinating speech articulation. *Nature* 384, 159-161.

Fahn, S., Elton, R.L., and the committee motUd. (1987). Unified Parkinson's Disease Rating Scale. In: S. Fahn, C.D. Marsden, and D.B. Calne (Eds.) *Recent developments in Parkinson's disease.* 153-164, New Jersey: Health Care Information.

Gentil, M., Chauvin, P., Pinto, S., Pollak, P., and Benabid, A.L. (2001). Effect of Bilateral Stimulation of the Subthalamic Nucleus on Parkinsonian Voice. *Brain and Language* 78, 233-240.

Gentil, M., Garcia-Ruiz, P., Pollak, P., and Benabid, A.L. (1999). Effect of stimulation of the subthalamic nucleus on oral control of patients with Parkinsonism. *Journal of Neurology, Neurosurgery & Psychiatry* 67, 329-333.

Gentil, M., Pinto, S., Pollak, P., and Benabid, A.L. (2003). Effect of bilateral stimulation of the subthalamic nucleus on Parkinsonian dysarthria. *Brain and Language* 85, 190-196.

Gentil, M., Tournier, C.L., Pollak, P., and Benabid, A.L. (1999). Effect of bilateral subthalamic nucleus stimulation and dopatherapy on oral control in Parkinson's disease. *European Neurology* 42, 136-40.

Grafton, S., Mazziotta, J.C., Prestry, S., Friston, K.J., Frackowiak, R.J.S., and Phelps, M.E. (1992). Functional anatomy of human procedural learning determined with regional cerebral blood flow and PET. *Journal of Neuroscience* 12, 2542-2548.

Grossman, M., Cooke, A., DeVita, C., Lee, C., Alsop, D., Detre, J., Gee, J., Chen, W., Stern, M.B., and Hurtig, H.I. (2003). Grammatical and resource components of sentence processing in Parkinson's disease: An fMRI study. *Neurology* 60, 775-781. Grossman, M., Lee, C., Morris, J., Stern, M.B., and Hurtig, H.I. (2002). Assessing resource demands during sentence processing in Parkinson's disease. *Brain and Language* 80, 603-616.

Guehl, D., Cuny, E., Benazzouz, A., Rougier, A., Tison, F., Machado, S., Grabot, D., Gross, C., Bioulac, B., and Burbaud, P. (2006). Side-effects of subthalamic stimulation in Parkinson's disease: Clinical evolution and predictive factors. *European Journal of Neurology* 13, 963-971.

Hariz, M.I., Johansson, F., Shamsgovara, P., Johansson, E. , Hariz, G.M., and Fagerlund, M. (2000). Bilateral subthalamic nucleus stimulation in a Parkinsonian patient with preoperative deficits in speech and cognition: Persistent improvement in mobility but increased dependency: A case study. *Movement Disorders* 15, 136-187.

Hartelius, L. & Svensson, P. (1994). Speech and swallowing symptoms associated with Parkinson's disease and multiple sclerosis: A survey. *Folia Phoniatrica and Logopaedia* 46, 9-17.

Haslinger, B., Erhard, P., Kämpfe, N., Boecker, H., Rummeny, E., Schwaiger, M., Conrad, B., and Ceballos-Baumann, A.O. (2001). Event-related functional magnetic resonance imaging in Parkinson's disease before and after levodopa. *Brain* 124, 558-570.

Jahanshahi, M., Jenkins, H.I., Brown, R.G., Marsden, C.D., Pasingham, R.E., and Brooks, D. (1995). Self-initiated versus externally triggered movements. I. An investigation using measurement of regional cerebral blood flow with PET and movement-related potentials in normal and Parkinson's disease subjects. *Brain* 118, 913-933.

Jenkins, I.H., Fernandez, W., Playford, E.D., Lees, A.J., Frackowiak, R.J.S., Passingham, R.E., and Brooks, D. (1992). Impaired activation of the supplementary motor area in Parkinson's disease is reversed when akinesia is treated with apomorphine. *Annals of Neurology* 32, 749-57.

Kenney, C., Simpson, R., Hunter, C., Ondo, W., Almaguer, M., Davidson, A. and Jankovic, J. (2007). Short-term and long-term safety of deep brain stimulation in the treatment of movement disorders. *Journal of Neurosurgery* 106, 621-625.

Klawans, H.L. (1986). Individual manifestations of Parkinson's disease after ten or more years of levodopa. *Movement Disorders* 1, 187-192.

Klostermann, F., Ehlen, F., Vesper, J., Nubel, K., Gross, M., Marzinzik, F., Curio, G., and Sappok, T. (2008). Effects of subthalamic deep brain stimulation on dysarthrophonia in Parkinson's disease. *Journal of Neurology, Neurosurgery & Psychiatry* 79, 522-529.

Kopell, B.H., Rezai, A.R., Chang, J.W., and Vitek, J.L. (2006). Anatomy and physiology of the basal ganglia: Implications for deep brain stimulation for Parkinson's disease. *Movement Disorders* 21, 238-246.

Krack, P., Batir, A., Van Bercom, N., Chabardes, S., Fraix, V., Ardouin, C., Koudsie, A., Dowsey-Limousin, P., Benazzouz, A., LeBas, J.F., Benabid, A.L., and Pollak, P. (2003). Five years follow-up of bilateral stimulation of the subthalamic nucleus in advanced Parkinson's disease. *New England Journal of Medicine* 349, 1925-1934.

Krause, M., Fogel, W., Mayer, P., Kloss, M., and Tronnier, V. (2004). Chronic inhibition of the subthalamic nucleus in Parkinson's disease. *Journal of Neurological Sciences* 219, 119-124.

Lee, C.S., Schulzer, M., Mak, E.K., Snow, B.J., Tsui, J.K., Calne, S., Hammerstad, J., and Calne, D.B. (1994). Clinical observations on the rate of progression of idiopathic Parkinsonism. *Brain* 117, 501-507.

Limousin, P., Krack, P., Pollak, P., Benazzouz, A., Ardouin, C., Hoffmann, D., and Benabid, A.L. (1998). Electrical stimulation of the subthalamic nucleus in advanced Parkinson's disease. *New England Journal of Medicine* 339, 1105-1111.

Liotti, M., Ramig, L.O., Vogel, D., New, P., Cook, C.I., Ingham, R.J., Ingham, J.C., and Fox, P.T. (2003). Hypophonia in Parkinson's disease: Neural correlates of voice treatment revealed by PET. *Neurology* 60, 432-440.

Marsden, C.D. (1994). Parkinson's disease. *Journal of Neurology, Neurosurgery & Psychiatry* 57, 672-681.

Moretti, R., Torre, P., and Antonello, R.M. (2003). Speech initiation hesitation following subthalamic nucleus stimulation in a patient with Parkinson's disease. *European Neurology* 49, 251-253.

Murphy, K., Corfield, D.R., Guz, A., Fink, G.R., Wise, R.J., Harrison, J., and Adams, L. (1997). Cerebral areas associated with motor control of speech in humans. *Journal of Applied Physiology* 83, 1438-1447.

Mutch, W.J., Strudwick, A., Roy, S.K., and Downie, A.W. (1986). Parkinson's disease: Disability, review, and management. *British Medical Journal* 293, 675-677.

Nakano, K., Tokushige, A., Kohno, M., Hasegawa, Y., Kayahara, T., and Sasaki, K. (1992). An autoradiographic study of cortical projections from motor thalamic nuclei in the macaque monkey. *Neuroscience Research* 13, 119-137.

Obeso, J.A., Rodriguez-Oroz, M., Lanciengo, J.L., Artieda, J., Gonzalo, N., and Olanow, C.W. (2000). Pathophysiology of the basal ganglia in Parkinson's disease. *Trends in Neurosciences* 23, 8-19.

Okuda, B., Kawabata, K., Tachibana, H., and Sugita, M. (1999). Cerebral blood flow in pure dysarthria: Role of frontal cortical hypoperfusion. *Stroke* 30, 109-113.

Olesen, J. (1971). Contralateral focal increase of cerebral blood flow in man during arm movement. *Brain* 94, 635-646.

Ostergaard, K. & Dunde, N.A. (2006). Evolution of Parkinson's disease during 4 years of bilateral deep brain stimulation of the subthalamic nucleus. *Movement Disorders* 21, 624-631.

Ozsancäk, C., Parais, A.M., and Auzou, P. (2002). Perceptual analysis of dysarthria: Presentation and validation of a clinical scale. Preliminary study. *Revue Neurologique (Paris)* 158, 431-438.

Paus, T., Petrides, M., Evans, A.C., and Meyer, E. (1993). Role of the human anterior cingulate cortex in the control of oculomotor, manual and speech responses: A positron emission tomography study. *Journal of Neurophysiology* 70, 453-469.

Péran, P., Rascol, O., Démonet, J.F., Celsis, P., Nespoulous, J.L., Dubois, B., and Cardebat, D. (2003). Deficit of verb generation in nondemented patients with Parkinson's disease. *Movement Disorders* 18,150-156.

Peters, S., Suchan, B., Rusin, J., Daum, I., Köster, O., Przuntek, H., Müller, T., and Schmid, G. (2003). Apomorphine reduces BOLD signal in fMRI during voluntary movement in Parkinsonian patients. *Neuroreport* 14, 809-812.

Pinto, S., Gentil, M., Fraix, V., Benabid, A.L., and Pollak, P. (2003). Bilateral subthalamic stimulation effects on oral force control in Parkinson's disease. *Journal of Neurology* 250, 179-187.

Pinto, S., Thobois, S., Costes, N., Le Bars, D., Benabid, A.L., Broussolle, E., Pollak, P., and Gentil, M. (2004). Subthalamic nucleus stimulation and dysarthria in Parkinson's disease: A PET study. *Brain* 127, 602-615.

Pinto, S., Ozsancäk, C., Tripoliti, E., Thobois, S., Limousin-Dowsey, P., and Auzou, P. (2004). Treatments for dysarthria in Parkinson's disease. *Lancet Neurology* 3, 547-556.

Pinto, S., Gentil, M., Krack, P., Sauleau, P., Fraix, V., Benabid, A.L., and Pollak, P. (2005). Changes induced by levodopa and subthalamic nucleus stimulation on Parkinsonian speech. *Movement Disorders* 20, 1507-1515.

Pinto, S., Mancini, L., Brehmer, R., Thornton, J., Jahanshahi, M., Yousry, T., Rothwell, J., and Limousin-Dowsey, P. (2006). Functional MRI during combined hand movement and speech production in Parkinson's disease. *Movement Disorders* 21(supplement 15), 615-616.

Playford, E.D., Jenkins, I.H., Passingham, R.E., Nutt, J., Frackowiak, R.S., and Brooks, D.J. (1992). Impaired mesial frontal and putamen activation in Parkinson's disease: A positron emission tomography study. *Annals of Neurology* 32, 151-161.

Ramig, L.O., Bonitati, C.M., Lemke, J.H., and Horii, Y. (1994). Voice treatment for patients with Parkinson's disease. Development of an approach and preliminary efficacy data. *Journal of Medical Speech-Language Pathology* 2, 191-209.

Rascol, O., Sabatini, U., Fabre, N., Brefel, C., Loubinoux, I., Celsis, P., Senard, J.M., Montastruc, J.L., and Chollet, F. (1997). The ipsilateral cerebellar hemisphere is overactive during hand movements in akinetic Parkinsonian patients. *Brain* 120, 103-110.

Rektorova, I., Barrett, J., Mikl, M., Rektor, I. & Paus, T. (2007). Functional abnormalities in the primary orofacial sensorimotor cortex during speech in Parkinson's disease. *Movement Disorders* 22, 2043-2051.

Remy, P., Zilbovicius, M.W., Leroy-Willig, A., Syrota, A., and Samson, Y. (1994). Movement- and task-related activations of motor cortical areas: A positron emission tomography study. *Annals of Neurology* 36, 19-26.

Rodriguez-Oroz, M.C., Obeso, J.A., Lang, A.E., Houeto, J.L., Pollak, P., Rehncrona, S., Kulisevsky, J., Albanese, A., Volkmann, J., Hariz, M.I., Quinn, N.P., Speelman, J.D., Guridi, J., Zamarbide, I., Gironell, A., Molet, J., Pascual-Sedano, B., Pidoux, B., Bonnet, A.M., Agid, Y., Xie, J., Benabid, A.L., Lozano, A.M., Saint-Cyr, J., Romito, L., Contarino, M.F., Scerrati, M., Fraix, V., and Van Blercom, N. (2005). Bilateral deep brain stimulation in Parkinson's disease: A multicenter study with 4 years follow-up. *Brain* 128, 2240-2249.

Roland, P.E., Larsen, B., Lassen, N.A., and Skinhodj, E. (1980). Supplementary motor area and other cortical areas in organization of voluntary movements in man. *Journal of Neurophysiology* 54, 118-136.

Romito, L.M., Scerrati, M., Contarino, M.F., Iacoangeli, M., Bentivoglio, A.R., and Albanese, A. (2003). Bilateral high frequency subthalamic stimulation in

Parkinson's disease: Long-term neurological follow-up. *Journal of Neurosurgical Sciences* 47, 119-128.

Rousseaux, M., Krystkowiak, P., Kozlowski, O., Ozsancäk, C., Blond, S., and Destée, A. (2004). Effects of subthalamic nucleus stimulation on Parkinsonian dysarthria and speech intelligibility. *Journal of Neurology* 251, 327-334.

Rowe, J., Stephan, K.E., Friston, K., Frackowiak, R., Lees, A., and Passingham, R. (2002). Attention to action in Parkinson's disease. Impaired effective connectivity among frontal cortical regions. *Brain* 125, 276-289.

Sabatini, U., Boulanouar, K., Fabre, N., Martin, F., Carel, C., Colonnese, C., Bozzao., L., Berry, I., Montastruc, J.L., Chollet, F., and Rascol, O. (2000). Cortical motor reorganization in akinetic patients with Parkinson's disease: A functional MRI study. *Brain* 123, 394-403.

Saint-Cyr, J.A., Trépanier, L.L., Kumar, R., Lozano, A.M., and Lang, A.E. (2000). Neuropsychological consequences of chronic bilateral stimulation of the subthalamic nucleus in Parkinson's disease. *Brain* 123, 2091-2108.

Samuel, M., Ceballos-Baumann, A.O., Blin, J., Uema, T., Boecker, H., Passingham, R.E., and Brooks, D.J. (1997). Evidence for lateral premotor and parietal overactivity in Parkinson's disease during sequential and bimanual movements. A PET study. *Brain* 120, 963-976.

Santens, P., DeLetter, M., Van Borsel, J., De Reuck, J., and Caemaert, J. (2003). Lateralized effects of subthalamic nucleus stimulation on different aspects of speech in Parkinson's disease. *Brain and Language* 87, 253-258.

Schüpbach, W.M.M., Chastan, N., Welter, M.L., Houeto, J.L., Mesnage, V., Bonnet, A.M., Czernecki, V., Maltête, D., Hartmann, A., Mallet, L., Pidoux, B., Dormont, P., Navarro, S., Cornu, P., Mallet, A., and Agid, Y. (2005). Stimulation of the subthalamic nucleus in Parkinson's disease: A 5-year follow-up. *Journal of Neurology, Neurosurgery & Psychiatry* 76, 1640-1644.Seitz, R.J. & Roland, P.E. (1992). Learning of sequential finger movements in man: A combined kinematic and positron emission tomography (PET) study. *European Journal of Neuroscience* 4, 154-165.

Tabbal, S.D., Revilla, F.J., Mink, J.W., Schneider-Gibson, P., Wernle, A.R., de Erausquin, G.A., Perlmutter, J.S., Rich, K.M., and Dowling, J.L. (2007). Safety and efficacy of subthalamic nucleus deep brain stimulation performed with limited intraoperative mapping for treatment of Parkinson's disease. *Neurosurgery* 61, 119-127.

Thobois, S., Dominey, P., Decety, J., Pollak, P., Gregoire, M.C., and Broussolle, E. (2000). Overactivation of primary motor cortex is asymmetrical in hemiparkinsonian patients. *Neuroreport* 11, 785-789.

Thobois, S., Mertens, P., Guenot, M., Bouvard, M., Broussolle, E., and Sindou, M. (2002). Subthalamic nucleus stimulation in Parkinson's disease. Clinical evaluation of 18 patients. *Journal of Neurology* 259, 529-534.

Törnqvist, A.L., Schalén, L., and Rehncrona, S. (2005). Effects of different electrical parameter settings on the intelligibility of speech in patients with Parkinson's disease treated with subthalamic deep brain stimulation. *Movement Disorders* 20, 416-423.

Turner, R.S., Grafton, S.T., McIntosh, A.R., DeLong, M.R., and Hoffman, J.M. (2003). The functional anatomy of Parkinsonian bradykinesia. *Neuroimage* 19, 163-179.

Urban, P.P., Wicht, S., Hopf, H.C., Fleischer, S., and Nickel, O. (1999). Isolated dysarthria due to extracerebellar lacunar stroke: A central monoparesis of the tongue. *Journal of Neurology, Neurosurgery & Psychiatry* 66, 495-501.

Urban, P.P., Wicht, S., Vukurevic, G., Fitzek, C., Fitzek, S., Stoeter, P., Massinger, C., and Hopf, H.C. (2001). Dysarthria in acute ischemic stroke: Lesion topography, clinicoradiologic correlation, and etiology. *Neurology* 56, 1021-1027.

Vingerhoets, F.J.G., Villemure, J.G., Temperli, P., Pollo, C., Pralong, E., and Ghika, J. (2002). Subthalamic DBS replaces levodopa in Parkinson's disease: Two-yearfollow-up. *Neurology* 58, 396-401.

Wang, E., Metman, L.V., Bakay, R.A., Arzbaecher, J., Bernard, B., and Corcos, D.M. (2006). Hemisphere-Specific Effects of Subthalamic Nucleus Deep Brain Stimulation on Speaking Rate and Articulatory Accuracy of Syllable Repetitions in Parkinson's Disease. *Journal of Medical Speech and Language Pathology*, 14, 323-334.

Wang, E., Verhagen, M.L., Bakay, R., Arzbaecher, J. , and Bernard, B. (2003). The effect of unilateral electrostimulation of the subthalamic nucleus on respiratory/phonatory subsystems of speech production in Parkinson's disease: A preliminary report. *Clinical Linguistics and Phonetics* 17, 283-289.

Wise, R.J., Greene, J., Buchel, C., and Scott, S.K. (1999). Brain regions involved in articulation. *Lancet* 353, 1057-1061.

Wu, T. & Hallett, M. (2005). A functional MRI study of automatic movements in patients with Parkinson's disease. *Brain* 128, 2250-2259.

Yu, H., Sternad, D., Corcos, D.M., and Vaillancourt, D.E. (2007). Role of hyperactive cerebellum and motor cortex in Parkinson's disease. *NeuroImage* 35, 222-33.

Zhang, J.G., Zhang, K., Ma, Y., Hu, W.H., Yang, A.C., Chu, J.S., Wu, S.T., Ge, M., Zhang, Y., and Wang, Z.C. (2006). Follow-up of bilateral subthalamic deep brain stimulation for Parkinson's disease. *Acta Neurochirurgica* 99, 43-47.

6

The neurobiological correlates of developmental dyslexia

SYLVIANE VALDOIS
CAROLE PEYRIN
MONICA BACIU

Abstract: Developmental dyslexia is a specific reading disability that is neurobiological in origin. We first summarise behavioural evidence suggesting that developmental dyslexia results from a phonological processing disorder. Atypical functioning in left perisylvian regions have been reported as the neural signature of this phonological disorder. The second section provides evidence for a visual attention (VA) span disorder as a second core deficit in developmental dyslexia. The VA span denotes the number of distinct visual elements which can be processed in parallel in a multi-element array. A reduction in the VA span size has been reported in a good number of dyslexic individuals and this disorder typically dissociates from phonological problems in the dyslexic population. Functional neuroimaging investigations have revealed atypical parietal activations in the dyslexic individuals with a VA span disorder. Further, evidence has been reported that behavioural dissociations between phonological and VA span disorders result in brain dysfunctions that are limited to the cerebral networks underlying the altered cognitive function.

1. INTRODUCTION

Developmental dyslexia is characterised by an unexpected difficulty in reading in children who otherwise possess the intelligence and motivation necessary for accurate and fluent reading. It is a specific learning disability that is neurobiological in origin. Actually, developmental dyslexia is considered as the most common neurobehavioural disorder affecting children, with prevalence rates ranging from 5% to 17% (see the "Rapport d'Expertise INSERM, 2007, for a review). Developmental dyslexia can be characterised at three different levels of description: the behavioural, cognitive and biological levels (Frith, 1997). At the behavioural level, developmental dyslexia expresses itself by poor reading performance. Difficulties are observed in text reading as well as single word identification, and performance is affected on all tasks requiring reading. This behavioural disorder can be explained by a cognitive dysfunction, itself secondary to a neurobiological dysfunction. It is thought to have a genetic origin (Ramus, 2006). Dyslexia is further sensitive to cultural and environmental influences which interact with both the cognitive and neurobiological levels.

Decades of intensive research in cognitive neuropsychology and neuroscience have resulted in suggestions for possible causes of developmental dyslexia. In most studies, developmental dyslexia was considered as a unitary syndrome resulting from a single cognitive disorder and a single brain dysfunction. Within this framework, the proposal of a phonological deficit as the cognitive basis of developmental dyslexia is largely accepted. Evidence for such a disorder and its cerebral correlates will be briefly reviewed in the first section of this chapter. The hypothesis that visual dysfunctions might be involved in developmental dyslexia has also been investigated. The implication of a visual dysfunction at the origin of developmental dyslexia is hotly debated. It is now well documented that visual processing is not grossly impaired in developmental dyslexia. Dyslexic individuals exhibit preserved abilities to identify and process single letters when presented either in isolation or in strings (Shovman & Ahissar, 2006; Hawelka & Wimmer, 2008). However, there is evidence that some aspects of visual processing are impaired in many dyslexic individuals. Low level visual disorders (i.e., poor contrast sensitivity at low spatial frequency and high temporal frequency or difficulties in movement speed processing), have been reported within the framework of the magnocellular theory of developmental dyslexia (Stein, 2003). Further, deficits in rapid stimulus sequence processing which have been interpreted within the sluggish attentional shifting theory framework have been found in developmental dyslexia (Hari & Renvall, 2001). However, these visual disorders typically co-occur with the phonological disorder that remains as the most plausible proximal cause of developmental dyslexia (Ramus, 2003). In spite of the success of the phonological hypothesis, reports of opposite patterns of performance in developmental dyslexia (i.e., phonological vs surface variants) and of good phoneme awareness skills in some dyslexic children challenge the view that a selective phonological core deficit is the source of reading disorders in all cases of developmental dyslexia. The double deficit hypothesis (Wolf & Bowers, 1999) was proposed to account for such a heterogeneity suggesting that some dyslexic children suffered for either a phonological or a rapid automatised naming disorder, or both. However, the cognitive mechanisms underlying difficulties in rapid automatised naming are still not well understood. Deficits in rapid automatic naming tasks have often been interpreted as resulting from slow lexical retrieval of letter names, thus reflecting a specific dimension of the phonological deficit (Ramus & Szenkovits, 2008). Other studies to the reverse have shown that the phonological and rapid automatised naming disorders independently contribute to reading acquisition (Powell et al., 2007) and developmental dyslexia (Wolf et al., 2002). The main point that remains unresolved is the identification of the cognitive mechanisms which are impaired in children with poor performance in rapid automatised naming. Furthermore, no study was conducted with the purpose of investigating the cerebral correlates of such disorders. As a consequence, the hypothesis of a rapid automatised naming disorder in developmental dyslexia will not be discussed in the present chapter. We will rather focus on the visual attention (VA) span deficit hypothesis of developmental dyslexia, recently proposed by our team in an attempt to account for developmental dyslexia as a multifactorial syndrome. Evidence for a double dissociation between the phonological and VA span disorders in children with developmental dyslexia will be provided in the second section of this chapter together with neuroimaging data on the cerebral correlates of the VA span disorder. Thanks to its dissociation from phonological problems, the VA span disorder appears as a potential second core disorder in developmental dyslexia. Evidence for two independent cognitive disorders related to different neurobiological dysfunctions revives the hypothesis of distinct and theoretically relevant subtypes of developmental dyslexia.

2. THE PHONOLOGICAL DEFICIT HYPOTHESIS

2.1. BEHAVIOURAL EVIDENCE FOR A PHONOLOGICAL DISORDER

There is now strong evidence in support of a phonological disorder as an underlying cause of developmental dyslexia (Vellutino et al., 2004). Studies conducted on large samples of dyslexic individuals consistently found that dyslexic readers performed below the level of normal readers on a number of tasks involving phonological processing. Difficulties were reported in the repetition of long and complex (e.g., including consonant clusters) pseudo-words and in tasks of phoneme fluency in which children are asked to name as many words as possible beginning with a pre-specified phoneme. Children with developmental dyslexia further exhibit poor performance in tasks of verbal short term memory (Jeffries & Everatt, 2004); they do not spontaneously encode phonological information in word recall tasks (Rack et al., 1985) and their performance tends to decrease with the task requirements, in particular with increasing memory load (Ramus & Szenkovitz, 2008). Difficulties in acquiring phoneme awareness were further reported in dyslexic children, showing their poor sensitivity to the constituent sounds in words (Bradley & Bryant, 1978; Morais, Cluytens, & Alegria, 1984). Lastly, persistent phonological difficulties have been found in well-compensated adult dyslexics (Bruck, 1992; Shaywitz et al., 1999) so that deficits in phonological processing continue to characterise dyslexic readers even in adolescence and adulthood.

In reading, specific difficulties in pseudo-word reading are considered as the hallmark of developmental dyslexia (Snowling, 2000). They are viewed as further evidence for a phonological disorder inasmuch as pseudo-word reading involves grapheme-to-phoneme conversion rules and phonemic blending. In support for the phonological deficit hypothesis, most theoretical models of reading (Ans et al., 1998; Coltheart et al., 2001; Harm & Seidenberg, 1999; Perry et al., 2007) assume that a phonological disorder results in poor pseudo-word reading and developmental dyslexia. The existence of a causal relationship between phonological disorders and reading acquisition problems is therefore theoretically-justified. However, the most compelling evidence for a causal relationship between phonological skills deficiencies and developmental dyslexia is provided by intervention and training studies. Indeed, several studies have documented that direct instruction designed to facilitate phoneme awareness and letter-sound mapping improves word identification (Ehri et al., 2001). All these findings are strong evidence for a core phonological disorder in developmental dyslexia. The phonological theory is further supported by studies examining the neurobiological underpinnings of developmental dyslexia.

2.2. THE NEUROBIOLOGICAL CORRELATES OF THE PHONOLOGICAL DISORDER

Most current studies of neural factors in developmental dyslexia use functional neuroimaging modalities that allow measuring changes in metabolic activity and blood flow in specific brain regions while participants are engaged in cognitive tasks. Because it is a non-invasive and safe method that can be used repeatedly, most studies used functional magnetic resonance imaging (fMRI) for identifying the cerebral dysfunctions in developmental dyslexia. Three main regions of the left-hemisphere have been consistently implicated in studies of individuals with developmental dyslexia (Démonet et al., 2004). Differences in activation patterns between normal and dyslexic readers have been reported in two perisylvian regions of the left hemisphere while participants were engaged in tasks involving phonological processing (such as rhyme judgment, verbal working memory or pseudo-word reading). Such differences have been reported in the inferior frontal areas - including Broca's area - implicated in phonological and articulatory processing and the inferior parietal lobule in which decline in fMRI activation have been reported in the left supra-marginal gyrus, a region important for phonological processing, and in the angular gyrus, most probably involved in grapheme-phoneme correspondences. The importance of these regions in developmental dyslexia is further supported by studies - based on the investigation of post-mortem brain specimens - showing that focal anomalies of the brain structure are more common in the left perisylvian regions in people with a history of dyslexia (Galaburda et al., 1985). Moreover, studies of developmental dyslexia in children or adults who received phonologically based remediation have demonstrated that reading improvement is associated with increased activation of previously underactivated left hemisphere brain regions (Aylward et al., 2003; Eden at al., 2004; Shaywitz et al., 2005; Simos et al., 2002). Temple and colleagues (2003) investigated brain plasticity in a group of 20 10-year-old dyslexic children who received an intensive phonology-based intervention during 8 weeks daily. Increased activity after remediation was observed in left hemisphere temporo-parietal cortex and inferior frontal gyrus, both regions that showed activity in the normal-reading children during fMRI when performing the rhyming task. These overall findings are evidence in support of the phonological theory of developmental dyslexia. They point to the perisylvian regions of the left-hemisphere, in particular the inferior frontal gyrus and inferior parietal lobule, as the cerebral correlates of the phonological disorder in developmental dyslexia.

A third brain region of the left hemisphere was consistently reported as showing reduced activity in dyslexic individuals (Démonet et al., 2004; Paulesu et al., 2001). This region located in the inferior part of the temporal lobe is known as the visual word form area (Cohen et al., 2000). It is in particular involved in letter perception and letter-string processing. Increased activation of this region nevertheless relates to the legality of the to-be-processed letter string - greater activity in response to words and legal pseudo-words than consonant strings or non-nameable symbol-strings -, thus suggesting that development of the visual word form area might in part depend on the individual phonological processing skills.

2.3. LIMITS OF THE PHONOLOGICAL HYPOTHESIS

In spite of its success, the phonological deficit hypothesis is challenged by reports of opposite patterns of performance in different subtypes of developmental dyslexia. The absence of phoneme awareness problems in at least some dyslexic children further challenge the view that a selective phonological core deficit is the source of reading disorders in all cases of developmental dyslexia. Case studies of developmental surface dyslexia have in particular been described who are characterised by selective difficulties in irregular word reading but preserved performance in pseudo-word reading, thus a performance pattern opposite to that reported in children with phonological dyslexia (Castles & Coltheart, 1996; Brunsdon, Coltheart & Nickels, 2005; Dubois et al., 2007; Hanley & Gard, 1995; Valdois et al., 2003). Moreover surface dyslexic individuals exhibit good phoneme awareness and good verbal short term memory skills against the hypothesis of an underlying phonological impairment. However, most studies failed to identify the cognitive disorder responsible for developmental surface dyslexia and the surface dyslexic's reading performance was described as similar to that of younger but normal readers so that it was concluded that children with surface dyslexia exhibited a developmental lag and that only those with phonological dyslexia reflected true developmental deviance (Manis et al., 1996; Sprenger-Charolles et al., 2000). Recent studies however suggest that a visual attention span disorder might be involved in developmental surface dyslexia independently of any phonological deficit (Valdois et al., 2003; Dubois et al., 2007).

3. THE VISUAL ATTENTION SPAN DEFICIT HYPOTHESIS

Learning to read in an alphabetic system involves learning the relationships between sequences of visual symbols (i.e., relevant orthographic units such as graphemes, syllables, whole words) and the corresponding units of sounds (i.e., relevant phonological units such as phonemes, syllables or whole words). Accordingly, it is undisputable that reading requires visual processing and that differences in visual processing would affect the reading process, limiting what could be learned and the level of efficiency the system could achieve (Seidenberg, 1992; Kwon, Legge & Dubbels, 2007).

3.1. THE MULTI-TRACE MEMORY MODEL OF POLYSYLLABIC WORD READING

In their theoretical model of reading, Ans et al. (1998) supported a multifactorial approach of developmental dyslexia in hypothesising that different subtypes of developmental dyslexia might result from distinct cognitive disorders. The multitrace memory model of polysyllabic word reading (MTM model, hereafter) indeed postulates that, in addition to the phonological component, a visual attentional component - called the visual attentional window - plays a crucial role in skilled reading and reading acquisition. Actually, the size of the visual attentional window determines the amount of orthographic information that is extracted from the input letter string during reading and becomes available for processing. The model, outlined in Figure 1, postulates that reading relies on two types of reading procedures, a global and an analytic procedure, that differ in the kind of visual attention and phonological processing they involve.

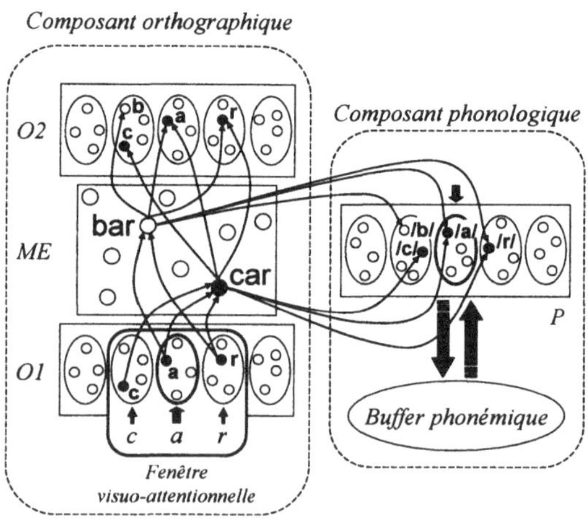

Figure 1: Schematic representation of the multitrace memory model of polysyllabic word reading. *O1, O2* = input and output orthographic layers; *EM* = Episodic Memory; *P* = phonological output layer.

First, the two reading procedures differ in the size of the visual attentional window through which information from the orthographic input is extracted. In global reading mode, the visual attentional window extends over the whole sequence of the input letter-string whereas it narrows down to focus attention successively on the different parts of the input when reading in analytic mode.

Thus, global processing typically requires a larger visual attentional window than analytic processing. In analytic processing the visual attentional window is reduced to the sublexical parts of the input string corresponding to relevant orthographic units. The size of these units can vary so that letters or graphemes, syllables or morphemes can be processed depending on reading experience and word characteristics. However, the visual attentional window is typically smaller when reading in analytic mode than in global mode in which the whole word string has to be simultaneously processed.

Second, the two reading procedures also differ with respect to phonological processing. In global mode, the entire phonological output of the input letter-string is generated in a single step. In analytic mode, phonological outputs corresponding to each focal sequence (i.e., letters within the visual attentional window) are successively generated and have to be maintained in verbal short-term memory until the end of processing. Most familiar words are processed as a whole by the network, whereas global processing typically fails for pseudo-words which are then processed analytically. It follows that performance on familiar words which typically involve large visual attentional windows but whose phonological counterpart is generated in a single step would be more sensitive to a reduction of the visual attentional window; in contrast and inasmuch as pseudo-word reading typically involves smaller visual attentional windows but is more demanding in verbal short term memory load, pseudo-word reading performance would be more sensitive to phonological processing disorders, in particular verbal short-term memory problems. Thus, the model suggests that a selective visual attentional window or phonological deficit might impact on reading acquisition and result in different subtypes of developmental dyslexia.

3.2. THE NOTION OF VISUAL ATTENTION SPAN

The notion of visual attention span was introduced as the psychological counterpart of the MTM model's visual attentional window (Bosse, Tainturier & Valdois, 2007). The visual attention (VA) span is defined as the amount of distinct visual elements which can be processed in parallel in a multi-element array. With respect to reading, the VA span refers to the number of orthographic units that can be processed simultaneously in a single fixation. In our previous studies (Bosse, Tainturier & Valdois, 2007; Prado et al., 2007; Lassus-Sangosse et al., 2008), the VA span was estimated using two tasks (see Figure 2) which required the report of a single letter or of all of the letters of briefly presented multi-letter strings. The tasks require letter names not letter sounds to be reported.

In global report, twenty 5-consonant strings are successively displayed. Each trial consists of a 5-consonant string displayed at the centre of the screen for 200 ms, a duration which corresponds to the mean duration of fixations in reading, long enough for an extended glimpse, yet too short for a useful eye movement (Figure 2a). Children have to name verbally as many letters as possible. In partial report, a vertical bar is presented for 50 ms at the offset of the letter string, indicating the position of the letter to be reported. Although a single letter has to be reported at each trial, all 5 consonants have to be simultaneously processed since information on the position of the to-be-reported letter is only available after the disappearance of the string. The VA span is estimated as the mean number of letters accurately reported at each trial in global report and over five successive trials in partial report. Its size was estimated around 4 letters in our previous experiments. This suggests that about 4 independent orthographic units can be simultaneously processed during a single fixation in reading (Prado et al., 2007).

The two report tasks we used to estimate the VA span in normal and dyslexic readers were designed to share some of their characteristics with reading without involving phonologically-based chunking mechanisms. In particular, the displayed letter strings were only composed of consonants and two subsequent consonants never corresponded to a French grapheme (e.g., PH, TH) or a frequent bigram in French (e.g., TR, PL, BR).

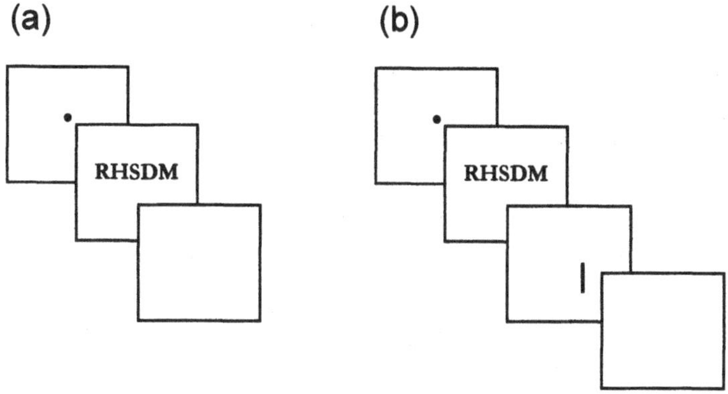

Figure 2: The global (a) and partial (b) report tasks.

Accordingly, each letter was processed as a single element independent of all the other ones in the string. The 5-consonant strings never matched the skeleton of a real word (e.g., FLMBR for FLAMBER "burn") thus preventing lexical access which might have contributed to improve performance in letter name recall.

Further, the potential influence on performance of verbal short term memory is rather unlikely. Indeed, while global report requires all five letter names to be reported verbally, a single cued letter has to be reported in partial report so that memory load is far reduced in this second task. It is noteworthy that in line with the literature (Pelli et al., 2006), our previous works suggest that, even in global report, performance is not primarily affected by verbal short term memory skills. Indeed, in a recent study done on a large sample of typically developing children (N=417) in 1st, 3rd and 5th grade (Bosse & Valdois, in press), we showed that VA span abilities predicted reading performance independently of the child phonemic awareness and verbal short term memory. Moreover, the VA span was typically reported as impaired in dyslexic children who demonstrated no associated verbal short term memory problems whereas it was preserved in those dyslexic children with poor phonological and verbal short term memory skills (Bosse et al., 2007; Valdois et al., 2003). Finally, Lassus-Sangosse and colleagues (2008) reported impaired performance in global report in dyslexic children who otherwise exhibited normal performance in a sequential report task - requiring the recall the letter names of 5 serially displayed consonants - which was more taxing in memory load. As a consequence, the global and partial report tasks primarily assess the visual and visual attentional processing skills required for processing visual letters in strings.

3.3. THE VA SPAN DISORDER IN DEVELOPMENTAL DYSLEXIA

Simulations conducted using the MTM network showed that a phonological disorder had no impact on visual attentional processing and reversely. These two kinds of processing are independent in the network, thus suggesting that a phonological disorder if associated to developmental dyslexia should most often dissociate from VA span disorders and vice versa. In support of this prediction, Valdois et al. (2003) reported two contrasted cases of developmental dyslexia showing that phonological and VA span disorders could dissociate in dyslexic individuals. In this study, the performance pattern of two teenagers Laurent and Nicolas was described. Laurent exhibited a phonological dyslexia profile characterised by poor pseudo-word reading whereas Nicolas had selective difficulties in irregular word reading, thus conforming to the surface dyslexia profile. The two participants were given tasks of phonological processing and VA span. Results showed that Laurent performed very poorly on all tasks of phoneme awareness and verbal short term memory but had a VA span similar to that of normal readers matched for chronological age. In contrast, Nicolas demonstrated very good performance on all phonological tasks but performed very poorly on the tasks of global and partial report, thus reflecting reduced VA span abilities. The study further revealed that Nicolas's performance on the VA span tasks not only differed from the performance of normal readers of the same chronological age but also from that of younger children matched on reading-level. Consequently, the poor performance of Nicolas on the VA span tasks could not be viewed as just reflecting his poor reading level. The absence of VA span disorder in Laurent who otherwise exhibited a reading level very similar to that of Nicolas also speaks against a consequence relationship. It follows that despite similar reading levels, these teenagers exhibit dissociated phonological and VA span processing skills, as expected within the MTM network.

Because case studies provide no information on the prevalence of each cognitive disorder in the dyslexic population, a large sample study was conducted on two populations of French and British dyslexic children whose reading performance, phoneme awareness and VA span abilities were assessed (Bosse et al., 2007). Results showed that phonological and VA span disorders dissociated in most (> 60%) dyslexic children. The proportion of children with a single VA span disorder was comparable to that of children with a single phonological deficit and a subgroup of children was characterised by a double deficit, exhibiting both a phonological and VA span disorder. Moreover, results showed that VA span abilities independently contributed to reading performance in developmental dyslexia. Indeed, VA span abilities were found to contribute to irregular word and pseudo-word reading in our dyslexic sample, after control for the influence of phonological processing skills or chronological age. Thus, a VA span disorder appears as contributing to the poor reading outcome of dyslexic individuals independently of their phonological abilities. Neuroimaging studies were conducted in order to identify the neurobiological correlates of this disorder.

3.4. THE NEUROBIOLOGICAL CORRELATES OF THE VA SPAN

The neural mechanisms involved in VA span were first assessed in a group of young adult normal readers who were submitted to two visual attentional tasks during fMRI examination (Peyrin et al., submitted). The participants were engaged in a task of flanked parafoveal letter processing and in a global report task similar to that used in our previous experiments but adapted to the fMRI requirements. In the flanked letter processing task, two stimuli were simultaneously displayed, one centred on the fixation point, the second randomly displayed in the left or right visual field. The stimuli were made up of either two letters or a letter and a geometrical figure. In the experimental condition, the eccentric stimulus was flanked by two "X" letters whereas it was presented in isolation in the control condition (see Figure 3a). The participants were asked to press a response key, each time and only when they detected an unmatched stimulus pair (made up of a letter and a geometrical figure).

In the experimental global report task (Figure 3b), strings of 5 consonants were displayed on the screen for 200 ms and the participants were asked to report silently as many letters as possible immediately after they disappeared. Five symbol strings were displayed during the control condition and the participants had to count silently from one to five after they disappeared.

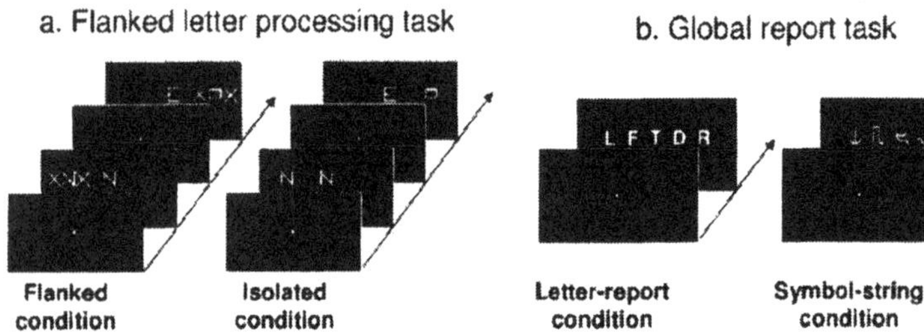

Figure 3: Example of the experimental tasks used under fMRI.

The activation patterns obtained during the experimental tasks were first compared to a baseline condition during which the participants just fixated a crosshair on the screen, second to the control conditions. Results revealed that, relative to the baseline, both tasks activated a large network of brain regions, including the superior and inferior parietal lobules. These parietal regions were more bilaterally activated during the global report task and more left-lateralised during flanked letter processing. Both tasks commonly activated the left superior parietal lobule. Comparison of the flanked and isolated letter processing conditions revealed greater activity in the left superior parietal lobule during flanked letter processing (Figure 4). Relative to symbol-string processing, the letter global report task elicited stronger activation within the angular/middle occipital gyrus of the left hemisphere.

The two tasks of flanked letter processing and letter global report thus primarily activate the parietal regions of the left hemisphere, in particular the superior parietal lobule. This localisation contrasts with that typically reported in relation with phonological processing (which primarily involves the left inferior frontal gyrus and the supramarginal gyrus).

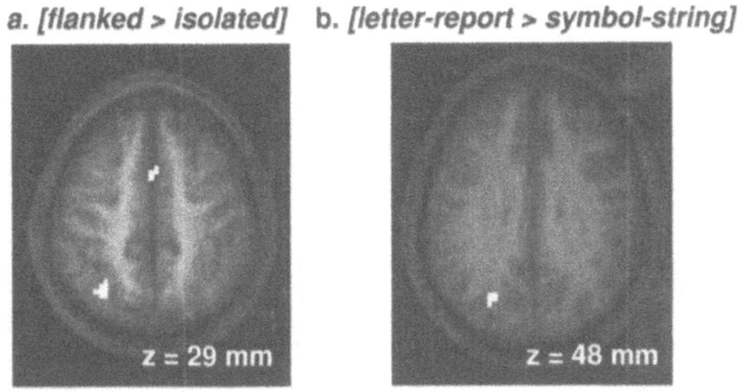

Figure 4: Cerebral regions specifically activated by contrasting interest conditions to control conditions for each task. (a) For the flanked letter processing task, the [flanked > isolated] contrast revealed greater activity in the left superior parietal lobule during flanked letter processing. (b) For the global report task, the [letter report > symbol-string] contrast elicited stronger activation within the angular gyrus of the left hemisphere during the global report of letters.

3.5. A PARIETAL DYSFUNCTION AS THE NEURAL CORRELATE OF THE VA SPAN DISORDER

The hypothesis that a parietal dysfunction might characterise dyslexic individuals with a VA span disorder was assessed in a single case study (Peyrin et al., submitted). The participant, FG, was a 22-year-old well-compensated dyslexic who exhibited poor performance in both irregular word and pseudo-word reading. FG showed good performance in tasks of pseudo-word repetition, phoneme deletion and spoonerisms, thus demonstrating preserved phonological processing skills. In contrast, he performed poorly on the tasks of letter report, thus reflecting a VA span disorder. FG thus demonstrated a VA span disorder but preserved phonological skills.

To highlight the cerebral dysfunction underlying his poor VA span, FG's brain activations were recorded while he was engaged in the flanked letter processing task during fMRI. His brain activations were further measured during a task of rhyme detection to check good functioning of the cerebral regions involved in phonological processing. Brain activity maps for the two experimental tasks compared to the baseline are reported in Figure 5 for FG and a control group of non-dyslexic young adults.

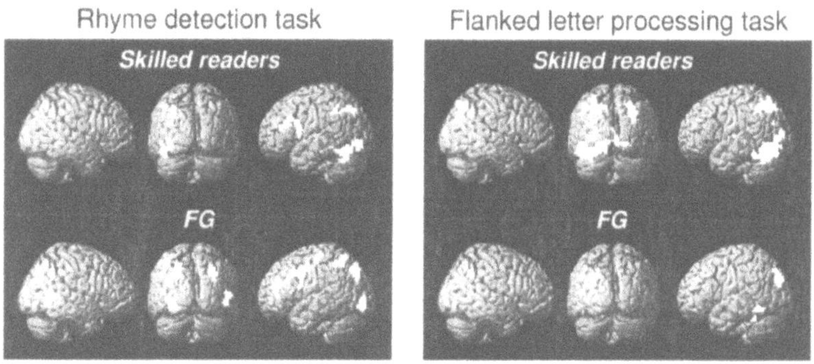

Figure 5: For skilled readers, the rhyme detection task specifically activated a large fronto-temporo-parietal network including the anterior and inferior part of the left inferior frontal gyrus (Broca's area, BA 44/45) and the flanked letter processing task activated a temporo-parietal network including the left inferior temporal cortex (BA 37), the bilateral extrastriate visual cortices (BA 18/19), the superior (BA 7) and inferior (BA 39/19, BA 40) parietal lobules. With respect to skilled readers, FG showed reduced activation within the left parietal areas (BA 7 and BA 39/19) and no significant activation within the right parietal areas during the flanked letter processing task.

FMRI data acquired from skilled readers showed that the rhyme detection task specifically activated a large cerebral network including the anterior part of the left inferior frontal gyrus and the left supramarginal gyrus. Similar to skilled readers, Broca's area and the left supramarginal gyrus were activated during the rhyming task in FG. During the flanked letter processing task, normal readers activated a large parieto-temporal network including the superior parietal lobule bilaterally and the left inferior parietal lobule. For FG, parietal activations were less extensive than for the control participants in the left superior parietal lobule (healthy readers: 247 voxels; FG: 66 voxels) and the right superior parietal lobule was not activated in contrast to normal readers. FG thus demonstrates decreased activity in parietal regions during the visual attentional task but preserved brain activity during rhyme judgement. His brain activation pattern thus parallels his behavioural pattern characterised by poor VA span but preserved phonological skills.

4. CONCLUSION

Substantial evidence has established that phonological skills deficiencies cause developmental dyslexia. Results of neuroimaging studies further suggest that defective activity in the perisylvian regions of the left hemisphere, in particular the left inferior frontal and supramarginal gyri, are the neurobiological markers of the phonological disorder highlighted at the behavioural level. However, although most research groups consider dyslexia as a unitary syndrome resulting from a core phonological disorder, the heterogeneity of the dyslexic population rather suggests that different subtypes of developmental dyslexia might result from distinct cognitive disorders themselves due to different types of cerebral dysfunctions. In line with this multifactorial approach, the hypothesis that a VA span disorder might contribute to the poor reading outcome of dyslexic readers was assessed through single case and large group studies. These studies demonstrated that phonological and VA span disorders dissociate in most dyslexic children. Investigations of the cerebral regions involved in VA span revealed the implication of a large network of parietal regions, including the superior parietal lobule bilaterally. A specific dysfunction of the superior parietal lobule was demonstrated in a young adult with developmental dyslexia who exhibited a VA span disorder in the absence of phonological problems at the behavioural level. This participant was further found to normally activate the left inferior frontal area and the left supramarginal gyrus during phonological processing. Overall and although additional studies are required for establishing a causal relationship between VA span abilities and reading performance in both typically developing and dyslexic children, these findings suggest that the heterogeneity of developmental dyslexia might reflect the existence of different subtypes of dyslexic individuals characterised by distinct cognitive and brain dysfunctions. Two subtypes are in particular suspected characterised by poor phonological abilities and dysfunction of the left inferior frontal gyrus and inferior parietal lobule for one subtype, and poor VA span abilities and dysfunction of the superior parietal lobules for the other one. These two subtypes do not necessarily correspond to the phonological and surface dyslexia subtypes as established from the dyslexic's reading patterns. Indeed, even if a single phonological disorder is expected to more straightforwardly affect pseudo-word reading, such a trouble can further slow down the acquisition of specific orthographic knowledge thus (at least temporarily) resulting in poor regular and irregular word reading as well. Similarly, poor VA span abilities would mainly affect irregular word reading but a severe reduction of the VA span is further expected to impact the processing of large orthographic units thus further resulting in poor pseudo-word reading.

REFERENCES

Ans, B., Carbonnel, S., and Valdois, S. (1998). A connectionist multi-trace memory model of polysyllabic word reading. *Psychological Review* 105, 678-723.

Aylward, E.H., Richards, T.L., Berninger, V.W., Nagy, W.E., Field, K.M., Grimme, A.C., Richards, A.L., Thomson, J.B., and Cramer, S.C. (2003). Instructional treatment associated with changes in brain activation in children with dyslexia. *Neurology* 61, 212-219.

Bosse, M.L., Tainturier, M.J., and Valdois, S. (2007). Developmental dyslexia: The visual attention span deficit hypothesis. *Cognition* 104, 198-230.

Bosse, M.L. & Valdois, S. (In Press). Influence of the visual attention span on child reading performance: a cross-sectional study. *Journal of Research in Reading*.

Bradley, L., & Bryant, N. R. (1978). Difficulties in auditory organisation as a possible cause of reading backwardness. *Nature* 271, 746-747.

Bruck, M. (1992). Persistence of dyslexics' phonological awareness deficits. *Developmental Psychology* 28, 874-886.

Brunsdon, R. Coltheart, M. & Nickels, L. (2005). Treatment of irregular word spelling in developmental surface dysgraphia. *Cognitive Neuropsychology* 22, 213-251.

Campbell, R., & Butterworth, B. (1985). Phonological dyslexia and dysgraphia in a highly literate subject: A developmental case with associated deficits of phonemic processing and awareness. *The Quarterly Journal of Experimental Psychology* 37, 435-475.

Castles, A., & Coltheart, M. (1996). Cognitive correlates of developmental surface dyslexia : a single case study. *Cognitive Neuropsychology* 13(1), 25-50.

Cohen, L., Dehaene, S., Naccache, L., Lehericy, S., Dehaene-Lambertz, G., Henaff, M. A., and Michel, F. (2000). The visual word form area: spatial and temporal characterization of an initial stage of reading in normal subjects and posterior split-brain patients. *Brain* 123, 291-307.

Coltheart, M., Rastle, K., Perry, C., Langdon, R., and Ziegler, J. (2001). DRC: A dual route cascaded model of visual word recognition and reading aloud. *Psychological Review* 108, 204-256.

Démonet, J.F., Taylor, M.J., and Chaix, Y. (2004). Developmental dyslexia. *The Lancet* 363, 1451-1460.

Dubois, M., Lafaye de Micheaux, P., Noël, M.P., and Valdois, S. (2007). Pre-orthographical constraints on visual word recognition: Evidence from a case study of developmental surface dyslexia. *Cognitive Neuropsychology* 24, 1-38.

Eden, G.F., Jones, K.M., Cappell, K., Gareau, L., Wood, F.B., Zeffiro, T.A., Dietz, N.A.E., Agnew, J.A., and Flowers, D.L. (2004). Neural changes following remediation in adult developmental dyslexia. *Neuron* 44, 411-422.

Ehri, L.C., Nunes, S.R., Willows, D.M., Schuster, B.V., Yaghoub Zadeh, Z., and Shanahan, T. (2001). Phonemic awareness instruction helps children learn to read: Evidence from the National Reading Panel's meta-analysis. *Reading Research Quarterly* 36, 250-287.

Frith, C. (1997). Brain, mind and behaviour in dyslexia. In: C. Hulme & M. Snowling (eds.) *Dyslexia: Biology, cognition and intervention*, 1-19, London: Whurr Publishers.

Galaburda, A.M., Sherman, G.P., Rosen, G.D., Aboitiz, F., and Geshwind, N. (1985). Developmental dyslexia: Four consecutive patients with cortical anomalies. *Annals of Neurology* 18, 222-233.

Hanley, J.R. & Gard, F. (1995). A dissociation between developmental surface and phonological dyslexia in two undergraduate students. *Neuropsychologia* 33, 909-914.

Harm, M. W. & Seidenberg, M. S. (1999). Phonology, reading acquisition, and dyslexia: insights from connectionist models. *Psychological Review* 106, 491-528.

Hawelka, S. & Wimmer, H. (2008). Visual target detection is not impaired in dyslexic readers. *Vision Research* 48 (6), 850-852.

Jeffries, S. & Everatt, J. (2004). Working memory: Its role in dyslexia and other specific learning difficulties. *Dyslexia* 10, 196-214.

Lassus-Sangosse, D., N'Guyen-Morel, M.A., and Valdois, S. (2008). Sequential or simultaneous visual processing deficit in developmental dyslexia. *Vision Research* 48, 979-988.

Morais, J., Cluytens, M., and Alegria, J. (1984). Segmentation abilities of dyslexics and normal readers. *Perceptual and Motor Skills* 58, 221-222.

Paulesu, E., Démonet, J.F., Fazio, F., McCrory, E., Chanoine, V., Brunswick, N., Cappa, S.F., Cossu, G., Habib, M., Frith, C.D., and Frith, U. (2001). Dyslexia: cultural diversity and biological unity. *Science* 291, 2165-2167.

Pernet, C. Valdois, S., Celsis, P., and Démonet, J.F. (2006). Lateral masking, levels of processing and stimulus category: A comparative study between normal and dyslexic readers. *Neuropsychologia* 44, 2374-2385.

Perry, C., Ziegler, J.C., and Zorzi, M. (2007). Nested incremental modeling in the development of computational theories: the CDP+ model of reading aloud. *Psychological Review* 114, 273-315.

Peyrin, C., Baciu, M., Pernet, C., Lamalle, L., Segebarth, C., Démonet, J.F. & Valdois, S. (submitted). Cerebral correlates of the visual attentional processes involved in reading: An fMRI Study in healthy skilled readers.

Peyrin, C., Lallier, M., Baciu, M., Démonet, J.F., Le Bas, J.F., and Valdois, S. (submitted). Dissociation of phonological and visual attentional processing in developmental dyslexia: fMRI evidence from two case reports.

Powell, D., Stainthorp, R., Stuart, M., Garwood, H., and Quinlan, P. (2007). An experimental comparison between rival theories of rapid automatized naming performance and its relationship to reading. *Journal of Experimental Child Psychology* 98, 46-68.

Prado, C., Dubois, M., and Valdois, S. (2007). The eye movements of dyslexic children during reading and visual search: impact of the visual span. *Vision Research* 47 (19), 2521-2530.

Rack, J. (1985). Orthographic and phonetic coding in normal and dyslexic readers. *British Journal of Psychology* 76, 325-340.

Ramus, F. (2006). Genes, Brain, and cognition: A roadmap for the cognitive scientist. *Cognition* 101, 247-269.

Ramus, F. & Szenkovits, G. (2008). What phonological deficit? *The Quarterly Journal of Experimental Psychology* 61, 129-141.

Shaywitz, S.E., Fletcher, J.M., Holahan, J.M., Shneider, A.E., Marchione, K.E., Stuebing, K.K., Francis, D.J., Pugh, K.R., and Shaywitz, B.A. (1999). Persistence of dyslexia: The Connecticut longitudinal study at adolescence. *Pediatrics* 104, 1351-1359.

Shaywitz, S.E. & Shaywitz, B.A. (2005). Dyslexia (specific reading disability). *Biological Psychiatry* 57, 1301-1309.

Shovman, M.M. & Ahissar, M. (2006). Isolating the impact of visual perception on dyslexics' reading ability. *Vision Research* 46, 3514-3525.

Simos, P.G., Fletcher, J.M., Bergman, E., Breier, J.I., Foorman, B.R., Castillo, E.M., Davis, R.N., Fitzgerald, M. and Papanicolau, A.C. (2002). Dyslexia-specific brain activation profiles become normal following remedial training, *Neurology* 58, 1203-1213.

Snowling, M. (2000). *Dyslexia* (second Edition). Oxford: Blackwell Publishing.

Stein, J. F. (2003). Visual motion sensitivity and reading. *Neuropsychologia* 41, 1785-1793.

Temple, E., Deutsch, G.K., Poldrack, R.A., Miller, S.L., Tallal, P., Merzenich, M.M., and Gabrieli, J.D.E. (2003). Neural deficits in children with dyslexia ameliorated by behavioural remediation: Evidence from functional MRI. *Proceedings of the National Academy of Science* 100, 2860-2865.

Valdois, S., Bosse, M.L., Ans, B., Carbonnel, S., Zorman, M., David, D., and Pellat, J. (2003). Phonological and visual processing deficits can dissociate in developmental dyslexia: Evidence from two case studies. *Reading and Writing: An Interdisciplinary Journal* 16, 541-572.

Vellutino, F. R., Fletcher, J. M., Snowling, M. J., and Scanlon, D. M. (2004). Specific reading disability (dyslexia): what have we learned in the past four decades? *Journal of Child Psychology and Psychiatry* 45, 2-40.

Wolf, M. & Bowers, P. G. (1999). The double-deficit hypothesis for the developmental dyslexias. *Journal of Educational Psychology* 91(3), 415-438.

Wolf, M., Goldberg O'Rourke, A., Gidney, C., Lovett, M., Cirino, P., and Morris, R. (2002). The second deficit: An investigation of the independence of phonological and naming-speed deficits in developmental dyslexia. *Reading and Writing: An Interdisciplinary Journal* 15, 43-72.

7

Brain imaging and cortical excitability in persistent developmental stuttering

MARTIN SOMMER
NICOLE SPINDLER
KATHRIN KNAPPMEYER
EVKE JANE HUNTER
VERONIKA GUTMANN
ALEXANDER WOLFF VON GUDENBERG
WALTER PAULUS

Abstract: Persistent developmental stuttering (PDS) is a frequent speech disorder affecting about 1 % of the post pubertal population, predominantly males. Early neurophysiological studies suggested impaired cerebral dominance in affected adults. More recent structural brain imaging studies on PDS point to a left hemispheric alteration of the Broca's area and the white matter in the adjacent Rolandic Operculum. Functional imaging studies suggest a right hemispheric motor and premotor overactivity in patients with PDS during speech and nonspeech tasks, possibly compensating for left-hemispheric structural alterations. Transcranial magnetic studies on brain excitability indicated normal interhemispheric inhibition between motor cortices and normal excitability within primary motor areas, suggesting that the altered patterns of cerebral activity reflect subcortical or higher order cortical association areas. We conclude with a tentative framework integrating these neurological and potential psychological factors contributing to PDS.

1. INTRODUCTION

Stuttering is a frequent speech fluency disorder. In up to 5 % of all children, stuttering sets in between 2-6 years of age, a period critical for language acquisition. Later on, the vast majority of these children experience a spontaneous recovery. Stuttering persists after puberty only in about 1 % of the general population, with a male to female ratio of about 4 to 1. Hereditary factors appear to influence the occurrence and the persistence of persistent developmental stuttering (PDS) (Yairi and Ambrose, 1999). This PDS has rather consistent core symptoms of sound and syllable repetitions and audible and inaudible sound prolongations as well as speech blocks. These primary symptoms are usually accompanied by highly variable secondary symptoms such as grimacing, movements of the extremities or avoidance behaviour (Bloodstein, 1995; Buchel and Sommer, 2004).

In adulthood, another form of speech dysfluency, so called neurogenic stuttering (de Nil et al., 2007) can abruptly set in after a defined brain damage, e.g. stroke or intracerebral hemorrhage or relating to drug usage and extrapyramidal diseases or progressive diseases like dementia. Types of dysfluency of this adult-onset stuttering differ to some extent from those of PDS (mainly sound-, syllable- and single-syllable word repetitions, blocks are rarely observed, less secondary behaviour), and the sex ratio is more balanced than in PDS (Ringo and Dietrich, 1995). While no single brain area could be delineated from a variety of case studies, brain damage to subcortical areas of the left hemisphere seems particularly prone to cause adult-onset stuttering (Ringo and Dietrich, 1995).

2. STUDIES ON THE ORIGIN OF STUTTERING

2.1. TIMING OF CORTICAL ACTIVATION AND REACTION TIMES

For childhood-onset stuttering and PDS, a hypothetical neurological basis (Travis, 1978) has long met significant scepticism (Plankers, 1999). Early cortical excitability studies focussed on dichotic listening and EEG analyses (Travis, 1978). They already suggested some impairment of hemispheric dominance in stuttering individuals, e.g. showing less right-ear advantage on dichotic listening tasks (Sussman and MacNeilage, 1975). Reaction time studies reported a longer reaction time in manual or vocal choice reaction time tasks (Woodruff Starkweather et al., 1984), irrespective of task complexity (Webster and Ryan, 1991).

Using Magnetoencephalography, Salmelin and colleagues (Salmelin et al., 2000) studied the precise timing of cerebral activity between the visual presentation of a word on a screen and the Go-Signal initiating overt reading of that word. While the group of healthy, fluent speaking control subjects activated the Broca area *before* the left hemisphere motor area, adults afflicted with PDS showed the reverse order and activated the Broca area *after* activation of the left hemisphere motor area. The interpretation was that motor activity is launched before the proper speech-relevant programs are transmitted, pointing to a signal transmission problem.

2.2. STRUCTURAL BRAIN IMAGING

With the advent of structural brain imaging an increasing number of studies on adults with PDS provided evidence for more variable gyrification in Broca's area (Brodman area 43/44) (Foundas et al., 2001), lack of asymmetry of the Planum temporale (Foundas et al., 2001), anomalous morphology of grey matter density in the superior temporal gyrus extending to the planum temporale and increased white matter density in right homologues of speech motor control areas (Beal et al., 2007), and left Rolandic Opercular white matter disturbance (Sommer et al., 2002; Chang et al., 2006).

For the latter finding we used Diffusion Tensor Imaging (DTI). This MRI technique measures water diffusion in each volume of brain (voxel). Within fibre bundles water diffuses not randomly, but preferentially along the direction of the fibres. The denser the fibres are packed, the more pronounced will be the directional preference of water diffusion. The fractional anisotropy ranges from 0 (isotropic, purely randomly directed diffusion) to 1 (anisotropy, perfect preference for one direction of diffusion) and probably reflects white matter density and integrity (Schmithorst et al., 2002).

We studied 15 adults afflicted with PDS (mean age 30.6, range 18–44 years) and 15 carefully selected control subjects with no personal or family history of stuttering or cluttering (mean age 30.0, range 23–43 years). The left Rolandic Operculum (Brodman area 43) was the only area in the brain (excluding the cerebellum, which was not in the field of view) which showed a reduced fractional anisotropy in the stuttering as compared to the control group (Sommer et al., 2002). There was no area with a higher than normal anisotropy in the stuttering group. Recently, this finding in adults was replicated in 9-12 year old boys. Here, three levels of fractional anisotropy were observed, with the group of boys who never stuttered showing the highest anisotropy in the Rolandic Operculum, and the group of boys who still stuttered showing the lowest fractional anisotropy there. A third group of boys who had recovered from childhood stuttering showed an intermediate anisotropy in this brain region (Chang et al., 2006). Since the Rolandic Operculum is a traffic junction or "hub" of fibres linking Broca' area, auditory and sensorimotor speech-relevant areas, it is conceivable that this results in an altered quantity or quality of signal transmission, thus contributing to a speech production prone to errors such as dysfluencies. In either of the two publications there was little overlap between groups with regard to fractional anisotropy.

For comparison, note that in adults suffering from dyslexia a reduced fractional anisotropy has been found bilaterally in temporo-parietal areas (Klingberg et al., 2000). This well matches the clinical symptomatology and is yet another example of subtle structural differences that potentially constitute a disease mechanism.

The *chicken or egg* question is a clear limitation of such cross-sectional structural imaging on adolescents or adults affected by a disease since early childhood. It cannot be excluded that a white matter alteration is a *consequence* and not a *cause* of a particular long-standing disorder such as stuttering or dyslexia. Structural plasticity has been clearly shown for grey matter (Draganski et al., 2004), similar evidence for white matter use-dependent plasticity is still lacking in adults but certainly conceivable. Imaging in children close to disease onset may be able to solve this *chicken or egg* question.

2.3. FUNCTIONAL BRAIN IMAGING

Functional brain imaging studies allow basically investigating language and speech processes. Referring to stuttering this offers differentiation of neural processes between PWS and PWNS and to differ between fluent and stuttered speech (for broader overview see de Nil, 2004). These functional imaging studies showed right sided overactivity of motor and premotor areas, these included dorsolateral regions (Brodmann areas 8 and 9), medial orbital (Brodmann 11) and medial prefrontal cortices (Brodmann 10) (Fox et al., 1996; Braun et al., 1997). In addition, these studies showed a reduced activity of auditory processing areas on the left side, including the superior temporal gyrus (Brodmann area 22), the inferior angular gyrus (Brodmann area 39) and the middle temporal gyrus (Brodmann area 21) (Fox et al., 1996; Braun et al., 1997). Brown et al. (2005) confirmed this by an ALE Meta-Analysis based on several recent studies of functional neuroimaging that similar areas are involved in stuttered as in fluent speech. However there was an over-activation of motor areas (primary motor cortex, supplementary motor area and cingulate motor area) and cerebellar vermis. Additionally frontal operculum, rolandic operculum and anterior insula were noticeable due to anomalous right- laterality in stutterers. No auditory activations in stutterers were detectable due to hearing one's one speech.

The significance of the right-hemispheric motor and premotor activity is still under debate. It could be causally related to stuttering (Fox et al., 2000), or it could be compensatory for left-hemispheric structural problems specified above (Braun et al., 1997; Sommer et al., 2002; Preibisch et al., 2003).

2.4. ELECTROPHYSIOLOGICAL STUDIES ON BRAIN FUNCTION

An established tool to assess the interplay between both hemispheres is the inter-hemispheric inhibition (IHI) measured using transcranial magnetic stimulation (TMS). IHI determines non-invasively and *in vivo* the interplay between primary motor cortices. IHI is altered in individuals with early musical training (Ridding et al., 2000), a condition known to depend on an early time window to gain fine sensori-motor proficiency (Elbert et al., 1995; Amunts et al., 1997; Hutchinson et al., 2003). IHI in the motor cortex was found to be stronger after activation of the dominant hemisphere – the one controlling the dominant hand (Bäumer et al., 2007). One hypothesis of stuttering suggests reduced hemisphere predominance for speech functions compared to unaffected persons (Travis, 1978). Therefore we hypothesized that IHI may be abnormal in adults afflicted with PDS, possibly reflecting the presumed compensatory role of right hemisphere motor and premotor areas.

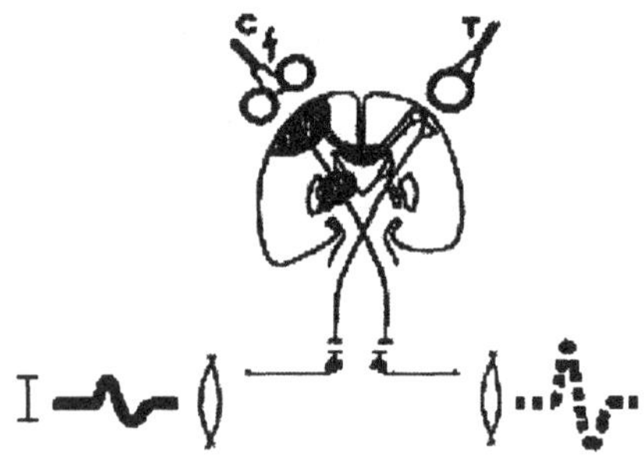

Figure 1: Inter-hemispheric inhibition tested by a conditioning stimulus (c) over one hemisphere followed by a test stimulus (t) over the other hemisphere. The amplitude of the motor evoked potential contralateral to the test pulse is reduced due to inter-hemispheric inhibition.

In a study currently under review, we assessed the inter-hemispheric inhibition (IHI) in a group of adults afflicted with PDS. We studied 15 subjects with PDS (mean age 28.7 SD 10.6) years, all right-handed with a mean Oldfield handedness score of 81.5 (SD 24.3) points. All subjects showed core symptoms of stuttering (repetitions and prolongations of sounds, speech blocks) (Bloodstein, 1995). 15 fluent-speaking subjects with no personal history of stuttering (mean age 26.7 (SD 4.6)) served as control subjects. All participants were male and right-handed

We used two TMS coils with the abductor digiti minimi muscle at rest and measured the modulation of the motor evoked potential (MEP) amplitude induced by a supra-threshold pulse to the test motor cortex by a preceding pulse applied to the other, conditioning motor cortex (Figure 1).

There was no significant between-group difference for either hemisphere. This data suggest that the interplay between the primary motor cortices of either hemisphere is normal in patients with PDS regarding to the function of the hand muscle chosen here.
Hand muscle representations are closely linked to facial muscle representations, and excitability changes in articulatory motor representations often extend to hand muscles (Tokimura et al., 1996; Willems et al., 2007; Gentilucci et al., 2008). Since this view has been challenged (Ziegler, 2003), though, it needs to be confirmed that our results obtained in hand muscles can be generalized to articulatory representations, e.g. tongue, lip or laryngeal muscles.

2.5. IS STUTTERING A FOCAL DYSTONIA?

In a classical definition, "focal, task-specific dystonia, of which writer's cramp and musician's s dystonia are examples, is characterised by excessive muscular activation during fine manipulative tasks" (Ridding et al., 1995). From a clinical point of view and facing the highly task-specific overactivation of articulatory muscles, PDS has been hypothesized to be a focal dystonia (Kiziltan and Akalin, 1996). We recently tested this hypothesis studying the intracortical excitability in PDS subjects. The intracortical excitability measures the balance between inhibitory and excitatory circuits in the motor cortex. Many movement disorders show a reduced intracortical inhibition, likely reflecting altered basal ganglia output. Focal dystonias such as writer's cramp or blepharospasm are one example (Ridding et al., 1995; Sommer et al., 2002), and so that it was reasonable to assume that intracortical inhibition might be reduced in PDS as well.
To address this question we studied 18 subjects with PDS (mean age 39.5 SD13.0) who all showed core symptoms of stuttering, i.e. repetitions and prolongations of sounds, speech blocks. We also assessed 18 speech-fluent control subjects with no personal history of stuttering (mean age 43.6 SD 14.). All participants had at least 80 of 100 points for right-handedness on the Oldfield handedness questionnaire (Oldfield, 1971).
For intracortical excitability we delivered conditioning-test paired transcranial magnetic stimulation (TMS) pulses that consisted of a

subthreshold conditioning stimulus (90% AMT) followed by a test pulse yielding motor evoked potentials (MEP)s in a small hand muscle (abductor digiti minimi) of ~1 mV after an interval of 1, 2, 3, 4, 5, 6, 7, 8, 10, 15, 20, or 30 ms. This study (Sommer et al., 2003) revealed no abnormality of intracortical excitability in PDS, which makes the analogy to focal dystonias less likely.

3. SYNTHESIS AND OUTLOOK

At least three core studies in recent years have provided evidence for subtle anatomical abnormalities in adults suffering from PDS. The grey matter of Broca's area shows more than normal gyrification and extra gyruses (Foundas et al., 2001), and there is reduced white matter consistency in the left Rolandic Operculum, a traffic junction or "hub" of fibres linking speech, auditory and motor relevant areas (Sommer et al., 2002; Chang et al., 2006). It is conceivable that the core symptoms of stuttering, i.e. repetitions, prolongations and speech blocks, arise on such a neurological ground. However, to confirm this hypothesis the *chicken or egg* issue needs to be settled. These anatomical studies provide a framework for explaining the physiological findings from functional imaging studies, mainly the right (pre)motor over-activity in PDS subjects which could be compensatory for a left hemispheric structural problem. Complementary findings post-treatment show increased activity of these left hemispheric areas and activation of adjacent areas of the left Rolandic Operculum (Neumann et al. 2003). The structural abnormalities may also explain the altered sequence of left-hemispheric activations (Salmelin et al., 2000). In this context it is reasonable to remind studies on reaction times and motor execution in stuttering subjects. These studies suggest subtle motor execution problems in PWS in domains beyond pure speech tasks. Therefore, careful analysis movement preparation, initiation and execution may provide a functional link between brain structure and clinical findings (Van Lieshout et al., 2004).

What the brain imaging findings do only partially account for is a) the secondary symptoms that are so variable from individual to individual, and b) the situation-dependent variability of stuttering severity. It is well

conceivable that the secondary symptoms represent a learned behaviour strongly modified by the interactions of the affected individual with his or her peers and parents. Here, compensatory or avoidance behaviours may come into play, as do the therapies aiming at modifying them.
We therefore suggest that the highly conserved core symptoms of PDS may arise on a neurological ground, possibly located in the left inferior frontal gyrus and the adjacent left Rolandic Operculum. On the other hand, the highly variable secondary symptoms may represent a learned behaviour and a mixture of partially conscious avoidance and coping strategies.

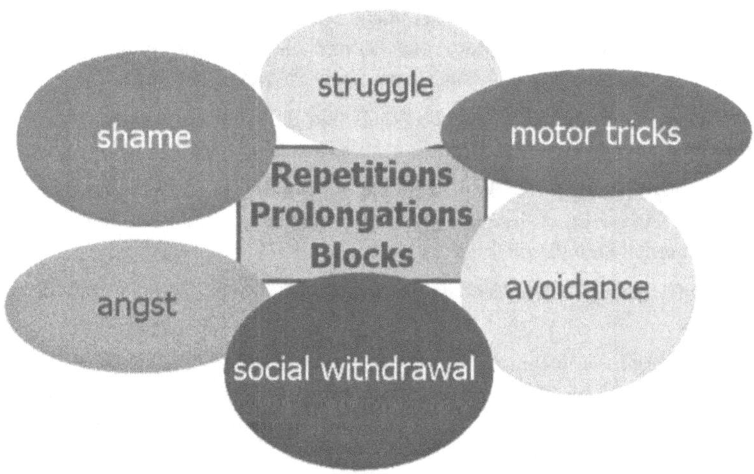

Figure 2: Model of universal, possibly neurogenic primary symptoms of persistent developmental stuttering (repetitions, prolongations, blocks) surrounded and partially hidden by highly variable secondary symptoms, possibly representing learned behaviour.

Further roads of study include the modulation of the primary symptoms by altering cortical excitability, the *chicken or egg* question, and the evaluation of therapies altering primary or secondary symptoms.

ACKNOWLEDGEMENTS

Part of the data reviewed here have been generated with the support of the DFG (Deutsche Forschungsgemeinschaft) grant SO 429/2-1 and SO 429/2-2, from the DFG Graduiertenkolleg GRK 632, from the Medical faculty of the University of Göttingen (Forschungsförderung), and from the Rose foundation.

REFERENCES

Amunts, K., Schlaug, G., Jäncke, L., Steinmetz, H., Schleicher, A., Dabringhaus, A., and Zilles, K. (1997). Motor cortex and hand motor skills: structural compliance in the human brain. *Human Brain Mapping* 5, 206-215.

Beal, D. Graccoc, V., Lafaillea, S., and De Nil, L. (2007). Voxel-based morphometry of auditory and speech-related cortex in stutterers. *Neuroreport* 18, 1257- 1260.

Bäumer, T., Dammann, E., Bock, F., Klöppel, S., Siebner, H.R., and Münchau, A. (2007). Laterality of interhemispheric inhibition depends on handedness. *Experimental Brain Research* 180, 195-203.

Bloodstein, O. (1995). *A handbook on Stuttering*. San Diego: Singular Publishing Group.

Braun, A.R., Varga, M., Stager, S., Schulz, G., Selbie, S., Maisog, J.M., Carson, R.E., and Ludlow, C.L. (1997). Altered patterns of cerebral activity during speech and language production in developmental stuttering. An H2 15O positron emission tomography study. *Brain* 120, 761-784.

Brown, S., Ingham, R., Ingham, J., Laird, A., and Fox, P. (2005). Stuttered and Fluent Speech Production: An ALE Meta-Analysis of Functional Neuroimaging Studies. *Human Brain Mapping* 25, 105- 117.

Buchel, C. & Sommer, M. (2004) What causes stuttering? *PLoS Biology* 2(2), E46.

Chang, S.E., Erickson, K., Ambrose, N., Hasegawa-Johnson, M., and Ludlow, C. (2006). Deficient white matter development in left hemisphere speech-language regions in children who stutter. *Society for Neuroscience Convention online (Atlanta, USA)*, Program No. 488.414.

De Nil, L. (2004). Recent developments in brain imaging research in stuttering. In: B. Maassen, R. Kent, H. Peters, P. van Lieshout, and W. Hulstijn (eds.) *Speech motor control in normal and disordered speech*, 113-137, Oxford (UK): Oxford University Press.

De Nil, L., Jokel, R., and Rochon, E. (2007). Stuttering associated with acquired neurological disorders: Review, assessment and intervention. In: E.G. Conture & R. F. Curlee (eds.) *Stuttering and Related Disorders of fluency*, 326-343, New York: Thieme Medical Publishers.

Draganski, B., Gaser, C., Busch, V., Schuierer, G., Bogdahn, U., and May, A. (2004). Neuroplasticity: changes in grey matter induced by training. *Nature* 427, 311-312.

Elbert, T., Pantev, C., Wienbruch, C., Rockstroh, B., and Taub, E. (1995). Increased cortical representation of the fingers of the left hand in string players. *Science* 270, 305-307.

Foundas, A.L., Bollich, A.M., Corey, D.M., Hurley, M., and Heilman, K.M. (2001). Anomalous anatomy of speech-language areas in adults with persistent developmental stuttering. *Neurology* 57, 207-215.

Fox, P.T., Ingham, R.J., Ingham, J.C., Zamarripa, F., Xiong, J.H., and Lancaster, J.L. (2000). Brain correlates of stuttering and syllable production. A PET performance-correlation analysis. *Brain* 123, 1985-2004.

Fox, P.T., Ingham, R.J., Ingham, J.C., Hirsch, T.B., Hunter Downs, J., Martin, C., Jerabek, P., Glass, T., and Lancaster, J.L. (1996). A PET study of the neural systems of stuttering. *Nature* 382, 158-162.

Gentilucci, M., Dalla and Volta, R. (2008). Spoken language and arm gestures are controlled by the same motor control system. *The Quarterly Journal of Experimental Psychology (Colchester)* 61(6), 944-57.

Hutchinson, S., Lee, L.H., Gaab, N., and Schlaug, G. (2003). Cerebellar volume of musicians. *Cerebral Cortex* 13, 943-949.

Kiziltan, G. & Akalin, M.A. (1996). Stuttering may be a type of action dystonia. *Movement Disorders* 11, 278-282.

Klingberg, T., Hedehus, M., Temple, E., Salz, T., Gabrieli, J.D.E., Moseley, M.E., and Poldrack, R.A. (2000). Microstructure of temporo-parietal white matter as a basis for reading ability: Evidence from diffusion tensor magnetic resonance imaging. *Neuron* 25, 493-500.

Neumann, K., Euler, H., Von Gudenberg, A., Giraud, A., Lanfermann, H., Gall, V., and Preibisch, C. (2003). The nature and treatment of stuttering as revealed by fMRI: A within- and between-group comparison. *Journal of Fluency Disorders* 28, 381- 410.

Oldfield, R.C. (1971). The assessment and analysis of handedness: the Edinburgh inventory. *Neuropsychologia* 9, 97-113.

Plankers, T. (1999). Speaking in the claustrum: the psychodynamics of stuttering. *International Journal of Psychoanalysis* 80, 239-256.

Preibisch, C., Neumann, K., Raab, P., Euler, H.A., von Gudenberg, A.W., Lanfermann, H., and Giraud, A.L. (2003). Evidence for compensation for stuttering by the right frontal operculum. *NeuroImage* 20, 1356-1364.

Ridding, M.C., Brouwer, B., Nordstrom, M.A. (2000). Reduced interhemispheric inhibition in musicians. *Experimental Brain Research* 133, 249-253.

Ridding, M.C., Sheean, G., Rothwell, J.C., Inzelberg, R., Kujirai, T. (1995). Changes in the balance between motor cortical excitation and inhibition in focal, task specific dystonia. *Journal of Neurology, Neurosurgery & Psychiatry* 59, 493-498.

Ringo, C.C. & Dietrich, S. (1995). Neurogenic stuttering: An analysis and critique. *Journal of Medical Speech-language Pathology* 3, 111-222.

Salmelin, R., Schnitzler, A., Schmitz, F., and Freund, H.J. (2000). Single word reading in developmental stutterers and fluent speakers. *Brain* 123, 1184-1202.

Schmithorst, V.J., Wilke, M., Dardzinski, F.J., and Holland, S.K. (2002). Correlation of white matter diffusivity and anisotropy with age during childhood and adolescence: a cross-sectional diffusion-tensor MR imaging study. *Radiology* 222, 212-218.

Sommer, M., Wischer, S., Tergau, F., and Paulus, W. (2003). Normal intracortical excitability in developmental stuttering. *Movement Disorders* 18, 826-830.

Sommer, M., Koch, M.A., Paulus, W., Weiller, C., and Büchel, C. (2002). Disconnection of speech-relevant brain areas in persistent developmental stuttering. *Lancet* 360, 380-383.

Sussman, H.M. & MacNeilage, P.F. (1975), Studies of hemispheric specialization for speech production. *Brain and Language* 2, 131-151.

Tokimura, H., Tokimura, Y., Oliviero, A., Asakura, T., and Rothwell, J.C. (1996). Speech-induced changes in corticospinal excitability. *Annals of Neurology* 40(4), 628-34.

Travis, L.E. (1978). The cerebral dominance theory of stuttering: 1931-1978. *Journal of Speech, Language, and Hearing Research* 43, 275-281.

Van Lieshout, P., Hulstijn, W., and Peters, H. (2004). Searching for the weak link in the speech production chain of people who stutter: A motor skill approach. In: B. Maassen, R. Kent, H. Peters, P. van Lieshout, W. Hulstijn (eds.) *Speech Motor Control in Normal and Disordered Speech*, 313-356, Oxford (UK): Oxford University Press.

Webster, W.G., and Ryan, C.R. (1991). Task complexity and manual reaction times in people who stutter. *Journal of Speech and Hearing Research* 34, 708-714.

Willems, R.M., Ozyürek, A., and Hagoort, P. (2007). When language meets action: the neural integration of gesture and speech. *Cerebral Cortex* 17(10), 2322-33.

Woodruff Starkweather, C., Franklin, S., and Smigo, T.M. (1984). Vocal and finger reaction times in stutterers and nonstutterers: differences and correlations. *Journal of Speech and Hearing Disorders* 27,193-196.

Yairi E & Ambrose NG (1999). Early childhood stuttering I: persistency and recovery rates. *Journal of Speech, Language, and Hearing Research* 42, 1097-1112.

Ziegler, W. (2003). Speech motor control is task-specific: Evidence from dysarthria and apraxia of speech. *Aphasiology* 17, 3-36.

8

The sensory-motor theory of semantics: Evidence from functional imaging[1]

UTA NOPPENEY

Abstract: This review discusses the contributions of functional imaging (fMRI/PET) to our understanding of how semantic concepts are represented and processed in the human brain. The sensory-motor theory of semantic memory suggests that semantic processing relies on reactivation of sensory-motor representations that were involved during original perception and action. More specifically, it attributes an apparent category-specific (e.g. tool vs animals) organization of semantics on anatomical segregation for different semantic features (e.g. action vs visual). Within this framework, we will review functional imaging evidence that semantic processing of tools and actions may rely on activations within the visuo-motor system.

1. INTRODUCTION

1.1. THE SENSORY-MOTOR THEORY OF SEMANTIC MEMORY

Since the seminal work of Warrington and Shallice (1984), numerous studies have reported neuropsychological patients showing unequal degrees of impairment across different domains of knowledge. The commonest manifestation of these so-called "category-selective deficits" is a selective deficit for concepts from the domain of living items with relative sparing of concepts from the domain of artefacts. Fewer studies have reported the opposite pattern that is a selective deficit for concepts

1 This article is an extended version of Noppeney, U. (2008) The neural systems of tool and action semantics: A perspective from functional imaging. Journal of Physiology - Paris

from the domain of artefacts (for review: (Capitani et al., 2003; Farah et al., 1996; Gainotti et al., 1995; Gainotti and Silveri, 1996; Hillis and Caramazza, 1991; Sacchett and Humphreys, 1992; Warrington and McCarthy, 1987; Warrington and Shallice, 1984)). These double dissociations of semantic deficits persist even when attempts are made to control general processing differences due to confounding variables such as familiarity, visual complexity or word frequency (Farah et al., 1996; Sartori et al., 1993). Hence, they appear to reflect some sort of semantic organisation at the neuronal level rather than an experimental artefact. However, the underlying organisational principles of semantic memory remain controversial. A number of cognitive models have been proposed:

The *category-specific model* (Caramazza and Shelton, 1998) proposes distinct neuronal systems that have specialized for processing items from different semantic categories (e.g. animals or artefacts) due to evolutionary pressures. Here, a functional segregation for different semantic categories may have emerged to allow for rapid identification and classification of animals as potential predators and plants as a source of food.

In contrast, the *conceptual structure account* (Tyler et al., 2000; Tyler and Moss, 2001) assumes a unitary distributed conceptual system that is structured according to correlations amongst semantic features (i.e. the degree to which semantic features co-occur in the environment). Selective semantic deficits are explained by differences in the structure of concepts across categories. Artefacts are defined by few and more distinctive features. In contrast, living items are characterized by many overlapping shared and highly intercorrelated features but only relatively few distinctive features. Hence, living items may place increased demands on integration and differentiation processes.

Finally, the *feature-based account* of semantic memory ((Warrington and Shallice, 1984); also referred to as the sensori-motor theory (Martin et al., 2000)) assumes that conceptual knowledge is represented in a large distributed network, indexing a range of semantic features (e.g. visual, auditory, action, functional properties (Allport, 1985)). Although category-specificity is not the underlying organisational principle, an apparent category-structure emerges because concepts rely differentially on sensory, action and verbally-learnt knowledge. In particular, category-specific semantic deficits for living and non-living items are explained by their differential associations with sensory and action features: While sensory features are important for distinguishing between living items, action semantics plays a critical role in the representation of inanimate items (especially tools) (Shallice, 1988; Warrington and Shallice, 1984). Hence, loss of sensory or action knowledge differentially disrupts the semantic representation of animate or inanimate objects respectively.

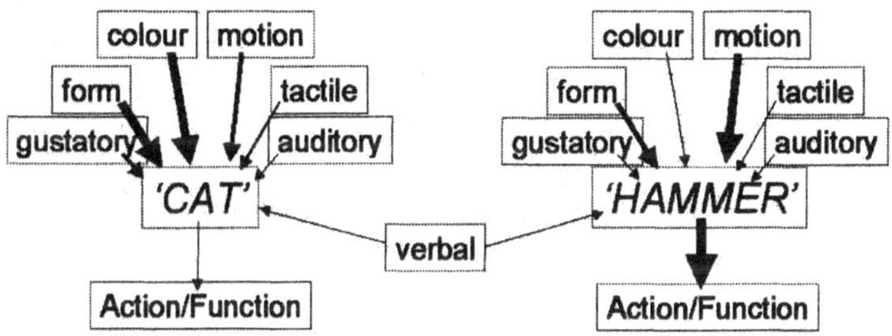

Figure 1: The feature based model of semantic memory. Illustration of the animate non-animate distinction. Arrow width indicates the contribution of a semantic feature to a particular semantic concept.

In terms of functional brain architecture, the sensory-motor theory of semantic memory (or sensory-motor theory) relates sensory (e.g. visual, auditory) and action (e.g. hand action, body motion) features to the input and output channels within the human brain (Martin et al., 2000; Martin and Chao, 2001). While sensory features may be subserved by brain regions close to or even overlapping with areas involved in perception (e.g. visual association areas), action semantics is hypothesized to be related to motor output regions (e.g. pre-motor cortex) as well as to brain areas involved in motion/action perception (e.g. areas adjacent to hMT+/V5). Thus, the neural systems representing/processing sensory or action semantic features may be 1) related to or 2) even identical with the regions that are engaged when the particular type of semantic knowledge has been originally acquired during sensory-motor experience. In case 1), there might be "semantic regions" that are selective for a particular type of semantic feature because of their afferent or efferent connections to sensory-motor regions. In case 2), "sensory-motor regions" themselves can sustain semantic representations or processes. From a cognitive perspective, the function of a so-called "sensory-motor region" would then depend on the particular task-context. From a neuronal perspective, it would depend on the brain regions it is interacting with. For instance, motion area hMT+/V5 might be involved in motion processing when being activated via forward (bottom up) connections from early visual areas but in semantic processes when being activated via backward (top down) connections from higher order semantic (e.g. anterior temporal cortex) or retrieval regions (e.g. prefrontal cortex) (Barsalou et al., 2003; Damasio, 1989; Damasio et al., 1996; Noppeney et al., 2006b; Pulvermuller, 2005). Here, a so-called "sensory-motor" region would be engaged in both sensory/motor processing and higher cognitive functions such as semantic processing.

In this paper, we will review functional imaging (fMRI, PET) studies investigating the neural systems supporting action and tool semantics. From the perspective of the sensory-motor theory of semantic memory, we will investigate whether the neural substrates underlying action and tool semantics are anatomically and functionally related to brain regions taking part in a visuo-motor action system. Hence, we will first review neurophysiological and functional imaging studies in non-human and human primates that have characterized the fronto-parietal circuitry underlying visuo-motor transformations. We will then review human functional imaging studies of the neural systems sustaining action and tool semantics. Collectively, these studies suggest that deep semantic processing of tool and action concepts relies on activations within the visuo-motor system as proposed by the sensory-motor theory of semantic memory.

1.2. THE VISUO-MOTOR SYSTEM AND ACTION SEMANTICS

1.2.1. THE VISUO-MOTOR SYSTEM

The visuo-motor system has been characterized initially by neurophysiological studies in non-human primates. These studies have suggested that distinct regions within the fronto-parietal circuitry may play a role in 1) visuo-motor transformations and 2) action matching, imitation and understanding (Rizzolatti and Luppino, 2001).

1) Visuo-motor transformations such as visual searching or grasping are thought to be mediated through interactions between the ventral premotor cortex and an anterior intraparietal area (AIP) that receives visual input and is connected with inferior temporal cortex (IT) (Rizzolatti and Craighero, 2004). In both AIP and ventral pre-motor cortex (in particular in the posterior bank of the ventral limb of the arcuate sulcus) canonical neurons have been found that fire when the monkey sees and grasps an object. In AIP, these visual-dominant neurons respond selectively to visual presentation of a particular class of three-dimensional objects (Murata et al., 2000). Hence, it has been suggested that AIP extracts and selects the relevant 3D features. These visual object properties (or affordances) may subsequently activate congruent motor prototypes in ventral premotor cortex and thus enable the appropriate action for a particular object (e.g. object grasping).

2) Action understanding may be sustained by a ventral pre-motor area (F5c, on the cortical convexity) and an anterior inferior parietal area (7b/PF) that is connected with the superior temporal sulcus (STS). In F5c and PF, neurons with mirror properties have been identified, i.e. these neurons discharge, when the monkey makes a particular action and when the monkey observes another individual making a similar action (Fogassi et al., 2005; Fogassi and Luppino, 2005; Rizzolatti et al., 2002; Rizzolatti and Craighero, 2004; Rizzolatti and Luppino, 2001). This action-selectivity depends primarily on the final goal of the action rather than particular kinematic characteristics. Thus, mirror neuron discharges are also observed when (i) the kinematics is altered (Fogassi et al., 2005; Fogassi and Luppino, 2005), (ii) the final hand-object interaction is hidden (Umilta et al., 2001) and (iii) only the sound of a particular action is presented (Kohler et al., 2002).

A recent fMRI study in the macaque has identified and further characterized multiple action representations within the frontal lobe that vary in their degree of abstraction (Nelissen et al., 2005). In particular, it has dissociated (i) caudal F5c that responds only when the agent is fully visible (e.g. the person together with the arm picking up the object), (ii) rostral F5ab (in the depth of the ventral limb of the arcuate sulcus) that is also activated by observation of an isolated arm and even an artificial device (though less effective) and (iii) 45B that is activated not only by actions but also by graspable objects.

A recent fMRI study in the macaque has identified and further characterized multiple action representations within the frontal lobe that vary in their degree of abstraction (Nelissen et al., 2005). In particular, it has dissociated (i) caudal F5c that responds only when the agent is fully visible (e.g. the person together with the arm picking up the object), (ii) rostral F5ab (in the depth of the ventral limb of the arcuate sulcus) that is also activated by observation of an isolated arm and even an artificial device (though less effective) and (iii) 45B that is activated not only by actions but also by graspable objects.

Thus, neurophysiological and functional imaging studies of non-human primates have implicated the fronto-parietal circuitry both in visuo-motor transformations and action observation. The F5-PF mirror neuron system may form the basis for action/intention understanding and imitation learning (Arbib and Bota, 2003; Rizzolatti and Arbib, 1998). While there is still some controversy about the homology between monkey and human mirror neuron areas, cytoarchitectonic and electrophysiological studies seem to suggest a similar fronto-parietal action system in humans. For instance, homologies have been proposed between human ventral premotor BA6 and caudal F5c in the macaque. Similarly, F5a (as designated by (Nelissen et al., 2005) may be the homologue of human BA44 (see (Petrides et al., 2005) for further discussion) and PF/AIP related to the anterior inferior parietal cortex in humans. These proposed homologies converge with recent functional imaging results in humans implicating the ventral pre-motor cortex and the anterior parietal cortex (supramarginal gyrus/AIP) in action observation, simulation, imitation and execution (Buccino et al., 2001; Buccino et al., 2004a; Buccino et al., 2004b; Decety et al., 1997; Grezes et al., 2003; Grezes and Decety, 2001; Iacoboni et al., 1999; Iacoboni et al., 2005; Jeannerod, 2001; Jeannerod and Frak, 1999; Johnson-Frey et al., 2003; Rizzolatti et al., 1996; Rushworth et al., 2003).

1.2.2. THE NEURAL SYSTEMS OF ACTION SEMANTICS

Consistent with the sensory-motor theory of semantic memory, a series of functional imaging studies have reported increased activation in the ventral premotor and the anterior inferior parietal cortex for retrieval of action semantics using verbal and non-verbal stimuli. Activation in the left ventral pre-motor cortex has been observed for generation of semantically related action words relative to naming of an object (Fiez et al., 1996; Grafton et al., 1997; Warburton et al., 1996). While these results may be confounded by internal verbalization and thus phonological retrieval, the seminal study by Martin et al. (1995) has revealed increased left premotor activation for generating an action (e.g. 'pencil' => 'write') associated with an object relative to its colour (e.g. 'pencil' => 'yellow') (Martin et al., 1995). Some studies (Perani et al., 1999a; Shapiro et al., 2006) have revealed increased pre-motor activation for lexical decisions on verbs relative to nouns (but see (Longe et al., 2007; Tyler et al., 2004) proposing an explanation in terms of morphological and syntactic mechanisms). Surprisingly, a recent study has shown selective activation along the (pre)-motor cortex in a somatotopic fashion for action words referring to face, arm or leg actions (e.g. 'lick', 'pick', 'kick') in a passive reading task (Hauk et al., 2004). Similarly, anterior inferior parietal activation has been observed for semantic decisions or similarity judgments on action (e.g. 'crush', 'screw') relative to non-action words (e.g. purple, crackle, success) (Noppeney et al., 2005) retrieval of an object's action relative to its function (Kellenbach et al., 2003) and listening to action-related relative to abstract sentences (Tettamanti et al., 2005).

In addition to AIP and ventral pre-motor areas, a left posterior middle temporal region (LPMT) has been associated consistently with action semantics. LPMT is activated for observing grasping movements relative to static objects (Perani et al., 2001; Rizzolatti et al., 1996), hands (Grezes et al., 1998) or random motion (Beauchamp et al., 2002; Bonda et al., 1996). Obviously, these activation differences may be due to specific kinematic characteristics of the stimuli at the perceptual level. However, LPMT activation was also increased for static pictures (e.g. a kettle pouring water into a cap) or sentences with implied motion/action relative to similar stimuli that did not imply motion (e.g. a kettle standing on a table) (Kourtzi and Kanwisher, 2000; Ruby and Decety, 2001; Senior et al., 2000). Moreover, in semantic decision or generation tasks, LPMT is activated for retrieval of action (e.g. "Do you twist this object?") relative to retrieval of visual semantics (e.g. "Is the object bigger than a kiwi?"), when the stimuli are written words or pictures referring to real world objects (Martin et al., 1995; Phillips et al., 2002b). Similarly, LPMT activation is increased for semantic tasks on spoken or written words (or sentences) referring to action/motion (e.g. "twist", "run") relative to visual (e.g. "red"), auditory (e.g. "pop") or abstract (e.g. "idea") semantic features (Noppeney et al., 2005; Wallentin et al., 2005) (see figure 2). Finally, Weisberg et al. (2007) have demonstrated that training a tool-like task with novel objects is associated with increased LPMT activation, though the time by condition interaction, i.e. the statistical comparison quantifying learning effects, was very small (for a related EEG study see also Kiefer et al., (2007)). Collectively, these studies demonstrate that LPMT is more engaged in action semantics relative to a range of other semantic types regardless of stimulus material (e.g. written words, sentences or pictures) or modality (auditory or visual, e.g. spoken or written words). Hence, the activations cannot be attributed to low level stimulus characteristics. Instead, these results characterize LPMT as a multimodal semantic region associated with action processing. As LPMT is just anterior (or overlapping) to motion area hMT+/V5, its role in action semantics might be engendered by its functional relation to action/motion perception mediated by afferents from area hMT+/V5. From a neurodevelopmental perspective, this raises the question whether early onset blindness that precludes visual experience of motion and enforces action experience via somatosensory-motor associations rather than visual motion perception, reduces or even abolishes the action-selective response in LPMT. Contrary to this conjecture, in both blind and sighted subjects, LPMT activation was increased for semantic decisions on spoken words referring to actions relative to words referring to visual, auditory or motion features (Noppeney et al., 2003). This remarkable resilience of LPMT action-selectivity to early visual deprivation might be explained by multimodal response characteristics of LPMT. For instance, action-selectivity may depend not only on afferent connections from motion area hMT+/V5 but also on its connectivity with motor areas. Alternatively, the semantic system develops not only due to experiential factors but also innately-specified neurobiological mechanisms.

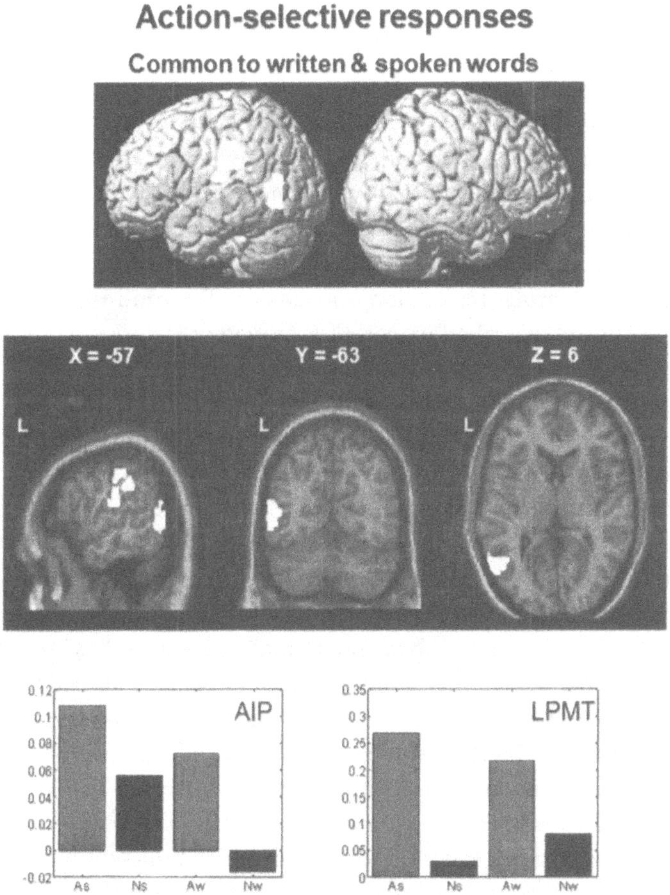

Figure 2: Action-selective responses common to spoken and written words; Top: Action-selective responses common to spoken and written words are rendered on a template of the whole brain and presented on coronal, axial and sagittal sections of a canonical brain. For illustrational purposes we have chosen: Extent threshold > 5 voxels. (modified from (Noppeney et al., 2005)) Bottom: Parameter estimates for action (grey) and non-action (black) conditions in AIP (co-ordinates: x = -57 y = -36 z = 30) and LPMT (co-ordinates: x = -57 y = -63 z = 6). As = Actionspoken, Ns = Non-Actionspoken, Aw = Actionwritten, Nw = Non-Actionwritten

1.3. CHARACTERIZATION OF ACTION-SELECTIVITY: HAND MANIPULATION & FUNCTIONAL KNOWLEDGE

1.3.1. THE DISTINCTION BETWEEN HAND ACTIONS AND WHOLE BODY MOVEMENTS

"Actions" can be classified as hand actions or whole body movements. A distinction between these two categories may be drawn at the perceptual and at the semantic level. At the perceptual level, it was suggested that hand manipulations are characterized by simple motion trajectories (Beauchamp et al., 2002). For instance, the movement for using a saw is primarily a simple translation movement. By contrast, whole body movements are described by complex motion trajectories. Thus, humans can independently move different body parts that are connected by articulated joints. Yet, it needs to be acknowledged that the motion trajectories of hand actions can be quite variable. Thus, writing with a pencil also involves multiple joints and evolves along a complex motion trajectory. Conversely, simple hand actions such as sawing may be associated posturing of the entire body. At the semantic level, hand actions are transitive actions and more strongly associated with tools and utensils. In contrast, whole body movements are intransitive actions and primarily linked with humans and animals. Based on these distinctions, the question arises whether regions within or beyond the action retrieval system respond more to hand actions than to whole body movements. At the perceptual level, this question has been addressed (Beauchamp et al., 2002) by comparing activations during observation of (i) natural simple tool movements (e.g. sawing), (ii) artificial simple tool movements (e.g. a rotating saw), (iii) natural complex human movements (e.g. running) and (iv) artificial simple human movements (e.g. a rotating human). While the right superior temporal sulcus (STS) showed an enhanced response to whole body movements, LPMT responded preferentially to hand movements – though this effect was very small. Using words rather than pictures, a recent study (Noppeney et al., 2005) intended to identify regions that responded selectively to particular action types i.e. hand actions or whole body movements at the semantic level. Subjects performed a semantic decision on hand action (e.g. Is it a hand action with/without a tool? Chisel, Knit, Tapping, Tickle) or body motions words (Is it a jumping movement? Leap, Swimming, Climb, Springing). Although AIP and LPMT showed enhanced responses for action relative to non-action words, they did not distinguish between hand actions and whole body movements. However, an area in the right STS, anterior to the region that responded selectively to movies of whole body movements, exhibited increased activation for whole body movements relative to hand actions (see also (James and Gauthier, 2003). In summary, studies of action observation and semantic retrieval provide converging evidence that LPMT activation is commonly increased for both, hand manipulation and whole body movements. There is some evidence that hand actions further enhance LPMT activation relative to whole body movements primarily at the perceptual level.

1.3.2. THE DISTINCTION BETWEEN MANIPULATION AND FUNCTIONAL KNOWLEDGE: KNOWING "HOW" AND KNOWING "WHAT FOR"

Tools or objects can be characterized by the motion features of an associated hand action (i.e. knowing "how" = manipulation knowledge) and by their function (i.e. knowing "what for" or the context of usage = functional knowledge). Although a particular type of manipulation can sometimes be associated with a specific function (e.g. a saw and a knife are associated with similar actions and have similar functions), the mapping between manipulation and functional properties is many to many. For instance, a piano and a record player subserve similar functions but are manipulated differently, while a piano and a typewriter fulfil different functions but are manipulated similarly. Neuropsychological studies (Buxbaum et al., 2000; Sirigu et al., 1991) have reported patients who could match items on the basis of their function but not on the basis of how they are manipulated and vice versa. More specifically, Sirigu et al. (1991) reported a herpes encephalitis patient that was impaired on functional knowledge with relative sparing of action knowledge. In contrast, Buxbaum et al. (2000) described two patients with large fronto-parietal or posterior parietal infarction that were primarily impaired on action knowledge with relative sparing of functional knowledge. This double dissociation suggests that the neural substrates of function and manipulation knowledge may be anatomically segregated and one might hypothesize that ventral premotor, AIP or LPMT respond to manipulation more than functional knowledge (though see alternative account that interprets the fronto-parietal system as a mechanical problem solving system based on object affordances (Hodges et al., 1999; Hodges et al., 2000). Consistent with this notion, no increased activation (Cappa et al., 1998; Mummery et al., 1998; Thompson-Schill et al., 1999) has been reported in any of these regions for retrieval of functional relative to visual semantics. A recent study (Kellenbach et al., 2003) directly compared retrieval of (i) an action associated with a manipulable object (e.g. 'Does using a saw involve a twisting or a turning movement?'), (ii) a function of a manipulable object (e.g. 'Is a saw used to put a substance on another object?') and (iii) a function of a non-manipulable object (e.g. a traffic light). This experimental design revealed distinct activation patterns in the cortical regions of the visuo-motor action system: In LPMT and ventral premotor cortex, activations were significantly increased for manipulable relative to non-manipulable objects. Only a small non-significant increase was observed for retrieval of action relative to functional knowledge (see also (Gerlach et al., 2002b), for converging results in the ventral pre-motor cortex). In contrast, in AIP, activation was increased for (i) manipulable objects relative to non-manipulable objects and (ii) action decisions relative to function decisions (see (Boronat et al., 2005) for similar results). Thus, while AIP showed an effect of stimulus (manipulable vs. non-manipulable objects) and task (action vs function retrieval), LPMT and the ventral pre-motor cortex showed only an effect of stimulus: Here, increased activation was elicited by manipulable objects irrespective of whether the task required action or function retrieval.

While Kellenbach et al. (2003) observed only action-selective but no function-selective activations, a recent functional imaging study (Canessa et al., 2007) found a double dissociation in line with the neuropsychological results: Subjects were presented with pictures showing pairs of manipulable objects (e.g. 'accordion' & 'pectoral expander') and asked whether the objects within each pair were used with the same manipulation pattern ('action knowledge') or in the same context ('function knowledge'). While the fronto-parietal system showed

increased activation for action relative to function knowledge, the lateral anterior inferior temporal and retrosplenial cortices showed the opposite pattern, i.e. increased activation for functional relative to action knowledge. This is in line with previous studies showing activation in the anterior temporal and medial parietal cortices for retrieval of encyclopaedic/verbally learnt semantic knowledge (e.g. deciding whether a food item comes from a tropical region (Noppeney and Price, 2003) or verifying general facts (Maguire and Mummery, 1999)).
Collectively, these results suggest that retrieval of action and function knowledge is sustained by two dissociable neural systems: Activation in the visuomotor system is primarily driven by action knowledge: In LPMT and the ventral pre-motor cortex, the action-selective response is automatically/implicitly invoked by manipulable objects irrespective of the specific task instructions, in AIP it is modulated by the particular task demands and enhanced for action relative to function retrieval. In contrast, retrieval of functional knowledge engages a parieto-temporal system that has previously been associated with retrieval of verbally-learnt or encyclopaedic knowledge and the integration of semantic features.

1.4. TOOL SELECTIVE RESPONSES

1.4.1. TOOL-SELECTIVITY IN THE VISUO-MOTOR ACTION SYSTEM

The feature-based theory has been developed to explain the intriguing category-selective deficits in neuropsychological patients. Rather than assuming category-specificity as an underlying organizational principle, it predicates category-selective effects on anatomical segregation for different types of semantics (e.g. action vs sensory features). In particular, it explains tools-selective effects by the association between tools and actions. Hence, one would expect that tool and action semantics activate overlapping brain systems: Indeed, many studies have consistently reported tool-selective activation in one or several regions of the visuo-motor action system: the left premotor cortex (Chao and Martin, 2000; Devlin et al., 2002; Gerlach et al., 2000; Gerlach et al., 2002a; Grabowski et al., 1998; Grafton et al., 1997; Kraut et al., 2002; Martin et al., 1996; Mecklinger et al., 2002), the left posterior middle temporal (Cappa et al., 1998; Chao et al., 1999; Chao et al., 2002; Chao and Martin, 2000; Damasio et al., 1996; Devlin et al., 2002; Lewis et al., 2005; Martin et al., 1996; Moore and Price, 1999; Mummery et al., 1996; Mummery et al., 1998; Perani et al., 1999b; Phillips et al., 2002a) and AIP (Cappa et al., 1998; Chao et al., 2002; Chao and Martin, 2000; Devlin et al., 2002; Noppeney et al., 2006b). These tool-selective activations have been observed irrespective of stimulus modality (e.g. sounds or pictures) or material (e.g. pictures or written words). Surprisingly, tool-selective responses in parietal cortex have been observed even without accompanying conscious knowledge. Thus, during binocular rivalry, tool pictures that subjects are unaware of due to inter-ocular suppression still elicit enhanced activations in the dorsal pathway (Fang and He, 2005). Taken together with the research on action semantics, these studies suggest that semantic category (e.g. tools versus animals) and semantic feature (e.g. action versus visual) may modulate the neural responses in overlapping brain systems. Indeed, independently manipulating stimulus-category (i.e. tools vs. fruits; (Phillips et al., 2002b)) and task instructions (i.e. attention to action vs visual features) in a 2X2 factorial design revealed that the tool and the action-selective effects modulate LPMT responses in an additive fashion: Tools relative to fruits activated LPMT irrespective of whether action or visual semantics is retrieved.

Conversely, retrieval of action relative to visual knowledge activated LPMT regardless of whether tools or fruits are presented (see Figure 3).

Thus, even when the stimuli were fruits, LPMT was more active when subjects made a semantic decision on an appropriate action (i.e. 'Can you peel it by hand') than on its real life size (i.e. 'Is it bigger than a lemon'). Similarly, AIP activation was increased for (i) manipulable objects relative to non-manipulable objects and (ii) action relative to function decisions (Kellenbach et al., 2003).

The studies reported so far implicate the visuo-motor system in both tools and action semantics. Thus, tool-selective responses may be mediated by their association with action features and an apparent category-specific organisation could emerge from a feature-based architecture. However, inconsistencies across studies also need to be noted. For instance, most studies have reported tool-selective responses only in a subset of these regions. Furthermore, manipulating task-context (e.g.

explicit vs. implicit semantic task) and object category (e.g. tools vs animals) in a multi-factorial design has demonstrated that tool-selective activations in the dorsal visuo-motor systems are profoundly context-sensitive and primarily detected for explicit semantic and in particular action retrieval tasks (Kellenbach et al., 2003; Noppeney et al., 2006b).

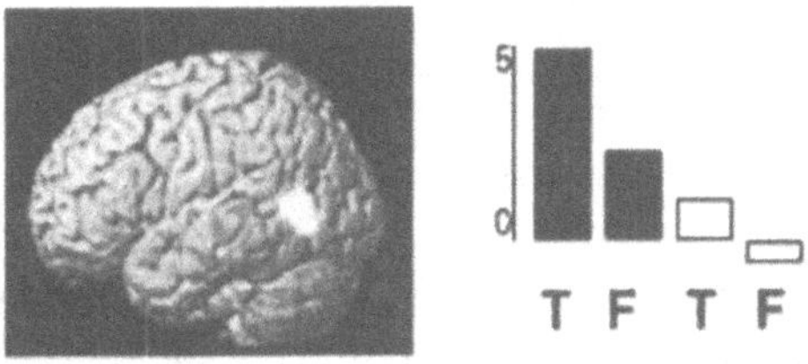

Figure 3: Additive effects of tool category and action retrieval in LPMT. Subjects were presented pictures or written words that referred to tools or fruits. In the activation conditions, they made a decision on action (e.g. Do you peel it by hand?) or visual semantics (e.g. Is it bigger than a kiwi?). In the baseline condition, they made a decision on the screen size of the stimulus (modified from (Phillips et al., 2002b)). Left: Activation for action > visual semantics masked with action semantics > baseline is rendered on an averaged normalised brain. Right: Parameter estimates for semantic conditions averaged over pictures and words relative to baseline are shown at the peak co-ordinate of action > visual semantics (x=-56 y=-60 z=0). T = Tools, F = Fruits; Black = Action, White = Visual.

The question therefore emerges, whether or not these action-selective activations are truly essential for implicit semantic processing that is involved in passive listening or reading. If the tool-selective responses in the visuo-motor system are indeed essential, they may simply be too small to be detected during implicit semantic tasks and only revealed when being amplified through attentional top-down modulation during explicit semantic tasks. Alternatively, the action-selective responses in the visuo-motor system might reflect particular task-induced processes such as action imagery or mechanical problem solving (Hodges et al., 1999), which are not necessarily involved in implicit semantic processing. Permanent (e.g. neuropsychology) or transient lesion (e.g. TMS) methods may help us to distinguish between these two possibilities: For instance, applying TMS to LPMT or ventral premotor cortex should be associated with impaired semantic processing and comprehension only if LPMT makes a critical functional contribution to action retrieval (see also (Pulvermuller et al., 2005) demonstrating a facilitatory effect of TMS over premotor cortex on lexical decisions of action words).

To summarize, consistent with the sensory-motor theory of semantic memory, tools that are more strongly linked with action features than animals, fruits or non-manipulable objects activate regions within the visuo-motor action system. However, these tool-selective responses are profoundly context-sensitive and primarily observed for explicit semantic tasks (i.e. deep semantic encoding). The semantic content by task context interactions may represent top-down modulation from higher order semantic or executive regions or task-induced processes such as action imagery or mechanical problem solving.

1.4.2. Dorso-ventral dissociation of tool-selective activations

In addition to activations in the visuomotor action system, tool-selective responses have been reported within the ventral occipito-temporal cortex: Within the fusiform, activations have been found medially for tools and laterally for animals. This raises the question whether the ventral occipito-temporal and dorsal temporo-parietal activations (i.e. LPMT, AIP) reflect similar cognitive processes or whether they emerge at different stages of tool categorization. Using stimulus or task manipulations, three recent studies have dissociated the functional roles of the dorsal visuo-motor system and the ventral occipito-temporal cortex in tool processing. Consistent with the neuropsychological literature (Humphreys and Forde, 2001) their results suggest that tool-selective responses can emerge at multiple processing levels during categorization of tools:

The first study (Chao et al., 2002) manipulated semantic category (animals vs tools) and visual experience (primed vs unprimed) in a picture naming task and demonstrated a priming induced response reduction non-selectively for tools and animals in the medial fusiform, but selectively for tools in LPMT. This unselective priming effect in the occipito-temporal area suggests that the "fusiform tool region" responds to both categories similarly.

The second study (Beauchamp et al., 2003) manipulated (i) semantic type (i.e. human motion vs tool motion) and (ii) stimulus display (real objects vs point light display) in a factorial design. Subjects categorized the stimuli as tools or humans. While LPMT showed a selective response for tool motion irrespective of stimulus display, the medial fusiform showed a tool-selective response primarily for real objects. Again, this suggests that LPMT is responsive to tools irrespective of stimulus modality, whereas the tool-selective responses in the medial fusiform depended on the stimulus display and is elicited primarily by pictures of objects.

The third study (Noppeney et al., 2006b) factorially manipulated (i) semantic category (tools vs animals), (ii) stimulus modality/material (pictures, spoken or written words) and (iii) task (explicit vs implicit semantic one-back-task) (see Figure 4). Subjects decided whether subsequent stimuli within a block were identical (= implicit semantic task, e.g. sparrow, sparrow), performed a similar action (= explicit action semantic task, e.g. stork, butterfly) or were of similar size in real life (= explicit visual semantic task, e.g. pigeon, rabbit).

From a methodological perspective, the study combined functional imaging with Effective Connectivity Analyses (i.e. Dynamic Causal Modelling) to investigate the neural mechanisms that mediate the tool-selective responses in multiple cortical regions. This approach dissociated two distinct mechanisms that engender tool-selectivity: In the ventral occipito-temporal cortex, category-selectivity was modality-dependent, observed primarily for pictures and mediated by bottom up effects. In the dorsal visuo-motor system, it was task-dependent, observed primarily for explicit semantic tasks and mediated by increased top-down influences of task-related prefrontal activity.

Collectively, the regionally distinct activation and connectivity patterns in the dorsal visuomotor system and the ventral occipito-temporal cortex suggest that these two category-selective systems may support different cognitive operations: The tool-selective responses in occipito-temporal regions is strongly influenced by stimulus-bound factors such as modality (pictures vs words), display (real objects vs point lights) or perceptual priming. These regions may therefore be engaged in structural processing of tools. In contrast, tool-selective responses in regions of the visuo-motor system were modulated by the task-context and observed primarily for explicit semantic tasks. These regions might play a role in explicit semantic processing that may involve additional processes such as action imagery. Thus, deep semantic processing of tools may rely on re-activating their associated action representations in the visuo-motor system via top down modulation from semantic retrieval (e.g. prefrontal cortex) or higher order semantic regions (e.g. anterior temporal regions).

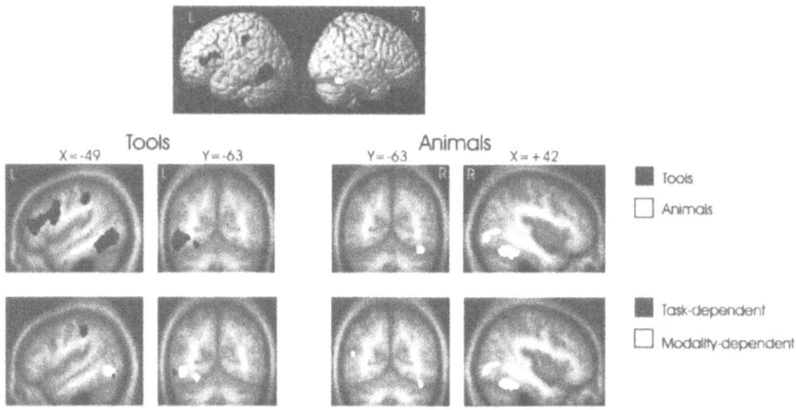

Figure 4: Dorso-ventral dissociation of category-selective activations. Top: Main effects of category: Tool- & animal-selective activations are rendered on an averaged normalised brain. Height threshold: $p<0.05$ corrected. Extent threshold: > 1 voxel, including only voxels that were activated for stimulus > fixation at $p < 0.001$ (uncorrected). Bottom: Main effects of category and category x task/modality interactions on coronal and sagittal slices of a structural image created by averaging the subjects' normalised images. Bottom: Main effects of category and category x task/-modality interactions on coronal and sagittal slices of a structural image created by averaging the subjects' normalised images. Row 1: Tools > Animals (Black); Animals > Tools (Light grey). Row 2: Tools > Animals for Semantic Decision > Implicit task (Black); (i) Tool- and animals selective activations for Pictures > Words (Light grey). Height threshold: $p<0.001$ uncorrected for illustration purposes. Extent threshold: > 19 voxels restricted to voxels that showed a significant effect of category-selectivity and stimulus > fixation. Modified from (Noppeney et al., 2006b).

The distinct activation patterns in the dorsal visuomotor system and the ventral occipito-temporal cortex converge with neuropsychological studies that revealed category-selective impairments at multiple processing levels ranging from structural to semantic (Humphreys and Forde, 2001).

In summary, tool-selectivity lies in the interaction of semantic content with either (i) stimulus-bound factors such as modality (= ventral occipito-temporal system) or (ii) task (= dorsal visuomotor system). From a cognitive perspective, category-selective responses therefore reflect either stimulus-bound structural processing or task-induced semantic operations. In terms of neural mechanisms, category-selective brain responses emerge from the patterns of interactions among brain regions. The two distinct classes of category-selectivity can be explained by differential top-down and bottom up influences for task and modality-dependent category-selective effects respectively. Thus, both functional imaging and neuropsychology suggest that some sort of category-selective organisation may be implemented at both, structural and semantic processing levels.

1.5. Conclusions and Future Directions

This section revisits several themes that have emerged from functional imaging studies of tool and action processing. First, we will evaluate the positive evidence that studies of tool and action semantics have provided for a sensory-motor theory of semantic memory. Second, we will review inconsistencies and null-results that may at first raise problems for a "simple-minded" feature-based theory. In particular, we will highlight that action and tool-selective activations are profoundly context sensitive. Third, these limitations will lead us to propose a neuroanatomical model of tool and action semantics that combines feature-based elements with higher order semantic convergence and retrieval/executive regions.

1.5.1. THE FEATURE-BASED MODEL OF SEMANTIC MEMORY: ACTION AND TOOL SEMANTICS

The feature-based model of semantic memory has primarily emerged from neuropsychology. It was developed to account for category-selective impairments of semantic memory (Shallice, 1988; Warrington and McCarthy, 1987; Warrington and Shallice, 1984). Rather than assuming a category-specific organisation, it explains category-specific deficits by 1) a functional segregation for different types of semantic features and 2) differential contributions of semantic features to distinct object categories. Translated into functional imaging, the feature-based model of semantic memory postulates that 1) there are brain regions with selective responses to different types of semantic features (e.g. action) and 2) these brain regions overlap with those that show a category-selective response (e.g. tools). In particular, we would expect that tools and action features show increased activation in overlapping brain regions. More closely related to the functional brain architecture, it has been suggested that the neural substrates underlying semantic features are 1) related to or 2) even identical with the regions that were engaged when the particular type of semantic knowledge was acquired during primary sensory-motor experience (Martin et al., 2000; Martin and Chao, 2001; Shallice, 1988; Shallice, 1996). Functional imaging studies of tools and action semantics provide at least partial evidence for the feature-based model: Semantic processing of tools and action features increased activation in the left posterior middle temporal gyrus (LPMT), the anterior inferior parietal and ventral premotor cortices that have previously been implicated in action imagery, observation and execution. Activation in this visuo-motor system was observed irrespective of stimulus material or modality. Hence, in the case of action and tool semantics, the functional imaging results show the expected congruency of 1) feature: action semantics, 2) category: tools and 3) sensory-motor region: visuo-motor system.

1.5.2. TASK BY STIMULUS INTERACTIONS AND THEIR NEURAL MECHANISM

So far, we have emphasized the consistency across studies. However, most studies have reported activation only in one of the regions within the fronto-parieto-temporal action system. More importantly, some studies (e.g. (Kellenbach et al., 2003; Noppeney et al., 2006b; Phillips et al., 2002b)) have highlighted that tool-selective activations are profoundly sensitive to the context as defined by the task-type (e.g. repetition, semantic decision) and the specific task-instructions (e.g. instructions for retrieval of an object's colour or a action, see also Barsalou et al., 2003). While deep semantic processing leads to robust activation in the fronto-parietal system, implicit semantic tasks do not elicit activations that can be detected consistently using stringent statistical criteria. Hence, semantic segregation needs to be considered within different task-contexts. For this, multi-factorial designs are required that allow us to 1) dissociate context-independent from context-sensitive effects and 2) characterize the interactions between semantic type and task-context. This approach may reveal "tool or action selectivity" as a semantic type/category by task interaction whereby the tool/action-selective role of a brain area is defined and modulated by the specific task-context. Investigating the retrieval of action semantics in a series of task-contexts and redefining tool/action selectivity as stimulus by task interaction may enable us to further characterize the particular functional contributions of different regions to tool and action processing.

In terms of neural mechanisms, task by stimulus interactions are consistent with the well established notion that functional specialisation emerges from changes in the interactions among brain areas (Friston and Price, 2001; Horwitz, 2003; McIntosh, 2000; Mesulam, 1990). More specifically, LPMT/AIP action-selectivity may not be a property of the region itself but emerges through its context-dependent interactions with other regions. While LPMT may be activated irrespective of stimulus category during reading, an action-selective response during explicit semantic decisions may emerge due to top-down modulation. Accordingly, the functional role played by any brain region is defined by its interactions with other brain regions. Although it is widely acknowledged that semantics is represented and processed in a distributed network (Barsalou et al., 2003; Martin and Chao, 2001; Noppeney, 2004; Pulvermuller, 2005; Rogers et al., 2004), only few functional imaging studies have investigated semantic processing formally from the perspective of functional integration (Mechelli et al., 2003; Noppeney et al., 2003; Noppeney et al., 2006b). For instance, a recent study (Noppeney et al., 2006b) has suggested that deep semantic processing of tools relies on re-activating the left anterior inferior parietal cortex via top-down modulation from prefrontal cortex. Thus, studies combining functional imaging with effective connectivity analyses will allow us to investigate how regionally semantic-selective responses emerge from interactions amongst brain regions. They also enable us to address the predictions made by the "sensory-motor" theory of semantics. In particular, they enable us to test whether identical brain regions sustain sensory/motor functions and semantic processing depending on their connectivity pattern. For instance, we can investigate whether V5/hMT+ is activated via forward connections from early visual areas during action observation, but via backward connections from prefrontal regions during semantic processing of action words.

1.5.3. A NEUROANATOMICAL MODEL OF ACTION AND TOOL SEMANTICS

To summarize, functional imaging studies have provided partial evidence for the sensory-motor theory of semantic memory by showing a congruency of 1) feature: action semantics, 2) category: tools and 3) sensory-motor region: visuo-motor system. Yet, the action-selective activations in the visuo-motor system have been shown to be profoundly context-sensitive; they were observed primarily for explicit semantic tasks and only inconsistently reported for implicit semantic processing. This raises the question whether the fronto-parietal action system plays a necessary or important role in shallow semantic processing of action and tool concepts during passive listening and reading. A series of neuro-psychological single case studies provides some support this view: Patients with large fronto-parietal lesions (e.g. due to vascular infarction in the territory of the left middle cerebral artery) show disproportionate semantic impairments for artefacts relative to living items (Gainotti et al., 1995; Warrington and McCarthy, 1987). However, these patients are extremely rare (e.g. a recent review describes only 6 patients with this neuropsychological pattern (Gainotti, 2000)). Furthermore, semantic deficits for artefacts are not limited to fronto-parietal lesions but can also be found in semantic dementia patients with bilateral anterior temporal atrophy as part of a general semantic deficit (Hodges et al., 1995; Hodges et al., 2006; Noppeney et al., 2006a; Snowden et al., 1989). Semantic dementia is characterized by a progressive deterioration of conceptual knowledge that can be observed irrespective of stimulus material (i.e. verbal vs non-verbal), modality of the stimulus (e.g. auditory vs visual) or modality of the required response (e.g. object naming vs object drawing vs object use) (Bozeat et al., 2000; Rogers et al., 2004). Semantic dementia patients exhibit a non-category-specific semantic impairment affecting both living things and tools. They are also impaired on using familiar tools, if the appropriate action associated with an object cannot be inferred from visual affordances but requires object identification. Collectively, the neuropsychological deficits of stroke and semantic dementia patients suggest that both, the fronto-parietal and anterior temporal cortices, make important but distinct functional contributions. Thus, semantic processing of action and tools concepts may rely on large-scale interactions between regions involved in action processing (e.g. fronto-parietal) and higher order semantic regions (e.g. anterior temporal cortex) (Damasio, 1989; Mesulam, 1990; Patterson et al., 2007). Yet, the specific functional role of the anterior temporal regions in action semantics remains unclear: It has been suggested that they function as convergence zones that are engaged in binding semantic features and enable retro-activation of the fronto-parietal action features through top-down modulation (Damasio, 1989). Alternatively, the anterior temporal regions "learn and abstract semantic relationships" during sensory-motor experience leading to an amodal code of semantic knowledge as objects' similarities and feature combinations. In the latter case, the anterior temporal cortices may sustain semantic knowledge in an amodal format and thus be sufficient for semantic processing (Rogers et al., 2004). Yet, the distinction between amodal semantic vs convergence area could be rather analytical than real: The two functional roles may actually form the extreme points of a continuum that is generated by dynamic interactions between anterior temporal and parietal cortices depending on the depth and focus of semantic processing. In the context of shallow implicit semantic processing, semantic activations may be confined to the anterior temporal lobe and not necessarily involve fronto-parietal cortices. In contrast, deep semantic encoding may lead to retroactivation of action representation in the parietal cortex through interactions with higher order association and multi-sensory integration regions (Beauchamp et al., 2004; Noppeney et al., 2008; Taylor et al., 2006). Furthermore, semantic activations are being amplified and modulated according to task context and goals of the subject through top-down modulation from semantic retrieval or executive regions such as the left prefrontal cortex. This perspective could explain why the tool- and action-selective activations in the fronto-parietal cortices are profoundly context-sensitive and primarily observed during deep semantic encoding tasks. To further investigate this hypothesis, future functional imaging and neuropsychological studies are needed that go beyond assessing semantic knowledge through explicit semantic decision and association tasks and also include implicit semantic conditions (e.g. using priming effects).

In conclusion, semantic processing of tool and action concepts may be construed as large-scale dynamic interactions between the fronto-parietal action system and higher order semantic (e.g. anterior temporal cortices) and executive/retrieval (e.g. prefrontal cortex) regions. To further elucidate these dynamic interactions, future functional imaging studies of tool and action semantics will need to 1) redefine tool and action selectivity as stimulus by task interactions using multi-factorial designs and 2) determine the underlying neural mechanisms and interaction patterns by combining functional imaging with connectivity analyses and modelling approaches e.g. Dynamic Causal Modelling.

ACKNOWLEDGEMENTS

This work was supported by the Deutsche Forschungsgemeinschaft and the Max Planck Society.

REFERENCES

Allport, D.A. (1985). Distributed memory, modular subsystems and dysphasia. In: S.K. Newman & R. Epstein (Eds.) *Current Perspectives in Dysphasia.* 32-60, Edinburgh: Churchill Livingstone.

Arbib, M., & Bota, M. (2003). Language evolution: neural homologies and neuroinformatics. *Neural Networks 16,* 1237-1260.

Barsalou, L.W., Simmons,W.K., Barbey, A.K., and Wilson, C.D. (2003). Grounding conceptual knowledge in modality-specific systems. *Trends in Cognitive Sciences* 7, 84-91.

Beauchamp, M.S., Lee, K.E., Argall, B.D., and Martin, A. (2004). Integration of Auditory and Visual Information about Objects in Superior Temporal Sulcus. *Neuron* 41, 809-823.

Beauchamp, M.S., Lee, K.E., Haxby, J.V., and Martin, A. (2002). Parallel visual motion processing streams for manipulable objects and human movements. *Neuron* 34, 149-59.

Beauchamp, M.S., Lee, K.E., Haxby, J.V., and Martin, A. (2003). FMRI responses to video and point-light displays of moving humans and manipulable objects. *Journal of Cognitive Neuroscience* 15, 991-1001.

Bonda, E., Petrides, M., Ostry, D., and Evans, A. (1996). Specific involvement of human parietal systems and the amygdala in the perception of biological motion. *Journal of Neuroscience* 16, 3737-44.

Boronat, C.B., Buxbaum, L.J., Coslett, H.B., Tang, K., Saffran, E.M., Kimberg, D.Y., and Detre, J.A. (2005). Distinctions between manipulation and function knowledge of objects: evidence from functional magnetic resonance imaging. *Cognitive Brain Research* 23, 361-373.

Bozeat, S., Lambon Ralph, M.A., Patterson, K., Garrard, P., and Hodges, J.R. (2000). Non-verbal semantic impairment in semantic dementia. *Neuropsychologia* 38, 1207-1215.

Buccino, G., Binkofski, F., Fink, G.R., Fadiga, L., Fogassi, L., Gallese, V., Seitz, R.J., Zilles, K., Rizzolatti, G., and Freund, H.J. (2001). Action observation activates premotor and parietal areas in a somatotopic manner: an fMRI study. *European Journal of Neuroscience* 13, 400-404.

Buccino, G., Lui, F., Canessa, N., Patteri, I., Lagravinese, G., Benuzzi,F ., Porro, C.A., and Rizzolatti, G. (2004a). Neural circuits involved in the recognition of actions performed by nonconspecifics: an FMRI study. *Journal of Cognitive Neuroscience* 16, 114-126.

Buccino, G., Vogt, S., Ritzl, A., Fink, G.R., Zilles, K., Freund, H.J., and Rizzolatti, G. (2004b). Neural circuits underlying imitation learning of hand actions: an event-related fMRI study. *Neuron* 42, 323-334.

Buxbaum, L., Veramonti, T., and Schwartz, M. (2000). Function and manipulation tool knowledge in apraxia: Knowing 'what for' but not 'how'. *Neurocase* 6, 83-97.

Canessa, N., Borgo, F., Cappa, S.F., Perani, D., Falini, A., Buccino, G., Tettamanti, M., and Shallice, T. (2007). The Different Neural Correlates of Action and Functional Knowledge in Semantic Memory: An fMRI Study. published online in *Cerebral Cortex*.

Capitani, E., Laiacona, M., Mahon, B., and Caramazza, A. (2003). What are the facts of semantic category-specific deficits? A critical review of the clinical evidence. *Cognitive Neuropsychology* 20, 213-262.

Cappa, S.F., Perani, D., Schnur, T., Tettamanti, M., and Fazio, F. (1998). The effects of semantic category and knowledge type on lexical-semantic access: a PET study. *NeuroImage* 8, 350-9.

Caramazza, A., and Shelton, J.R. (1998). Domain-specific knowledge systems in the brain the animate-inanimate distinction. *Journal of Cognitive Neuroscience* 10, 1-34.

Chao, L.L., Haxby, J.V., and Martin, A. (1999). Attribute-based neural substrates in temporal cortex for perceiving and knowing about objects. *Nature Neuroscience* 2, 913-9.

Chao, L.L., and Martin, A. (2000). Representation of manipulable man-made objects in the dorsal stream. *NeuroImage* 12, 478-84.

Chao, L.L., Weisberg, J., and Martin, A. (2002). Experience-dependent modulation of category-related cortical activity. *Cerebral Cortex* 12, 545-551.

Damasio, A.R. (1989). Time-locked multiregional retroactivation: a systems-level proposal for the neural substrates of recall and recognition. *Cognition* 33, 25-62.

Damasio, H., Grabowski, T.J., Tranel, D., Hichwa, R.D., and Damasio, A.R. (1996). A neural basis for lexical retrieval [published erratum appears in Nature 1996 Jun 27; 381(6595):810]. *Nature* 380, 499-505.

Decety, J., Grezes, J., Costes, N., Perani, D., Jeannerod, M., Procyk, E., Grassi, F., and Fazio, F. (1997). Brain activity during observation of actions. Influence of action content and subject's strategy. *Brain* 120, 1763-77.

Devlin, J.T., Moore, C.J., Mummery, C.J., Gorno-Tempini, M.L., Phillips, J.A., Noppeney, U., Frackowiak, R.S., Friston, K.J., and Price, C.J. (2002). Anatomic constraints on cognitive theories of category specificity. *NeuroImage* 15, 675-85.

Fang, F., and He, S. (2005). Cortical responses to invisible objects in the human dorsal and ventral pathways. *Nature Neuroscience* 8, 1380-1385.

Farah, M.J., McMullen, P.A., and Meyer, M.M. (1996). The living nonliving dissociation is not an artefact: Giving an a priori implausible hypothesis a strong test. *Cognitive Neuropsychology* 13, 137-154.

Fiez, J.A., Raichle, M.E., Balota, D.A., Tallal, P., and Petersen, S.E. (1996). PET activation of posterior temporal regions during auditory word presentation and verb generation. *Cerebral Cortex* 6, 1-10.

Fogassi, L., Ferrari, P.F., Gesierich, B., Rozzi, S., Chersi, F., and Rizzolatti, G. (2005). Parietal lobe: from action organization to intention understanding. *Science* 308, 662-667.

Fogassi, L., and Luppino, G. (2005). Motor functions of the parietal lobe. *Current Opinion in Neurobiology* 15, 626-631.

Friston, K.J., and Price, C.J. (2001). Generative models, brain function and neuroimaging. Scand. *Journal of Psychology* 42, 167-177.

Gainotti, G. (2000). What the locus of brain lesion tells us about the nature of the cognitive defect underlying category-specific disorders: a review. *Cortex* 36, 539-559.

Gainotti, G., Giustolisi, L., Daniele, A., and Silveri, M.C. (1995). Neuroanatomical correlates of category-specific semantic disorders: A critical survey. *Memory* 3, 247-264.

Gainotti, G., and Silveri, M.C. (1996). Cognitive and anatomical locus of lesion in a patient with a category-specific semantic impairment for living beings. *Cognitive Neuropsychology* 13, 357-389.

Gerlach, C., Law, I., Gade, A., and Paulson, O.B. (2000). Categorization and category effects in normal object recognition. A PET study. *Neuropsychologia* 38, 1693-1703.

Gerlach, C., Law, I., Gade, A., and Paulson, O.B. (2002a). The role of action knowledge in the comprehension of artefacts - a PET study. *NeuroImage* 15, 143-152.

Gerlach, C., Law, I., and Paulson, O.B. (2002b). When action turns into words. Activation of motor-based knowledge during categorization of manipulable objects. *Journal of Cognitive Neuroscience* 14, 1230-1239.

Grabowski, T.J., Damasio, H., and Damasio, A.R. (1998). Premotor and prefrontal correlates of category-related lexical retrieval. *NeuroImage* 7, 232-43.

Grafton, S.T., Fadiga, L., Arbib, M.A., and Rizzolatti, G. (1997). Premotor cortex activation during observation and naming of familiar tools. *NeuroImage* 6, 231-6

Grezes, J., Armony, J.L., Rowe, J., and Passingham, R.E. (2003). Activations related to "mirror" and "canonical" neurones in the human brain: an fMRI study. *NeuroImage* 18, 928-937.

Grezes, J., Costes, N., and Decety, J. (1998). Top-down effect of strategy on the perception of human biological motion: A PET investigation. *Cognitive Neuropsychology* 15, 553-582.

Grezes, J., and Decety, J. (2001). Functional anatomy of execution, mental simulation, observation, and verb generation of actions: a meta-analysis. *Human Brain Mapping* 12, 1-19.

Hauk, O., Johnsrude, I., and Pulvermuller, F. (2004). Somatotopic representation of action words in human motor and premotor cortex. *Neuron* 41, 301-307.

Hillis, A.E., and Caramazza, A. (1991). Category-specific naming and comprehension impairment: a double dissociation. *Brain* 114, 2081-94.

Hodges, J.R., Bozeat, S., Lambon Ralph, M.A., Patterson, K., and Spatt, J. (2000). The role of conceptual knowledge in object use evidence from semantic dementia. *Brain* 123 *(9)*, 1913-1925.

Hodges, J.R., Davies, R.R., and Patterson, K. (2006). Semantic dementia, or, a little knowledge is a dangerous thing. In: B. Miller & B. Boeve (Eds.) *The behavioural neurology of dementia.*

Hodges, J.R., Graham, N., and Patterson, K. (1995). Charting the progression in semantic dementia: implications for the organisation of semantic memory. *Memory* 3, 463-495.

Hodges, J.R., Spatt, J., and Patterson, K. (1999). "What" and "how": evidence for the dissociation of object knowledge and mechanical problem-solving skills in the human brain. *The Proceedings of the National Academy of Sciences US* 96, 9444-9448.

Horwitz, B. (2003). The elusive concept of brain connectivity. *NeuroImage* 19, 466-470.

Humphreys, G.W., and Forde, E.M. (2001). Hierarchies, similarity, and interactivity in object recognition: "category-specific" neuropsychological deficits. *Behavioral and Brain Sciences* 24, 453-76.

Iacoboni, M., Molnar-Szakacs, I., Gallese, V., Buccino, G., Mazziotta, J.C., and Rizzolatti, G. (2005). Grasping the intentions of others with one's own mirror neuron system. *PLoS Bioloty* 3, e79.

Iacoboni, M., Woods, R.P., Brass, M., Bekkering, H., Mazziotta, J.C., and Rizzolatti, G. (1999). Cortical mechanisms of human imitation. *Science* 286, 2526-2528.

James, T.W., & Gauthier, I. (2003). Auditory and action semantic features activate sensory-specific perceptual brain regions. *Current Biology* 13, 1792-1796.

Jeannerod, M. (2001). Neural simulation of action: a unifying mechanism for motor cognition. *NeuroImage* 14, 103-109.

Jeannerod, M., and Frak, V. (1999). Mental imaging of motor activity in humans. *Current Opinion in Neurobiology* 9, 735-739.

Johnson-Frey, S.H., Maloof, F.R., Newman-Norlund, R., Farrer, C., Inati, S., and Grafton, S.T. (2003). Actions or hand-object interactions? Human inferior frontal cortex and action observation. *Neuron* 39, 1053-1058.

Kellenbach, M., Brett, M., and Patterson, K. (2003). Action speak louder than functions. The importance of manipulability and action in tool representation. *Journal of Cognitive Neuroscience* 15, 30-46.

Kiefer, M., Sim, E.J., Liebich, S., Hauk, O., and Tanaka, J. (2007). Experience-dependent plasticity of conceptual representations in human sensory-motor areas. *Journal of Cognitive Neuroscience* 19, 525-542.

Kohler, E., Keysers, C., Umilta, M.A., Fogassi, L., Gallese, V., and Rizzolatti, G. (2002). Hearing sounds, understanding actions: action representation in mirror neurons. *Science* 297, 846-848.

Kourtzi, Z., and Kanwisher, N. (2000). Activation in human MT/MST by static images with implied motion. *Journal of Cognitive Neuroscience* 12, 48-55.

Kraut, M.A., Moo, L.R., Segal, J.B., and Hart, J.Jr. (2002). Neural activation during an explicit categorization task: category- or feature-specific effects? *Brain Research and Cognitive Brain Research* 13, 213-220.

Lewis, J.W., Brefczynski, J.A., Phinney, R.E., Janik, J.J., and DeYoe, E.A. (2005). Distinct cortical pathways for processing tool versus animal sounds. *Journal of Neuroscience* 25, 5148-5158.

Longe, O., Randall, B., Stamatakis, E.A., and Tyler, L.K. (2007). Grammatical categories in the brain: the role of morphological structure. *Cerebral Cortex* 17, 1812-1820.

Maguire, E.A., and Mummery, C.J. (1999). Differential modulation of a common memory retrieval network revealed by positron emission tomography. *Hippocampus* 9, 54-61.

Martin, A., and Chao, L.L. (2001). Semantic memory and the brain: structure and processes. *Current Opinion in Neurobiology* 11, 194-201.

Martin, A., Haxby, J.V., Lalonde, F.M., Wiggs, C.L., and Ungerleider, L.G. (1995). Discrete cortical regions associated with knowledge of color and knowledge of action. *Science* 270, 102-105.

Martin, A., Ungerleider, L.G., and Haxby, J.V. (2000). Category-specificity and the brain: The sensory / motor model of semantic representations of objects. In: M.S. Gazzaniga (ed.) *The Cognitive Neurosciences*, 1023-1037, Cambridge, MA: MIT Press.

Martin, A., Wiggs, C.L., Ungerleider, L.G., and Haxby, J.V. (1996). Neural correlates of category-specific knowledge. *Nature* 379, 649-652.

McIntosh, A.R. (2000). Towards a network theory of cognition. *Neural Networks* 13, 861-870.

Mechelli, A., Price, C.J., Noppeney, U., and Friston, K.J. (2003). A dynamic causal modeling study on category effects: bottom-up or top-down mediation? *Journal of Cognitive Neuroscience* 15, 925-934.

Mecklinger, A., Gruenewald, C., Besson, M., Magnie, M.N., and von Cramon, D.Y. (2002). Separable neuronal circuitries for manipulable and non-manipulable objects in working memory. *Cerebral Cortex* 12, 1115-1123.

Mesulam, M.M. (1990). Large-scale neurocognitive networks and distributed processing for attention, language, and memory. *Annals of Neurology* 28, 597-613.

Moore, C.J., and Price, C.J. (1999). A functional neuroimaging study of the variables that generate category-specific object processing differences. *Brain* 122, 943-962.

Mummery, C.J., Patterson, K., Hodges, J.R., and Price, C.J. (1998). Functional neuroanatomy of the semantic system: divisible by what? *Journal of Cognitive Neuroscience* 10, 766-777.

Mummery, C.J., Patterson, K., Hodges, J.R., and Wise, R.J. (1996). Generating 'tiger' as an animal name or a word beginning with T: differences in brain activation. *Proeedings of the Royal Society London Biological Sciences* 263, 989-95.

Murata, A., Gallese, V., Luppino, G., Kaseda, M., and Sakata, H. (2000). Selectivity for the shape, size, and orientation of objects for grasping in neurons of monkey parietal area AIP. *Journal of Neurophysiology.* 83, 2580-2601.

Nelissen, K., Luppino, G., Vanduffel, W., Rizzolatti, G., and Orban, G.A. (2005). Observing others: multiple action representation in the frontal lobe. *Science* 310, 332-336.

Noppeney, U. (2004). The feature-based model of semantic memory. In: R. Frackowiak, K. Friston, C.D. Frith, R. Dolan, C. Price, S. Zeki, J. Ashburner, and W. Penny (Eds.) *Human Brain Function,* 533-547, London: Elsevier.

Noppeney, U., Friston, K., and Price, C. (2003). Effects of visual deprivation on the organisation of the semantic system. *Brain* 126, 1620-1627.

Noppeney, U., Josephs, O., Hocking, J., Price, C., and Friston, K. (2008). The effect of prior visual information on recognition of speech and sounds. *Cerebral Cortex* 18(3), 598-609.

Noppeney, U., Josephs, O., Kiebel, S., Friston, K., and Price,C . (2005). Action selectivity in parietal and temporal cortex. *Brain Research and Cognitive Brain Research* 25, 641-649.

Noppeney, U., Patterson, K., Tyler, L., Moss, H.E., Stamatakis, E.A., Bright, P., Mummery, C.J., and Price,C. (2006a). Temporal lobe lesions and semantic impairment: A comparison of Herpes Simplex Virus Encephalitis and Semantic dementia. *Brain.*

Noppeney, U., and Price, C.J. (2003). Functional imaging of the semantic system: Retrieval of sensory-experienced and verbally-learnt knowledge. *Brain and Language* 84, 120-133.

Noppeney, U., Price, C.J., Penny, W.D., and Friston, K.J. (2006b). Two distinct neural mechanisms for category-selective responses. *Cerebral Cortex* 16, 437-445.

Patterson, K., Nestor, P.J., and Rogers, T.T. (2007). Where do you know what you know? The representation of semantic knowledge in the human brain. *Nature Reviews Neuroscience* 8, 976-987.

Perani, D., Cappa, S.F., Schnur, T., Tettamanti, M., Collina, S., Rosa, M.M., and Fazio, F. (1999a). The neural correlates of verb and noun processing. A PET study. *Brain* 122, 2337-2344.

Perani, D., Fazio, F., Borghese, N.A., Tettamanti, M., Ferrari, S., Decety, J., and Gilardi, M.C. (2001). Different brain correlates for watching real and virtual hand actions. *NeuroImage* 14, 749-58.

Perani, D., Schnur, T., Tettamanti, M., Gorno-Tempini, M., Cappa, S.F., and Fazio, F. (1999b). Word and picture matching: a PET study of semantic category effects. *Neuropsychologia* 37, 293-306.

Petrides, M., Cadoret, G., and Mackey, S. (2005). Orofacial somatomotor responses in the macaque monkey homologue of Broca's area. *Nature* 435, 1235-1238.

Phillips, J.A., Humphreys, G.W., Noppeney, U., and Price, C.J. (2002a). The neural substrates of action retrieval:An examination of semantic and visual routes to action. *Vision and Cognition* 9(4), 662-684.

Phillips, J.A., Noppeney, U., Humphreys, G.W., and Price, C.J. (2002b). Can segregation within the semantic system account for category- specific deficits? *Brain* 125, 2067-2080.

Pulvermuller, F. (2005). Brain mechanisms linking language and action. *Nature Reviews Neurosciences* 6, 576-582.

Pulvermuller, F., Hauk, O., Nikulin, V.V., and Ilmoniemi, R.J. (2005). Functional links between motor and language systems. *European Journal of Neuroscience* 21, 793-797.

Rizzolatti, G., and Arbib, M.A. (1998). Language within our grasp. *Trends in Neurosciences* 21, 188-194.

Rizzolatti, G., and Craighero, L. (2004). The mirror-neuron system. *Annual Reviews of Neuroscience* 27, 169-192.

Rizzolatti, G., Fadiga, L., Matelli, M., Bettinardi, V., Paulesu, E., Perani, D., and Fazio,F. (1996). Localization of grasp representations in humans by PET: 1. Observation versus execution. *Experimental Brain Research* 111, 246-252.

Rizzolatti, G., Fogassi, L., and Gallese, V. (2002). Motor and cognitive functions of the ventral premotor cortex. *Current Opinion in Neurobiology* 12, 149-154.

Rizzolatti, G., and Luppino, G. (2001). The cortical motor system. *Neuron* 31, 889-901.

Rogers, T.T., Lambon Ralph, M.A., Garrard, P., Bozeat, S., McClelland, J.L., Hodges, J.R., and Patterson, K. (2004). Structure and deterioration of semantic memory: a neuropsychological and computational investigation. *Psychological Review* 111, 205-235.

Ruby, P., and Decety, J. (2001). Effect of subjective perspective taking during simulation of action: a PET investigation of agency. *Nature Neuroscience* 4, 546-550.

Rushworth, M.F., Johansen-Berg, H., Gobel, S.M., and Devlin, J.T. (2003). The left parietal and premotor cortices: motor attention and selection. *NeuroImage* 20 (Suppl.1), 89-100.

Sacchett, C., and Humphreys, G.W. (1992). Calling a squirrel a squirrel but a canoe a wigwam: A categry-specific deficit for artifactual objects and body parts. *Cognitive Neuropsychology* 5, 3-25.

Sartori, G., Job, R., and Miozzo, M. (1993). Category-specific naming impairments? Yes. *Quarterly Journal of Experimental Psychology* 46(A), 489-504.

Senior, C., Barnes, J., Giampietro, V., Simmons, A., Bullmore, E.T., Brammer, M., and David, A.S. (2000). The functional neuroanatomy of implicit-motion perception or representational momentum. *Current Biology* 10, 16-22.

Shallice, T. (1988). *From Neuropsychology to Mental Structure.* Cambridge: Cambridge University Press.

Shallice, T. (1996). The language-to-object perception interface: evidence from neuropsychology. In: P. Bloom, M. Peterson, L. Nadel, and M. Garrett (Eds.) *Language & Space,* 531-552, MIT Press.

Shapiro, K.A., Moo, L.R., and Caramazza, A. (2006). Cortical signatures of noun and verb production. *Proceedings of the National Academy of Sciences U.S.A.* 103, 1644-1649.

Sirigu, A., Duhamel, J.R., and Poncet, M. (1991). The role of sensorimotor experience in object recognition. A case of multimodal agnosia [published erratum appears in Brain 1992 Apr;115(Pt 2):645]. *Brain* 114, 2555-2573.

Snowden, J., Goulding, P., and Neary, D. (1989). Semantic Dementia: A form of circumscribed brain atrophy. *Behavioural Neurology* 2, 167-182.

Taylor, K.I., Moss, H.E., Stamatakis, E.A., and Tyler, L.K. (2006). Binding crossmodal object features in perirhinal cortex. *Proceedings of the National Academy of Sciences U.S.A.* 103, 8239-8244.

Tettamanti, M., Buccino, G., Saccuman, M.C., Gallese, V., Danna, M., Scifo, P., Fazio, F., Rizzolatti, G., Cappa, S.F., and Perani, D. (2005). Listening to action-related sentences activates fronto-parietal motor circuits. *Journal of Cognitive Neuroscience* 17, 273-281.

Thompson-Schill, S.L., Aguirre, G.K., D'Esposito, M., and Farah, M.J. (1999). A neural basis for category and modality specificity of semantic knowledge. *Neuropsychologia* 37, 671-676.

Tyler, L.K., Bright, P., Fletcher, P., and Stamatakis, E.A. (2004). Neural processing of nouns and verbs: the role of inflectional morphology. *Neuropsychologia* 42, 512-523.

Tyler, L.K., and Moss, H.E. (2001). Towards a distributed account of conceptual knowledge. *Trends in Cognitive Science* 5, 244-252.

Tyler, L.K., Moss, H.E., Durrant-Peatfield, M.R., and Levy, J.P. (2000). Conceptual structure and the structure of concepts: A distributed account of category-specific deficits. *Brain and Language* 75, 195-231.

Umilta, M.A., Kohler, E., Gallese, V., Fogassi, L., Fadiga, L., Keysers, C., and Rizzolatti, G. (2001). I know what you are doing. a neurophysiological study. *Neuron* 31, 155-165.

Wallentin, M., Lund, T.E., Ostergaard, S., Ostergaard, L., and Roepstorff, A. (2005). Motion verb sentences activate left posterior middle temporal cortex despite static context. *Neuroreport* 16, 649-652.

Warburton, E., Wise, R.J., Price, C.J., Weiller, C., Hadar, U., Ramsay, S., and Frackowiak, R.S. (1996). Noun and verb retrieval by normal subjects. Studies with PET. *Brain* 119, 159-179.

Warrington, E.K., and McCarthy, R.A. (1987). Categories of knowledge. Further fractionations and an attempted integration. *Brain* 110, 1273-1296.

Warrington, E.K., and Shallice, T. (1984). Category specific semantic impairments. *Brain* 107, 829-54.

Weisberg, J., van Turennout, M., and Martin, A. (2007). A neural system for learning about object function. *Cerebral Cortex* 17, 513-521.

9

Pointing is 'special'

HÉLÈNE LŒVENBRUCK
MARION DOHEN
CORIANDRE VILAIN

Abstract: Deixis, or pointing, is the ability to draw the viewer/listener's attention to an object, a person, a direction or an event. Pointing is involved at different stages of human communication development, in multiple modalities: first with the eyes, then with the finger, then with intonation and finally with syntax. It is ubiquitous and probably universal in human interactions. The *'special'* role of index-finger pointing in language acquisition suggests that all pointing modalities may share a common cerebral network. This chapter aims at better grounding linguistic pointing in somatosensory as well as cerebral domains and at suggesting that it shares features with other pointing modalities. It is shown that manual and ocular pointings seem to recruit left posterior parietal and frontal cortices. Then vocal pointing is presented in details, for both production and perception. It is suggested that integrated multisensory representations may be needed in order to produce and perceive prosodic pointing and that these representations require the activation of associative cerebral areas. The results of a previous study support this hypothesis by showing that prosodic pointing seems to recruit a left temporo-parieto-frontal network whereas grammaticalized syntactic pointing mainly involves frontal regions. The involvement of the left parietal lobe is also apparent in our preliminary fMRI study of the perception of prosodic pointing. Finally, the exploratory results of a new study of multimodal pointing (digital, ocular, prosodic and syntactic) are presented. The common left parietal activation in ocular, digital and prosodic pointing is discussed in the framework of the link between gesture and language.

1. INTRODUCTION

1.1. WHAT IS SO SPECIAL ABOUT POINTING?

Recent research works suggest that deixis, ostension or pointing is at the root of human communication (e.g. Bates et al., 1975; Bruner, 1975; Corballis, 1991; Hewes, 1981; Kita, 2003; Rolfe, 1996; Tomasello et al., 2007). Pointing is the ability to draw the viewer/listener's attention to an object, a person, a direction or an event. Pointing is a communicative device which orients the attention of another person so that an object/person/direction/event becomes the shared focus of attention. It serves to single out, to individuate what will become the referent. In linguistics, deixis is defined as the way language expresses reference to points in time, space or events (Fillmore, 1997). In its narrow sense, it refers to the contextual meaning of deictic words, which include pronouns (me, you), place deictics (here, there), time deictics (now, then) and demonstratives (this, that). In its broad sense, deixis is a referential operation, i.e. it provides a mean to highlight relevant elements in the discourse, to designate, identify or even select an element. It is therefore tightly linked with topicalization, focus and extraction (see e.g. Berthoud, 1990; Jackendoff, 2002). Therefore, pointing, in its broad sense, can be conveyed in several ways: gesturally, with specific hand gestures, or verbally, with specific phonatory and articulatory movements (prosodic deixis) or through the use of a specific syntactic construction (syntactic deixis).

Pointing is 'special[1]' because it is...

... ubiquitous,

A pointing gesture is most often performed with the index finger and arm extended in the direction of the interesting object and with the other

---

1 The expression "Pointing is special" refers to the debate on the specialised nature of speech. This debate originates from Chomsky's (1957, 1966) position concerning the special nature of the human language faculty. This position has been taken over by researchers from the Haskins Laboratories, and in particular by Alvin Liberman, who wrote "On Finding that Speech Is Special" in 1982. During the summer school, the "speech-is-special" stance was the object of many questions and debates, driven by the Haskins Lab. alumnus Rudolph Sock.

fingers curled inside the hand (Butterworth, 2003). The 'canonical' index finger pointing is *ubiquitous* in everyday interactions, in most cultures of the world. It is observed in oral as well as signed communication. In some sign languages, index pointing is used linguistically for referential indexing. Noun phrases, for instance, may be associated with loci in space. Reference to a previously mentioned noun is performed by pointing again to its specific locus (Klima & Bellugi, 1988).

... universal,

Index finger pointing has been claimed to be a universal ability shared by all human beings (e.g. Povinelli & Davis, 1994). In some cultures, index finger pointing can be replaced with lip pointing (in the Barai in Papua New Guinea, see Wilkins, 2003). But pointing gestures, be they conveyed with the index-finger, the hand, or even the lip or the chin, remain a key *universal* communication tool in humans.

... has a long historical past,

Although its scientific study is relatively recent, index-finger pointing did not emerge in the XXth century. Traces of it can be found in early European art. The most famous paintings of points are those of Leonardo da Vinci, dating back from the late XVth century (such as the Virgin of the Rocks, 1483-1486, with the angel Uriel pointing towards baby John-the-Baptist; or St John the Baptist, 1513-1516, with his right hand pointing up toward heaven). But even earlier points can be found, like in the Bayeux Tapestry, which was embroidered towards the end of the XIth century, and which tells the 1066 Norman invasion of England (e.g. William of Normandy, on his ducal throne, pointing at Harold making an oath; or men pointing at the ominous Halley's comet). Furthermore pointing was not only used in European culture. Sculptures of pointing buddhas can be found in XVIIIth century Burmese art, for instance.

... performed by evolved animals,

It has long been claimed that pointing is a human-specific ability and that great apes, for instance, do not point (e.g. Povinelli et al., 2003). Works by Leavens, Hopkins and colleagues show, however, that chimpanzees in captivity can in fact point at unreachable food (Leavens et al., 2005). They sometimes use 'canonical' index finger pointing, but most often, they point with all fingers extended. And, like human infants, chimpanzees point spontaneously, without explicit training.

Therefore, although pointing does not seem to be specific to human primates – since apes, and other animals (think of the vocal reference calls of the vervet monkeys), may well be capable of it – it seems to be a *sophisticated social* behaviour, used by animals capable of some degree of imitation and inter-individual communication (Pollick & de Waal, 2007). Some researchers have even suggested that the index-finger pointing ability might be related to the thumb-index finger opposition and the pincer grip capacity (Butterworth, 2003).

... multimodal,

Pointing involves multiple modalities: it can be manual or digital (with the index finger), labial, facial (chin), ocular, and vocal.

As described above, pointing is most often, at least in Western cultures, *digital,* i.e. it is conveyed with an extended index finger. It is also very often *manual,* i.e. the whole extended hand is used to point. But when the hand is used, the handshape may vary (open flat hand held palm up, or palm facing laterally, thumb: see Kendon, 1996). Pointing can also be performed with protruded lips. *Labial* pointing has been observed in several communities in all inhabited continents (the Kuna indians in Panama, the Arrernte in Australia, the Awtuw and Barai in Papua New Guinea, the Ewe in Ghana, the Navajo in North America; cf. Wilkins, 2003). In fact, as Kendon (1996) notes, many different body parts can be used to perform pointing (head, lip, chin, elbow, foot, arm and hand).

Ocular pointing or deictic gaze is also frequent. It is the ability to (alternately) look at the 'object' then at the viewer's eyes. It is an invitation for the viewer to look at the object which becomes the shared focus of attention. A wonderful example of ocular pointing is the famous painting by Georges de la Tour, "Le Tricheur à l'as de carreau" (The cheat with the ace of diamonds, 1635). According to our interpretation of this painting, the woman standing next to the cheater gazes at him, thereby designating him for the woman sitting at her left. The sitting lady understands the ocular point, as she responds with a digital point.

Vocal pointing is what is sometimes called deixis or focus. In French, as in many languages, vocal deixis can be conveyed by syntactic extraction, using a deictic presentation form such as in the example below:

C'est Madeleine qui m'amena

*(**It's** Madeleine **who** brought me along.)*

It can also be conveyed by prosodic focus, i.e. by using a specific intonational contour on the pointed item, such as in the example below:

MADELEINE$_F$ m'amena.

(MADELEINE$_F$ brought me along.)

The effect of this intonational contour, which will be described in more detail in section 2.1., is to highlight the pointed item ('Madeleine'), the rest of the utterance bearing a flat, post-focal contour.

... involved in stages of language development

Ocular pointing (or deictic gazes, at 6 - 9 months) and, later, index finger-pointing (deictic gestures, at 9 - 11 months) have been shown to be two key stages in infant cognitive development that are correlated with stages in oral speech development.

Pointing with the eye is first observed at 8 to 9 months, mutual attention takes place between the adult and the baby. When the adult looks at something, the baby follows his/her gaze and looks in the same direction. At this stage, babies therefore have the ability to look where someone else is looking. Conversely, the baby seems to invite the adult to look at an object, by alternately looking at the object then at the adult's eyes. Quite early in development, babies can therefore use gaze to manipulate the attention of their carer.

Then, at 9 to 11 months, when infants start to be able to understand a few words, they produce pointing gestures, most often *index-finger pointing*. The emergence of pointing is a good predictor of first word-onset, and gesture production is related to gains in language development between 9 and 13 months (Bates et al., 1979; Butcher & Goldin-Meadow, 2000; Caselli, 1990). As explained in Butterworth (2003), pointing not only serves to single out the object but also to build a connection between the object and the speech sound. Finger pointing therefore seems clearly associated with lexicon construction.

Then at 16 to 20 months, during the transition from the one-word stage to the two-word stage, *combinations of words and deictic gestures* can be observed (such as a pointing gesture to a location and pronouncing 'dog', to indicate that a dog is there). Furthermore, the number of gestures and gesture-word-combinations produced at 16 months are predictive of total vocal production at 20 months (Morford & Goldin-Meadow, 1992; Capirci et al., 1996; Goldin-Meadow & Butcher, 2003;

Volterra et al., 2005). Finger pointing therefore clearly seems associated with morphosyntax emergence.

As for *vocal pointing*, only a few studies have examined the development of *prosodic focus* and *syntactic extraction* in children.

Concerning the *acoustic realisation of prosody*, pre-school children have been shown to master contrastive focus in English, in absence of any formal teaching (Hornby & Hass, 1970). Little is known about the development of prosodic focus in French, but the ability to realise adult-like pitch movements emerges quite early (Konopczinsky, 1986). Also, it has been shown that adult-like syllable lengthening is realised by young children (from 2 years of age) on accented vowels (Konopczinsky, 1986).

As concerns *articulatory production of prosodic pointing*, what is known is that lexical stress in English is differently realised in young children than in adults (Goffman & Malin, 1999; Connaghan et al., 2001). Children aged 3 to 6 years tend to produce larger movements, with reduced velocities, and increased durations, characteristics of slowly and carefully articulated speech. In a recent video study on French, Ménard et al. (2006) showed that French-speaking children (aged 4 and 8) do not differentiate articulatory and acoustic patterns across focused and unfocused syllables as much as adult speakers do. To summarise the findings, although the production of prosodic focus, or vocal pointing, seems to be mastered quite early (as early as 3 years of age) in the acoustic domain, and without formal teaching, its articulatory correlates seem to be acquired much later. But what seems lacking in children is not the capacity to hyper-articulate focused phrases, but to hypo-articulate surrounding phrases. The delay in articulatory performance could thus be related to general articulatory proficiency rather than to specific linguistic mastery. Since manual pointing emerges spontaneously before the end of the first year, it could be that acoustic correlates of prosodic focus are in fact mastered much earlier than 3 years of age.

The development of syntax in young children has been extensively studied by Tomasello and colleagues, among others (see also Brown, 1971; Sheldon, 1974; Tavakolian, 1981; MacWhinney & Pléh, 1988; McKee et al., 1998; Kidd & Bavin, 2000). In a study of the speech of English-speaking children between 1;9 and 5;2 years of age, Diessel & Tomasello (2000) showed that the earliest and most frequent relative clauses that children learn occur in *presentational constructions* that are propositionally simple.

They express a single proposition in two finite clauses, such as: "Here's a tiger **that's** gonna scare him" or "That's the sugar **that** goes in there". According to the authors, one of the factors that might explain why relative clauses emerge in these presentational constructions is the prefabricated character of the main clause. Interestingly, the main clause contains a deictic pronoun (i.e. this, that, here, there, it). Diessel & Tomasello argued that *"the early use of relative constructions involves a very simple procedure by which the child combines a prefabricated (main) clause (i.e. a clause of the type That's X, There's X, It's X) with a second component [...]."* (p.144). They observed presentational constructions in children aged 2 and younger (1;11). They quoted a study by Jisa and Kern (1998) on French children (aged 5;0-5;11) who also reported extensive use of presentational constructions in young children.

To sum up, pointing is involved at several stages of human communication development. It seems to be one of the first communicative tools used by babies. It is a key part of the shared attention mechanism in child-adult interaction. It seems to emerge spontaneously, in stages, and in association with oral productions. The crucial role of index-finger pointing in language development and the involvement of multiple forms of pointing at different stages of human communication development, first with the eyes, then the finger, then intonation and finally syntax, suggest that all pointing modalities may share a common cerebral network. The aim of this chapter is to better ground linguistic pointing in somatosensory and cerebral domains and to show that it shares features with other pointing modalities.

First, we will discuss the results of several studies in the literature related to manual and ocular pointing that can provide clues on the cerebral correlates of these two pointing modalities and can shed light on the potential general pointing network.

Then we will focus on oral linguistic pointing. Among the two forms of linguistic pointing, prosodic focus will be described in particular, since it bears interesting physiological characteristics. Its acoustic and articulatory correlates will be given in detail. It will be shown that prosodic focus is signalled using very specific acoustic and articulatory features and that speakers use reliable strategies to organise phonation and articulation together in order to convey prosodic pointing. On the perception side, results from auditory-visual experiments will be

presented that indicate that the phonatory and articulatory patterns are not just productive habits but that they are in fact well recovered by listeners and viewers. It will be suggested that integrated representations (acoustic, articulatory, proprioceptive) may be needed in order to produce prosodic pointing adequately and that these multisensory representations may be formed via the activation of associative cerebral areas. It will be hypothesised that these areas should also be involved during the perception of prosodic focus. Two preliminary fMRI studies of the production and perception of prosodic focus will be presented. Finally, we will present the first results of an fMRI study on the different pointing modalities that suggest that manual, ocular and prosodic pointing may well be grounded in a same cerebral network.
The organisation of the chapter is as follows. In section 1.2., a review of the literature provides elements for a description of the cerebral networks of manual and ocular pointings. These networks are the grounding red thread for the study of oral pointing presented in section 2. A summary of several works carried out in our laboratories on the production and perception of prosodic pointing, both in the acoustic and articulatory (or visible) domains, is provided in sections 2.1. and 2.2. This summary is then used to make hypothesis on the potential cerebral correlates of prosodic pointing in both production and perception. Results of a previous work on the cerebral correlates of the production of prosodic and syntactic pointing are provided in section 2.3.1. A work-in-progress on the cerebral correlates of the auditory-visual perception of prosodic focus is presented in section 2.3.2. Finally, preliminary results of an fMRI study of pointing in different modalities (manual, ocular, prosodic, syntactic) are presented in section 3. The implications of these findings are discussed in the conclusion.

1.2. MANUAL AND OCULAR POINTING

As explained above, the crucial role of pointing in communication, be it with the eyes, the finger, intonation or syntax, suggests that all pointing modalities may be grounded in a common cerebral network. The first question we want to address is: what are the cerebral correlates of manual and ocular pointing? Several observations provide preliminary answers to this question. The first set of observations deals with the role of the posterior parietal regions of both hemispheres in manual pointing tasks. It has been suggested that the spatial representations formed in the posterior parietal and premotor frontal regions could provide *"perceptual-premotor interfaces for the organization of movements* (e.g. *pointing, locomotion) directed towards targets in personal and extrapersonal space"* (Vallar, 1997, p.1401). Patients with left unilateral neglect have been shown to present deficits in pointing tasks (e.g. Edwards & Humphreys, 1999) while PET studies on normal subjects show activation within the left and/or right inferior parietal lobule (IPL) during pointing tasks (e.g. Lacquaniti et al., 1997; Kertzman et al., 1997). The role of the right and left posterior/inferior parietal regions in pointing tasks may further be related to data on brain-damaged deaf signers. Bellugi and colleagues presented a study of deaf signers of American Sign Language (ASL), two of which presented lateralized parietal lesions, one in the right hemisphere and the other in the left (Bellugi et al., 1989). Space in ASL is handled in two ways. The first is topographic: in the description of the layout of objects in space, spatial relations among signs reproduce the actual spatial relations among the objects. The second is deictic: space is used for referential indexing (as explained in the introduction). The right-lesioned signer had difficulty in the use of space for topography: room description was distorted spatially, with left side of signing space neglected. In the use of space for syntax, however, the entire signing space was covered and consistent reference to spatial loci was preserved. By contrast, the left-lesioned signer produced room descriptions without spatial distortions but made errors in the deictic use of space.

More recently a study on *finger pointing and looking* suggests that pointing with the finger and pointing with the eye seem to recruit a common left lateralized network including the frontal eye field and the posterior parietal cortex (Astafiev et al., 2003). In this study, the manual pointing task included a preparation phase and an execution phase. During the preparation phase, the subjects had to prepare to point at a cued location with the right index finger. During the execution phase, the subjects were asked to point towards the target as soon as the target flashed. The saccade task also included preparation and execution phases. Since the instruction was to (prepare to) look at a cued location, it can thus, according to us, be assimilated to ocular pointing. *In saccade preparation,* a transient sensory response to the cue was observed in the bilateral occipital cortex, a sustained response was observed in the bilateral frontal cortex, at the junction of precentral and superior frontal sulci, i.e. in the human frontal eye field (FEF) and a sustained response was observed along the horizontal segment of the intraparietal sulcus (IPS). *In pointing preparation,* bilateral FEF and IPS activations were observed, just as in saccade preparation. These results therefore suggest that the posterior parietal cortex and the frontal cortex contain regions that code preparatory signals for pointing independently of the effector used (eye, index-finger). They are consistent with previous fMRI experiments that reported common activity in the IPS and FEF for visually guided saccades and pointing movements (Connolly et al., 2000; Simon et al., 2002). Additional left hemisphere activation was observed for the manual pointing task, in the angular gyrus, the supramarginal gyrus, the superior parietal lobule, the dorsal precentral gyrus, and the superior temporal sulcus. The authors checked that the left-lateralization held, even when the left hand was used. Therefore manual pointing-specific responses were observed in the left lateral and medial posterior parietal and frontal cortex. Similar posterior parietal and superior frontal activations were observed for eye as well as arm pointing tasks by Hagler et al., 2007. But no evidence was found for manual-pointing-specific maps.

To summarise, recent neuroimaging studies provide clues to the description of the cerebral networks involved in manual and ocular pointing. They suggest that posterior parietal cortex and frontal cortex are bilaterally activated in ocular and manual pointing tasks. Additional left lateralized activation in the medial posterior parietal cortex could be specific to manual pointing. The question we want to address now is whether a similar network is involved in linguistic pointing. First, we will review several studies carried out in our laboratory that indicate what the speaker's somatosensory representations might be for linguistic pointing as well as to what extent the listener/viewer is able to decode audiovisual signals of vocal pointing. This will enable us to make hypothesis as to which regions the cerebral network for the production and perception of vocal pointing may include.

2. WHAT DO WE KNOW ABOUT VOCAL POINTING?

As mentioned in the introduction, vocal pointing in French (or deixis) can be conveyed by syntactic extraction or prosodic focus (Berthoud, 1990). Prosodic focus, as will be shown in the following, involves specific intonational and articulatory patterns. Syntactic extraction involves the use of a cleft form (*"c'est .... qui"*, "it's ... who"). It may or not be accompanied by prosodic focus. It should be mentioned here that there are two types of prosodic focus in French: *contrastive focus* which selects a constituent in the paradigmatic dimension and *intensification focus* which makes a contrast along the syntagmatic axis (Séguinot, 1976). This chapter is only concerned with *contrastive* prosodic focus and the term 'prosodic focus' will be used hereafter to refer to this type of focus.

Compared with a broad focus or non-deictic rendition of an utterance, *prosodic* focus involves precise acoustic and articulatory modifications, whereas *syntactic* extraction may simply use additional words, but no specific somatosensory change. We will first describe what we know about the somatosensory characteristics of *prosodic* focus, namely its acoustic and articulatory correlates. We will also examine how prosodic focus is perceived visually. This will lead to conjectures on the cerebral regions involved in the production and perception of prosodic pointing.

2.1. ACOUSTIC CORRELATES

Acoustic correlates of contrastive prosodic focus have been extensively described (see e.g. Astésano, 2001; Astésano et al., 2004; Dahan & Bernard, 1996; Delais-Roussarie et al., 2002; Di Cristo, 1998; Di Cristo & Jankowski, 1999; Dohen & Lœvenbruck, 2004; Jun & Fougeron, 2000; Rossi, 1999; Touati, 1987). Prosodic deixis in French involves an increase in fundamental frequency (F0) on the focused constituent as well as a lengthening of the focal constituent. It is also associated with an F0 lowering on the pre-focal constituent and a deaccentuation of post-focal constituents. Figure 1 illustrates the effect of prosodic focus on F0. Figure 1a shows the spectrogram and F0 for the neutral rendition of the sentence *"[MADELEINE]AP [m'amena]AP"* (MADELEINE brought me along). Figure 1b shows the same utterance with a focused subject. F0 raising on the first syllable of the Accentual Phrase[2] 'Madeleine' and post-focal deaccentuation are clearly visible. Metrical and rhythmical aspects of prosodic focus have also been studied. Following Di Cristo, Astésano (2001) postulates that the emphatic initial accent in contrastive focus is the 'hyper' realisation of the metrical, secondary initial accent in French. In that view, the initial contrastive accent shares common phonetic features with the metrical initial accent: both have similar infra-syllabic lengthening, with significant lengthening of the onset over the rhyme, and similar overall F0 configurations, which clearly distinguish them from final accents. However, these acoustic correlates are twice as large for the emphatic initial accent as for the metrical initial accent, confirming that it is a 'hyper' version of the initial accent (Astésano et al., 2007). In addition to the increase in duration of the focused phrase (typically of the focused syllable onset), an anticipatory increase in duration of the pre-focal syllable can sometimes be observed (Dohen & Lœvenbruck, 2004).

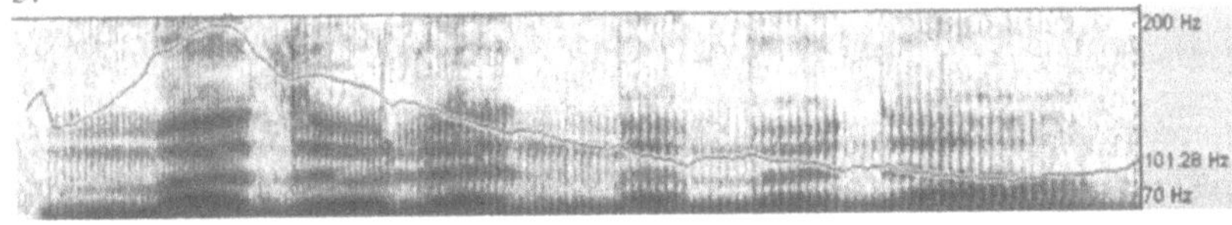

Figure 1: a) Spectrogram with superimposed F0 trace for a neutral rendition of the sentence "Madeleine m'amena". **b)** Focused rendition of the same sentence. The increased F0 peak on the first syllable /ma/ is typical of a focused phrase. The post-focal F0 trace falls to reach a flat floor. The second (highest) F0 peak observed in the neutral rendition (typical of the end of an Accentual Phrase) is suppressed.

2 For the definition of an Accentual Phrase (AP) in French, see Jun & Fougeron (2000). The AP has the default tonal representation /LHi LH*/, with an initial high tone Hi (also described as the peak of the 'accent secondaire'), a final high tone H*, realised on the phrase-final full syllable (peak of the 'accent primaire'), and two low L tones realised on the syllable preceding the H-toned syllable.

But there is no decrease in the duration of the post-focal items (no dephrasing). Restructuring of the focused Accentual Phrase is sometimes observed: it can be grouped with other phrases into one Intonational Phrase or divided into several Accentual Phrases.

2.2. ARTICULATORY CORRELATES, INCLUDING VISIBLE CUES

Summarised results of two research works on French, carried out in our laboratory, are presented here. The first one concerned tongue movements and was carried out using an electromagnetometer. The second set of studies examined lip and other facial movements. It used video and optical recordings. Perceptual tests checked whether the articulatory cues are perceived visually.

2.2.1. TONGUE MOVEMENT

Articulatory movements of the tongue were tracked using an electromagnetometer during the production of prosodic focus in several conditions (Lœvenbruck, 1999). Detailed methods are provided in Appendix A.1. A preliminary F0 analysis showed that, in all focused utterances, the F0 peak was carried by the phrase-initial /la/ syllable. The articulatory characteristics of the phrase-initial /la/ syllable in the neutral conditions were thus compared with those of the focus conditions. Articulatory analyses, shown in Figure 2, consisted in measuring maximal tongue displacement and peak velocity within the syllable.
The displacement data presented in Figure 3a show that, for this speaker, the tongue displacement in the /la/ syllable is larger in focused than in unfocused conditions, when the syllable belongs to a word that is not utterance initial. This means that the tongue movement is larger under focus in these sentence positions. When the word is utterance-initial, the tongue displacement is not larger when the syllable is focused. This is probably due to the fact that word-initial syllables in utterance-initial position are often articulated with more amplitude, even in unfocused contexts (see e.g. Fougeron & Keating, 1997; Tabain, 2003).

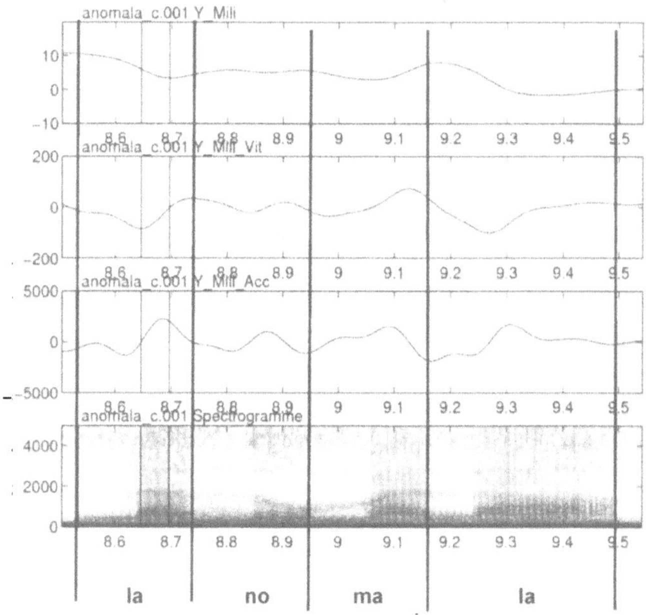

Figure 2: Articulatory labels for the first syllable of [lanomala] in 'Elle annihilait l'anomala en l'éloignant'. Top: tongue-middle vertical position (in mm); Middle: velocity (mm/s); Bottom: acceleration (mm/s^2). The dark vertical lines are acoustic landmarks for syllables [la], [no], [ma] and [la]. The disconnected lines are articulatory labels within the first syllable [la].

The results of the duration data, presented in Figure 3b, show that, for this speaker, the duration of the /la/ syllable is longer in focused than in unfocused conditions, when the syllable is not utterance initial. For utterance initial syllables, there is no increase in duration when the syllable is focused. This is probably due to the fact that word-initial syllables (particularly the onsets) in utterance-initial position are often lengthened, even in unfocused conditions (see Tabain, 2003).

a. 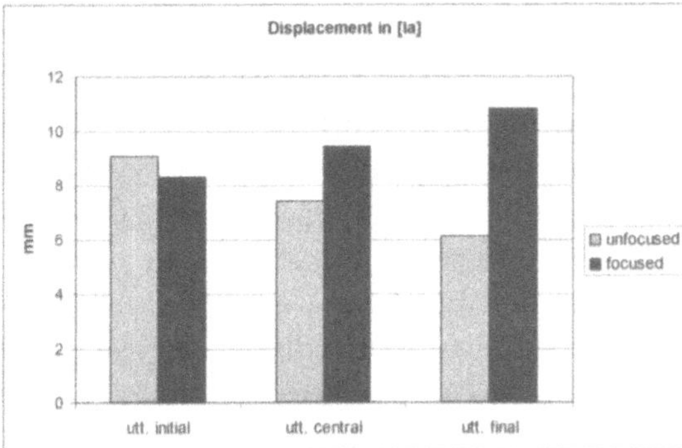

b. 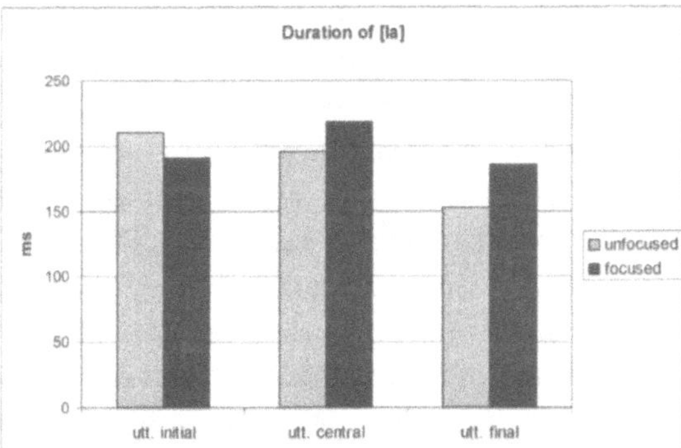

Figure 3: a) Tongue vertical displacement (mm) for /la/ in unfocused (light bars) and focused (dark bars) conditions, as a function of the position of the phrase in the utterance. **b)** Duration of /la/ in unfocused and focused conditions.

2.2.2. LIP CUES

In a second set of studies, movements of the lips were tracked during the production of vocal pointing (prosodic contrastive focus) using different measurement techniques.

a. The video study

The results summarised below are detailed in Dohen et al. (2004) and Dohen & Lœvenbruck (2005). The aim was to examine the possible articulatory visible correlates of contrastive focus in French. Data were collected for two speakers (A & B) for reiterant (A) and real speech (A &

B) using a very accurate lip-tracking device (descriptions can be found in Audouy, 2000). It appeared that contrastive focus was characterized by an increase (hyper-articulation) in inter-lip area and in inter-lip area peak velocity for the focal phrase. The amount of hyper-articulation was however highly speaker-dependent. Speaker A hyperarticulated much more than speaker B. Due to corpus constraints, protrusion could be analysed for speaker B only. It was also hyper-articulated and to a greater extent than inter-lip area. In addition, it appeared that speaker B hypo-articulated the post-focal sequence (reduced inter-lip area, inter-lip area velocity and protrusion) while speaker A barely did. Durational measurements were also conducted since duration can be a visual cue as well. These measurements showed that the focused syllables were significantly lengthened for both speakers, the first phoneme of the focused phrase being even more significantly lengthened. For speaker A, it was also observed that the last syllable of a phrase was significantly lengthened and hyper-articulated when the following phrase was focused. This was related to an anticipation strategy. We concluded from these observations that there is a global tendency towards hyperarticulating the focused phrase but that other visible cues are produced and that they appear to be speaker dependent. This is why, in order to be able to identify potential generic strategies, it seemed important to extend this study to a greater number of speakers.

Visual only perception tests were also conducted using the videos of speakers A and B (Dohen & Lœvenbruck, 2005). These tests showed that contrastive focus could be perceived through the visual modality alone and that the visual cues used for perception corresponded at least in part to those identified in the production studies. For both speakers, a few stimuli were well perceived even though the visible correlates described above (i.e. focal hyper-articulation and lengthening, with or without post-focal hypo-articulation) were not present. This suggested that other more subtle facial correlates may intervene. Studies on other languages have indeed shown that other facial movements such as eyebrow movements (Krahmer et al., 2002; Grandström & House, 2005) or head movements (Hadar et al., 1983; Cerrato & Skhiri, 2003; Munhall et al., 2004) or both (Graf et al., 2002) could intervene. Cavé et al. (1996) also showed that, in French, F0 variations and eyebrow movements could be linked. This is why it also seemed necessary to enlarge the set of facial movements measured by the use of a complementary technique.

b. The 3D motion capture (Optotrak) study

The aim of this second study, detailed in Dohen et al. (2006), was to further explore the articulatory visible correlates of contrastive focus in French, by extending the preliminary study in two directions. The first extension consisted in including a greater number of speakers in order to identify possible generic strategies. The preliminary study showed that one speaker's way to single out the focused phrase was to locally increase inter-lip area and its derivative as well as duration. The other speaker's behaviour was spread across the entire utterance. It consisted in creating a contrast within the utterance, by slightly hyper-articulating and lengthening the focused phrase as well as hypo-articulating the post-focal sequence.

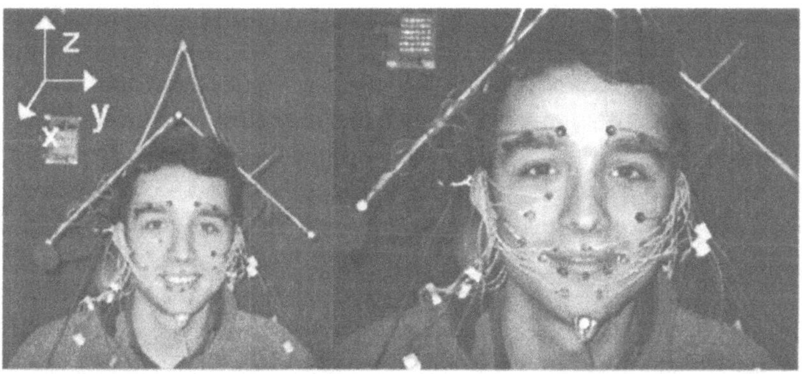

Figure 4: Optotrak measurement device: experimental setup. The 24 IREDs glued to the speaker's face are visible, as well as the 4 additional IREDs attached to a head rig for head motion correction. The x, y, z axes used for the articulatory measurements are shown. See Appendix A.2.

The first aim of this second study was thus to determine whether the two behaviours observed are shared by other speakers or if more variability is at stake. The second addition to the preliminary study consisted in extending the set of facial measurements by the use of a complementary recording technique. Results of the perceptual tests in the preliminary study suggested that other facial correlates than lip parameters may play a role in focus perception. The second study made use of an optical technique that allowed for the monitoring the positions of several markers on the face. Details on the experimental paradigm, the recording procedure and the data processing can be found in Appendix A.2. Five native speakers of French (B, C, D, E and F) were recorded using a 3D optical tracking system: Optotrak (IRED tracking system using markers glued to the speaker's face), which is less accurate on lip contours than the system used in *a.* but provides more facial data. Figure 4 gives an idea of the experimental setup used.

Articulatory and durational analysis

Figure 5 provides a visual overview of the results. Table 1 groups detailed intra- and inter-utterance contrasts (percent changes for each speaker and each parameter).

Speaker B – This speaker significantly lengthened and hyper-articulated (except lip spreading) the focused phrase. He also hypo-articulated the post-focal phrase(s). The strongest contrasts were measured for lip protrusion and duration and the smallest contrasts for jaw movements.

Speaker C – This speaker significantly lengthened and hyper-articulated the focused phrase. A slight hypo-articulation of the post-focal phrase(s) was also observed but only for jaw movements and lip opening. This speaker anticipated focus on the preceding phrase (slight lengthening and hyper-articulation for jaw movements and lip opening limited to the directly preceding phrase). The strongest contrasts were measured for lip protrusion and duration.

Speaker D – This speaker significantly lengthened and hyper-articulated (except lip spreading) the focused phrase. A post-focal hypo-articulation was measured for lip opening and lip protrusion. This speaker anticipated focus by hyper-articulating (only lip opening) the directly preceding phrase. The strongest contrasts were measured for lip protrusion and the smallest contrasts for lip spreading.

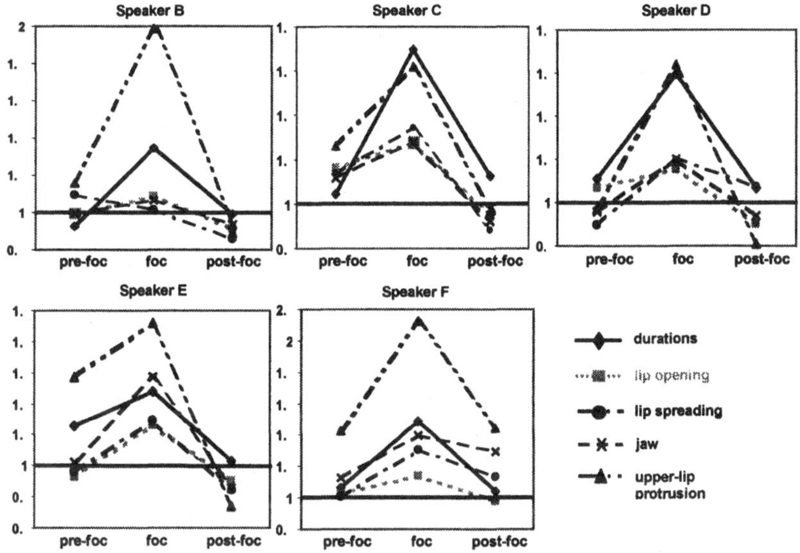

Figure 5: Durational and articulatory measurements for all five speakers: normalised values corresponding to the pre-focal (pre-foc), focal (foc) and post-focal (post-foc) sequences (the dark horizontal lines correspond to the neutral case, i.e. 1).

Speaker E – This speaker significantly lengthened and hyper-articulated the focused phrase. He also hypo-articulated the post-focal phrase(s) and anticipates focus by hyper-articulating (only lip protrusion) the directly preceding phrase. The strongest contrasts were measured for lip protrusion and the smallest contrasts for lip opening and lip spreading.
Speaker F – This speaker significantly lengthened and hyper-articulated the focused phrase. He also anticipated focus by hyper-articulating (only lip protrusion) the directly preceding phrase. The strongest contrasts were measured for lip protrusion and the smallest for lip opening.

Analysis of the other facial data

Eyebrow movement (raising) – There appeared to be a link between eyebrow raising and the production of prosodic contrastive focus only for three out of five speakers (B, C & E). This eyebrow raising was however not systematic and did not occur whenever focus is produced.

Speaker B was the one for which the combined productions (synchronous eyebrow raising and focus production) were the most frequent. The amplitudes of the movements are however very small (largest movement: 2mm). The other speakers either never raised their eyebrows, or did it randomly with no particular link to focus production.

Table 1: Results from the Optotrak study for each speaker (B, C, D, E and F) and each parameter: duration (Dur), vertical jaw movements (Jaw), lip opening (LO), lip spreading (LS) and upper lip protrusion (LP). The table provides the percent changes for the focused phrase compared to the rest of the utterance (intra-utterance contrast) and to the same phrase in the neutral version (inter-utterance contrast). The statistical significance threshold was fixed at p=0.01. 'ns' corresponds to a non-significant change.

	speaker		B	C	D	E	F
Intra-utterance contrast	Dur		+38.7%	+30.5%	+25.3%	+16.8%	+43.8%
	Jaw		+9.9%	+14.9%	+12.5%	+31.5%	+18.5%
	LO		+13.8%	+16.8%	+5.1%	+17.4%	+13.5%
	LS		ns	+17%	ns	+19.4%	+23.2%
	LP		+62.8%	+25%	+37.4%	+39.4%	+69.1%
Inter-utterance contrast	Dur	foc	+20.9%	+34.1%	+29.8%	+23.9%	+49%
		pre-foc	ns	+4.7%	+8.1%	+16.4%	+9%
		post-foc	ns	ns	ns	ns	ns
	Jaw	foc	+6.6%	+14%	+9.9%	+28.5%	+39.5%
		pre-foc	ns	+6%	ns	ns	ns
		post-foc	-6.5%	-8.7%	ns	-6.2%	+23.9%
	LO	foc	+8.7%	+13.9%	+7.6%	+13.3%	+13.6%
		pre-foc	ns	+6.3%	+5.7%	-4.1%	ns
		post-foc	-8.9%	-2.2%	-4.5%	-3.4%	ns
	LS	foc	ns	+17.3%	ns	+14.5%	+30%
		pre-foc	ns	ns	ns	ns	ns
		post-foc	-15.6%	ns	ns	-5.8%	ns
	LP	foc	+98.4%	+30.9%	+32%	+46%	+112.4%
		pre-foc	+25.1%	ns	ns	+24.4%	+53.7%
		post-foc	-8.1%	ns	-10%	-13%	+41.6%

Head movement – Speaker B was the only one for whom a correlation between head nods and focus production was observed. The correlation was not systematic, however, and the amplitudes and temporal alignment of the movements were highly variable. The other speakers also moved their heads but the movements were not correlated with focus production.

Perception tests

Visual perception tests were carried out on a selection of recordings from four of the speakers. These showed that focus could be correctly detected visually in 66.4% of the cases (chance level 33.3%) and suggested that the articulatory and facial visual cues identified above are well perceived visually.

c. Summary of findings on the articulatory signalling of focus

The production study described above along with that described in the previous section show that there are potential visible articulatory correlates to prosodic contrastive focus in French. One of our main conclusions is the fact that focus affects the whole utterance and not only the specific focused phrase. A number of articulatory gestures are affected by focus. The way and the extent to which these articulatory gestures are affected depend on the speaker. However, two main strategies emerge, an absolute one and a differential one:

Absolute visual signalling strategy: the focused constituent is lengthened and hyper-articulated to a large extent (inter-lip area, protrusion and jaw movements). Previous studies (Dohen & Lœvenbruck, 2005) showed that the peak velocities were also increased which signals an increase of the underlying articulatory effort during the gestures (Nelson, 1983). The speakers using this strategy therefore concentrate their efforts on the hyper-articulation of the focused phrase. Some speakers also slightly anticipate focus.

Differential visual signalling strategy: in this case, the focused phrase is also lengthened and hyper-articulated but to a smaller extent. Focus is sometimes anticipated. Additionally, the post-focal sequence is hypo-articulated compared to the neutral case. A visible contrast is thus created within the utterance: the focal hyper-articulation is not very distinct but is reinforced by the post-focal hypo-articulation.

We further observed that the visible articulatory parameter that was the most hyper-articulated under focus was protrusion. This is consistent with the finding that lip protrusion is the most visible lip feature (Benoît et al., 1994). It is a robust feature which is long-anticipated in the articulation of the preceding phonemes (Cathiard, 1994). We also found that there could be a link between prosodic contrastive focus and head (nod) and/or eyebrow (raising) movements. However this link is far from being systematic, particularly for the head movements. There are important inter- and intra-speaker variations in the movement amplitude and in its synchronisation with the acoustic signal.

d. Contribution of articulatory and facial visual cues to global perception

Combined auditory-visual perception studies detailed in Dohen & Lœvenbruck (under revision) analysed the potential contribution of visual information in global auditory-visual perception of prosodic contrastive focus in French. Whispered speech was used to 'naturally' degrade part of the acoustic prosodic cues (no fundamental frequency for whispered speech) and thereby the auditory only perception performances. This rendered the measurement of a potential visual advantage possible by avoiding a ceiling effect. The studies showed that the visual information available from articulatory and facial movements was combined to auditory information especially when auditory information was not sufficient to make a straight-forward perceptual judgment (whispered speech). It therefore appears that articulatory and facial cues to prosodic focus are not only produced but that these cues can be used in the perception process.

Altogether, these results suggest that speakers use reliable strategies to organise phonation and articulation adequately in order to convey prosodic pointing. On the perception side, the visual only and auditory-visual perception tests show that these phonatory and articulatory patterns are recovered by listeners/viewers and used for prosodic pointing detection. Our conjecture is that integrated (acoustic, articulatory, proprioceptive) representations may be needed in order to produce prosodic pointing adequately and that these representations may be formed via the activation of associative cerebral areas, such as temporal and/or parietal regions. The fact that manual and ocular pointing both recruit the (associative) posterior parietal cortex adds to the motivation to explore the cerebral correlates of prosodic pointing.

2.3. CEREBRAL CORRELATES OF VOCAL POINTING

2.3.1. PRODUCTION FMRI STUDY

The fMRI production study summarized below is described in more details in Lœvenbruck et al. (2005). The aim was to examine the cerebral correlates of vocal pointing in French, conveyed by prosodic focus and syntactic extraction. Sixteen healthy, male, right-handed native speakers of French were examined. The stimuli consisted of visually presented sentences in French. Three isosyllabic sentences were presented, one for each condition:
- baseline condition: "Madeleine m'amena"
(Madeleine brought me around).
- prosodic deixis condition: "MADELEINE m'amena"
(MADELEINE brought me around), to elicit contrastive focus on the agent.
- syntactic deixis condition: "C'est Mad'leine qui m'am'na"
(It's Mad'leine who brought me 'round).
The number of syllables in the sentence was maintained equal to 6, using schwa deletion. The methods are described in Appendix A.3.
The results of the fixed effect group and random effects analyses are reported here. Figure 6 represents the functional activations obtained for the main effects with the fixed effect analysis. The pattern of activations common to the two deixis conditions (each compared to the baseline) included Broca's region (BA 45, 47), the left insula and the premotor cortex (BA 6) bilaterally. Prosodic deixis additionally activated the left anterior cingulate gyrus (BA 24, 32), the left supramarginal gyrus (LSMG, BA 40) and the left postero-superior temporal gyrus (Wernicke's area, BA 22). The (prosodic deixis - syntactic deixis) contrast yielded significant activation in the left posterosuperior temporal gyrus and the LSMG. The results of the random effect analysis, using the same statistic-cal significance threshold ($p< .001$ corrected), for the same contrasts did not provide significant activations. With a less stringent significance

threshold however ($p<.05$ non corrected), the contrasts provide a similar pattern of activations as the one obtained with the fixed effect analysis.
This fMRI study shows activation of Broca's region in the deixis conditions compared to the baseline. The Left Inferior Frontal Gyrus (LIFG) was therefore activated during verbal pointing at the agent of the action, through prosody or syntax. This activation is consistent with functional neuroimaging studies on complex syntactic processing (Caplan et al., 2000; Friederici, 2002; Just et al., 1996). These studies have shown the involvement of the LIFG in plausibility judgments about syntactically complex constructions, which require intricate tracking of thematic roles. Our findings are also in line with studies on the observation and mental imagery of action which show LIFG activation during action tracking (Binkofski et al., 2000; Grafton et al., 1996; Iacoboni et al., 1999; Rizzolatti et al., 2007). According to Rizzolatti and colleagues, the role of the LIFG in speech would have evolved from a 'basic mechanism originally not related to communication: the capacity to recognize actions' (Rizzolatti & Arbib, 1998). In addition, Dogil and colleagues' fMRI study on the production of prosodic features at the syllable and phrase levels has also revealed left IFG activation (Mayer et al., 2002; Dogil et al., 2002). Taken together, these observations support the claim that the role of the LIFG is that of an action-structure parser, which, in morphosyntactic encoding and decoding, handles the parsing of the predicate and its arguments, or the attentional monitoring of "who does what to whom".
The left insula was also found activated in both (deixis – baseline) contrasts. The involvement of the left precentral gyrus of the insula in articulatory planning during speech has already been shown (Dronkers, 1996). As described above, prosody has acoustic and articulatory correlates. The production of prosodic focus may require more accurate planning of the movements of the larynx, the tongue and the jaw, which could explain why the prosodic deixis condition yields significant activation of the left insula when compared with the baseline (same words to articulate, but a more stringent prosody). Similarly, the syntactic deixis condition (compared to the baseline) likely requires more accurate articulatory planning, given the larger number of consonant clusters involved (due to schwa deletion).

The activation of the LSMG and of Wernicke's area in the prosodic deixis condition alone suggests that, when deixis is already encoded by syntax, no additional recruitment of the inferior parietal lobule and Wernicke's area is necessary. As mentioned in section 2, several studies suggest that the inferior parietal regions in both hemispheres function as sensory integrators which form representations necessary in the organisation of motor actions, such as linguistic or non-linguistic pointing at targets. The left hemisphere would have a linguistic predominance.

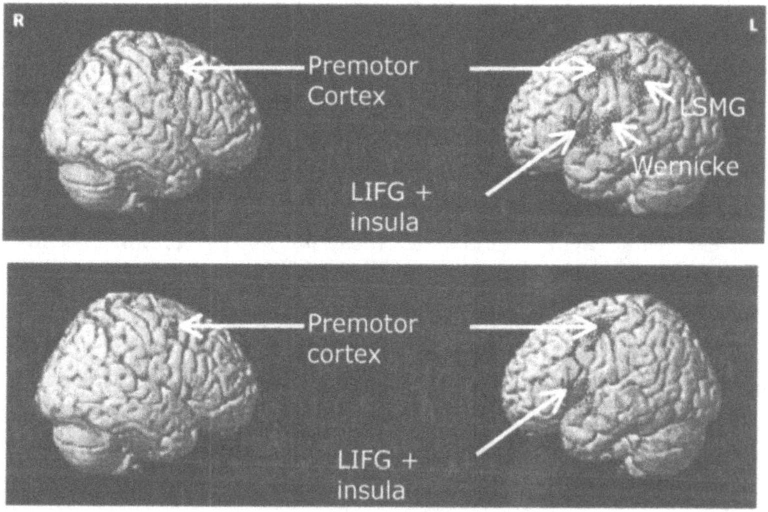

Figure 6: Activations in the prosodic deixis contrast (top) and syntactic deixis contrast (bottom). Both contrasts provide activations of frontal regions. Only the prosodic contrast shows temporal and parietal activations.

In speech, a left temporo-parieto-frontal network might be recruited in the organisation of verbal motor actions from auditory representations. Our results, with the activations of the LSMG, the LIFG and Wernicke's area in prosodic deixis, are in line with this hypothesis. Like visually-guided manual pointing, prosodic pointing may need multisensory representations to be formed via superior temporal and inferior parietal regions to organise articulation and phonation adequately. We therefore suggest that non-grammaticalized linguistic deixis recruits the temporo-parieto-frontal network and that grammaticalized deixis (syntactic deixis) is handled solely by the LIFG.

2.3.2. PERCEPTION FMRI STUDY

The production study described above suggests that associative brain areas are recruited for the production of vocal pointing. As demonstrated in section 2.2., the articulatory and phonatory patterns produced by speakers are also perceived by listeners/viewers. It can therefore be hypothesised that the cerebral network recruited for the production of vocal pointing is at least partly also recruited for its perception. This is what the study presented hereafter aims at testing.

Although, the acoustic and articulatory correlates of prosodic focus have been quite extensively studied (as recalled in section 2.), it remains unclear what neural processes underlie its perception. Meanwhile studies have shown that prosodic processing in general cannot be restricted to the right hemisphere (see Baum & Pell, 1999 for a review). Two studies have analysed the processing of prosodic focus (or closely related prosodic phenomena). The first one (Wildgruber et al., 2004) aimed at contrasting affective vs linguistic prosody. The linguistic prosodic task was an indirect informational focus detection task (find the most suitable answer to a specific question). For the linguistic prosodic task, the authors found bilateral activations of the primary and secondary auditory cortices, of the anterior insular cortex and of the frontal operculum (BA 6/44/47), right hemisphere activation of the dorso-lateral-frontal regions and left hemisphere activations of the inferior frontal cortex. The second study which examined the processing of prosodic focus (Tong et al., 2005) aimed at differentiating the processing of 'intonation' (question/affirmation discrimination) and that of contrastive stress. It additionally compared English and Chinese. For the processing of contrastive stress, the authors put forward bilateral activation of the intra-parietal sulcus (BA 40/7), right hemisphere activation of the medial frontal gyrus (BA 9/46) and left hemisphere activations of the supramarginal gyrus and the posterior medio-temporal gyrus (BA 21/20/37).

Moreover, as we have shown above (in section 2.2.), even though the perception of prosodic focus was often considered as uniquely auditory, it is possible to perceive prosodic focus visually and the visual modality can enhance perception when prosodic auditory cues are degraded (Dohen & Lœvenbruck, under revision). This finding emphasises the necessity to consider the perception of prosodic contrastive focus and speech prosody in general as multimodal. The perception fMRI study presented here aims at analysing the neural processing of prosodic focus from a multimodal point of view.
fMRI recordings were conducted for 12 native speakers of French at the ATR Brain Activity Imaging Center (Japan). Subjects were scanned while they were performing a prosodic focus detection task for three modalities (audio only A, visual only V and audiovisual AV). The stimuli were subject-verb-object (SVO) structured sentences uttered in both normal and whispered speech. In some cases, S was under prosodic contrastive focus. The speaker was a female native speaker of French. After seeing/hearing/seeing and hearing each stimulus, subjects were asked to tell whether they had perceived a correction (i.e. contrastive focus) or not. A detailed description of the stimuli and of the fMRI procedure (paradigm and data collection and analysis) can be found in Appendix A.4.

Behavioral results

Table 2 provides the percentages of correct answers for all conditions. It appears that subjects performed the task correctly: they were able to identify focus cases from non-focus cases (the percentages of correct answers were well above chance, in all conditions).

Table 2: Mean percentages of correct answers and standard deviations (sd) across all subjects for each modality (chance level: 50%).

modality	normal speech		whispered speech	
	% correct	sd	% correct	sd
AV	98.4	2.0	89.6	6.5
A	97.4	3.0	69.9	12.8
V	86.4	7.5	88	8.6

Preliminary fMRI results

The analysis of the fMRI data is still underway and the results presented here are only preliminary. A preliminary analysis was conducted for the focus vs no focus contrast for the auditory and auditory-visual modalities. It appeared that auditory alone (A) detection of prosodic focus involved the right associative auditory cortex and fusiform gyrus (BA 19) as well as the left middle frontal gyrus (BA 6/46) and inferior temporal gyrus (BA 37) and the cerebellum bilaterally. For the auditory-visual modality, we found bilateral activations of the middle and inferior frontal gyri (BA 40), the middle temporal gyrus (BA 21), the inferior parietal lobule (BA 40) and the fusiform gyrus (BA 37) as well as left activation of the supramarginal gyrus (BA 40).

It appears that for all modalities, prosodic focus detection or processing involves bilateral activations of associative brain areas. Auditory perception of prosodic focus (vs no focus) appears to be essentially processed in associative areas right superior temporal gyrus and left inferior temporal gyrus (BA 37). Multimodal (AV) perception of prosodic focus involves bilateral activations of temporal and parietal associative areas as well as inferior and middle frontal regions. This illustrates the underlying necessity of associating various types of information to detect focus (especially auditory and articulatory) and supports the assumption that the articulatory and phonatory patterns produced by the speaker are integrated in perception.

Similar activations of a complex neural network in the processing of focus have been observed in two recent ERP studies (Bornkessel et al., 2003; Magne et al., 2005). The implication of the left parietal lobe in the auditory-visual perception of prosodic pointing is interesting, in the light of our fMRI study of the production of prosodic pointing, and of the studies on manual and ocular pointing.

3. MULTIMODAL POINTING

The aim of this multimodal fMRI study was to investigate the cerebral correlates of pointing in several modalities (Lœvenbruck et al., 2007). To test the hypothesis that multimodal pointing could involve a continuum of cerebral regions, we designed an fMRI paradigm including four conditions: 1) index finger pointing, 2) eye pointing, 3) prosodic focus, 4) syntactic extraction.

Subjects and material

Fifteen healthy right-handed volunteers, aged 18-55 years, native speakers of French were examined. Stimuli consisted of two types (1 and 2) of images consisting of a girl (Lise) and a boy (Jules) next to each other and alternatively located on the right and on the left side of the screen. Type 1 images showed the girl holding a book, while the boy did not; Type 2 images showed the reverse. In the middle of all images, a fixation cross was displayed. A blank screen with a mid-centered black cross preceded each stimulus. The tasks consisted of verbal and non-verbal pointing to a character. Control conditions were included. The same question: "Est-ce que Lise tient le livre?" (Does Lise hold the book?) was used for all tasks. Subjects were instructed: (a) to confirm the question when type 1 images were presented (control), (b) to point to Jules when type 2 images were presented (contrastive pointing). The tasks were the following: During *prosodic pointing*, subjects uttered «JULES tient le livre» (JULES holds the book), with contrastive focus on "Jules". During *syntactic pointing*, they uttered «C'est Jules qui tient le livre» (It is Jules who holds the book), with syntactic extraction of "Jules". During *digital pointing*, they pointed with the right index finger to Jules. During *ocular pointing*, subjects looked in the direction of Jules.

The controls were the following: In prosodic and syntactic controls, subjects neutrally uttered: «Lise tient le livre » (Lise holds the book). In digital control, they performed a downward finger movement. In ocular control, they made a downward eye movement. The detailed methods are presented in Appendix A.5.

Preliminary fMRI results

Patterns of activation were examined for 15 subjects for each of the following contrasts:

- digital pointing tasks vs digital control
- ocular pointing tasks vs ocular control
- prosodic pointing tasks vs prosodic control
- syntactic pointing tasks vs syntactic control

Preliminary results of the random effect group analysis are reported.

Figure 7 represents functional activations during each pointing condition vs its control.

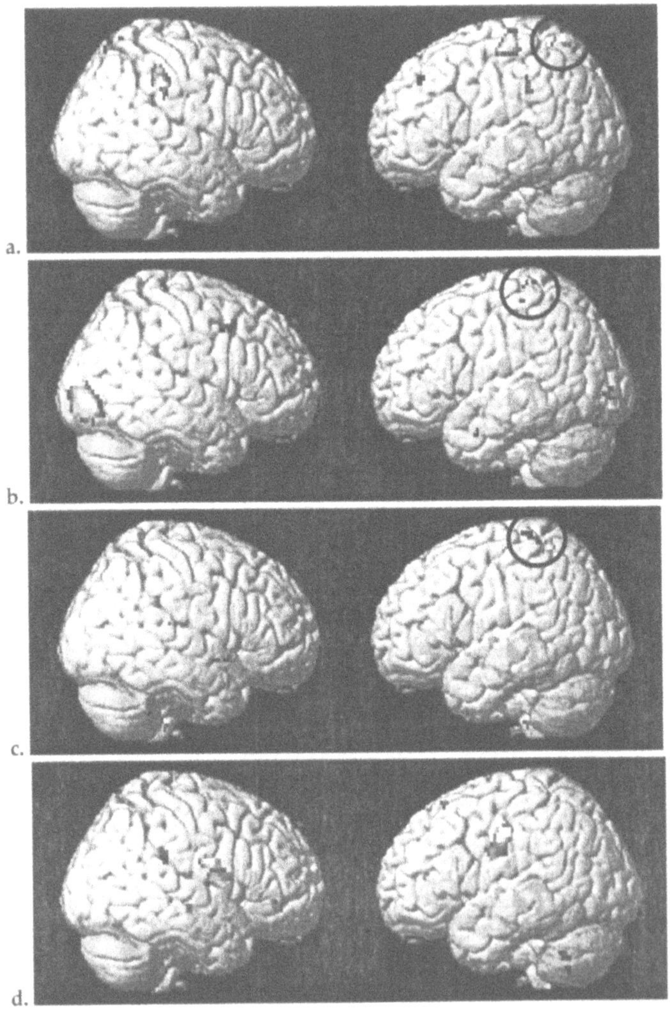

Figure 7: Activations during each pointing condition vs its control, rendered on a sagittal template, in a. digital- b. ocular- c. prosodic- d. syntactic-modes. The left hemisphere is on the right, the right one on the left

Digital pointing (vs its control) yielded bilateral activation of the superior parietal lobule (BA 7), with a left hemisphere dominance. There was bilateral activation of the supramarginal gyrus (BA 40), with a right hemisphere dominance. There was left frontal cortex activation (BA 4 ,6). *The ocular condition* activated the left hemisphere predominantly in the post central gyrus (BA 3) and the frontal lobe bilaterally (BA 4, 6). The occipital gyrus (BA 17, 18) was activated bilaterally. *The prosodic condition* recruited the superior parietal lobule (BA 7) bilaterally, with a left dominance. The supramarginal gyrus activation did not reach signify-cance, contrary to our previous finding on covert prosody (see section 2.3.1.). The left postcentral gyrus was activated (BA 2, 3). Perisylvian regions (BA 47, 13, 42) were activated bilaterally. *The syntactic condition* activated the right supramarginal gyrus (BA 40) and did not recruit the left parietal lobule. Right perisylvian regions (BA 44, 47, 21) were activated, as well as the premotor cortex (BA 6) bilaterally.

To summarise, this preliminary analysis revealed that the left superior parietal lobule (BA 7 or its neighbour BA 3) was activated in all three digital, ocular and prosodic pointing but not in syntactic pointing. These results indicate that pointing in different modalities may recruit the left superior parietal lobule, ocular pointing being more anterior than prosodic pointing, itself more anterior than digital pointing.

These results are in accordance with the results from our behavioural studies which suggest that speakers may use multisensory represent-tations in order to produce prosodic pointing adequately, just like they do to produce a manual or ocular gesture. These representations may be formed via the activation of associative parietal areas. The lack of parietal activation in syntactic pointing could be due to the absence of on-line multisensory construction in syntactic pointing, compared with prosodic pointing. Syntactic pointing uses a grammaticalized "frozen" construction and may not need integrated representations to be formed. This fMRI study therefore suggests that the left superior parietal lobule could be a potential substrate for pointing with the finger, the eye, and the larynx.

4. CONCLUSION

We have shown that pointing is a critical device to explore the potential common neural networks at play in gesture and language. The role of manual (or digital) pointing in language acquisition strongly suggests indeed that vocal pointing and pointing in other modalities may well be grounded in a common cerebral network.

We have argued from several neuroimaging studies on manual and ocular pointing that these two modalities seem to recruit a network including the left posterior parietal and frontal cortices.

Behavioural studies in our laboratory have shown that prosodic vocal pointing is a sophisticated behaviour that requires accurate laryngeal and articulatory control. Perception studies have revealed that the potential articulatory visible cues to prosodic vocal pointing are in fact visually perceived. In other words, viewers can decipher these sophisticated signals. We have claimed that speakers may need multisensory representations to produce prosodic pointing adequately and that these representations may involve the activation of associative parietal regions, close to the regions involved in manual and ocular pointings.

The results of a first study on covert vocal pointing, including prosodic pointing (i.e. focus) and syntactic pointing (i.e. syntactic extraction) have been presented. It was shown that covert prosodic pointing does recruit left parietal regions, whereas syntactic pointing mainly involves frontal region. The involvement of the left parietal lobe was confirmed by a recent fMRI study of the perception of prosodic pointing. Finally we presented the preliminary results of a new study of multimodal pointing (digital, ocular, overt prosodic and syntactic pointing). They seem to reveal a common pattern of left parietal activation in ocular, digital and prosodic pointing. A grammaticalization process has been suggested to explain the lack of parietal activation in syntactic pointing. Altogether these fMRI studies are in line with our conjecture that linguistic on-line pointing (prosodic focus) is grounded in the same cerebral network as gestural (manual and ocular) pointings. More analyses are underway to consolidate these results. If they come out as robust, then they will contribute to the debate on the gestural origin of language.

ACKNOWLEDGEMENTS

Many researchers were involved in the different works presented here. In alphabetical order, they are C. Abry, M. Baciu, A. Callan, D. E. Callan, F. Carota, M.–A. Cathiard, H. Hill, L. Lamalle, P. Perrier, C. Pichat, C. Savariaux, J.-L. Schwartz, C. Segebarth. We thank them all sincerely.

REFERENCES

Astafiev, S. V., Shulman, G. L., Stanley, C. M., Snyder, A. Z., Van Essen, D. C., and Corbetta, M. (2003). Functional Organization of Human Intraparietal and Frontal Cortex for Attending, Looking, and Pointing. *Journal of Neuroscience* 23, 4689-4699.

Astésano, C. (2001). *Rythme et accentuation en français: invariance et variabilité stylistique*, PhD Thesis, L'Harmattan édition et diffusion.

Astésano, C., Magne, C., Morel, M., Coquillon, A., Espesser, R., Besson, M., and Lacheret A. (2004). Marquage acoustique du focus contrastif non codé syntaxiquement en français. *Proceedings of the XXVièmes Journées d'Etudes sur la Parole*, 126–129. Fez (Morocco).

Astésano C., Bard E.G., and Turk A. (2007). Structural influence on initial accent placement in French. *Language and Speech* 50(3), 423-446.

Audouy, M. (2000). *Traitement d'images vidéo pour la capture des mouvements labiaux*. Final engineering report, Institut National Polytechnique de Grenoble.

Bates, E., Camaioni, L., and Volterra V. (1975). The acquisition of performatives prior to speech. *Merrill-Palmer Quarterly* 21, 205-226.

Bates, E., Benigni, L., Bretherton, I., Camaioni, L., and Volterra, V. (1979). *The emergence of symbols: cognition and communication in infancy*. New York: Academic Press.

Baum, S. R., and Pell M. D. (1999). The neural bases of prosody: Insights from lesion studies and neuroimaging. *Aphasiology* 13(8), 581-608.

Bellugi, U., Poizner, H., and Klima E.S. (1989). Language, modality and the brain. *Trends in Neurosciences* 12(10), 380-388.

Benoît, C., Mohamadi, T., and Kandel S. (1994). Effects of Phonetic Context on Audio-Visual Intelligibility of French. *Journal of Speech and Hearing Research* 37, 1195-1203.

Berthoud, A.-C. (1990). Deixis, thématisation et détermination. *La deixis. Colloque en Sorbonne*. M.-A. Morel & L. Danon-Boileau (eds.), 527-542, PUF.

Binkofski, F., Amunts, K., Stephan, K.M., Posse, S., Schormann, T., Freund H.-J., Zilles, K., and Seitz R. (2000). Broca's region subserves imagery of motion: a combined cytoarchitectonic and fMRI study. *Human Brain Mapping* 11, 273-285.

Bornkessel, I., Schlesewsky, M., and Friederici A.D. (2003). Contextual information modulates initial processes of syntactic integration: The role of inter- versus intrasentential predictions. *Journal of Experimental Psychology: Learning Memory and Cognition* 29, 269-298.

Brown H.D. (1971). Children's comprehension of relativized English sentences. *Child Development* 42, 1923–1936.

Bruner, J. (1975). The ontogenesis of speech acts. *Journal of Child Language* 2, 1–19.

Butcher, C. & Goldin-Meadow, S. (2000). Gesture and the transition from one- to two-word speech: when hand and mouth come together. In: D. McNeill (Ed.) *Language and gesture*, 235-257, Cambridge: Cambridge University Press.

Butterworth, G. (2003). Pointing is the royal road to language. In: S. Kita (ed.) *Pointing, where language, culture, and cognition meet*, 9-34, Mahwah, NJ: Lawrence Erlbaum Associates Publishers.

Capirci, O., Iverson, J. M., Pizzuto, E., and Volterra V. (1996). Gestures and words during the transition to two-word speech. *Journal of Child language* 23, 645- 673.

Caplan, D., Alpert, N., Waters, G., and Olivieri A. (2000). Activation of Broca's area by syntactic processing under conditions of concurrent articulation. *Human Brain Mapping* 9, 65-71.

Caselli, M.C. (1990). Communicative gestures and first words. In: V. Volterra & C.J. Erting (eds.), *From gesture to language in hearing and deaf children*, 56-57, New York: Springer-Verlag.

Cathiard, M.-A. (1994). *La perception visuelle de l'anticipation des gestes vocaliques : cohérence des évènements audibles et visibles dans le flux de la parole*, Unpublished PhD dissertation, Université Pierre Mendès France, Grenoble (France).

Cavé, C., Guaïtella, I., Bertrand, R., Santi, S., Harlay, F., and Espesser, R. (1996). About the Relationship between Eyebrow movements and F0 Variation. *Proceedings of ICSLP 1996* 4, 2175-2179.

Cerrato, L., & Skhiri, M. (2003). Analysis and measurement of communicative gestures in human dialogues. *Proceedings of AVSP 2003*, 251-256.

Cheney, D.L. & Seyfarth R.M. (1981). Selective forces affecting the predactor alarm calls of vervet monkeys. *Behaviour* 76, 25-61.

Chomsky, N. (1957). *Syntactic Structures*. The Hague: Mouton.

Chomsky, N. (1966). *Cartesian linguistics*. New York: Harper Row.

Connaghan, K.P., Moore, C.A., Reilly K.J., Almand K.B., and Steeve R.W. (2001). Acoustic and physiologic correlates of stress production across systems, *Poster presented at the American Speech-Language-Hearing Association*, New Orleans, L.A.

Connolly, J.D., Goodale, M.A., Desouza J.F., Menon R.S., and Vilis T. (2000). A comparison of frontoparietal fMRI activation during anti-saccades and antipointing. *Journal of Neurophysiology* 84, 1645–1655.

Corballis, M.C. (1991). *The lopsided ape: Evolution of the generative mind*. New York: Oxford University Press.

Dahan, D. & Bernard, J.-M. (1996). Interspeaker Variability in Emphatic Accent Production in French. *Language and Speech* 39(4), 341-374.

Delais-Roussarie, E., Rialland, A., Doetjes, J., and Marandin, J.-M. (2002). The Prosody of Post Focus Sequences in French. *Proceedings of Speech Prosody 2002*, Aix-en-Provence (France), 239-242.

Di Cristo, A. (1998). Intonation in French. In: D. Hirst & A. Di Cristo (eds.) *Intonation Systems: a Survey of Twenty Languages*, 195-218, Cambridge University Press.

Di Cristo, A. & Jankowski, L. (1999). Prosodic Organisation and Phrasing after Focus in French. *Proceedings of ICPhS 1999*, San Francisco (USA), 1565-1568.

Diessel, H. & Tomasello, M. (2000). The development of relative clauses in spontaneous child speech. *Cognitive Linguistics* 11, 131-151.

Dogil, G., Ackermann, H., Grodd, W., Haider, H., Kamp, H., Mayer, J., Riecker, A., and Wildgruber, D. (2002). The Speaking Brain. *Journal of Neurolinguistics* 15(1), 59-90.

Dohen, M., Lœvenbruck, H., Cathiard, M.-A., and Schwartz J.-L., 2004. Visual perception of contrastive focus in reiterant French speech. *Speech Communication* 44, 155-172.

Dohen, M. & Lœvenbruck, H. (2004). Pre-focal Rephrasing, Focal Enhancement and Post-focal Deaccentuation in French. *Proceedings of the 8th International Conference on Spoken Language Processing* 1, Jeju island (Korea), 785-788.

Dohen, M. & Lœvenbruck, H. (2005). Audiovisual Production and Perception of Contrastive Focus in French: a multispeaker study. *Proceedings of Interspeech 2005*, 2413-2416.

Dohen, M., Lœvenbruck, H., and Hill H. (2006). Visual correlates of prosodic contrastive focus in French: description and inter-speaker variability. *Proceedings of Speech Prosody 2006* 1, Dresden (Germany), 221-224.

Dohen, M. & Lœvenbruck, H. (under revision). Interaction of audition and vision for the perception of prosodic contrastive focus. *Language and Speech*.

Dronkers, N. F. (1996). A new brain region for coordinating speech articulation. *Nature* 384, 159-161.

Edwards, M.G. & Humphreys, G.W. (1999). Pointing and grasping in unilateral visual neglect: effect of on-line visual feedback in grasping. *Neuropsychologia* 37(8), 959-973.

Erickson, D. (submitted). Effects of contrastive emphasis on jaw opening.

Fillmore, C. J. (1997). *Lectures on deixis.* Stanford: Center for the Study of Language and Information.

Fougeron, C. & Keating, P. A. (1997) Articulatory strengthening at edges of prosodic domains. *Journal of the Acoustic Society of America* 101, 3728-3740.

Friederici, A.D. (2002). Towards a neural basis of auditory sentence processing. *Trends in Cognitive Sciences* 6(2), 78-84.

Goffman, L. & Malin, C. (1999). Metrical Effects on Speech Movements in Children and Adults. *Journal of Speech, Language, and Hearing Research* 42 (4), 1003-1015.

Goldin-Meadow, S. & Butcher, C. (2003). Pointing toward two-word speech in young children. In: S. Kita (ed.) *Pointing: Where language, culture, and cognition meet,* 85-107, Mahwah, NJ: Earlbaum Associates.

Grafton, S.T., Arbib, M.A., Fadiga L., and Rizzolatti, G. (1996). Localization of grasp representations in humans by positron emission tomography. 2. Observation compared with imagination. *Experimental Brain Research* 112(1), 103-111.

Graf, H.P., Cosatto, E., Strom, V., and Huang, F.J. (2002). Visual Prosody: Facial Movements Accompanying Speech. *Proceedings of the 5th IEEE International Conference on Automatic Face and Gesture Recognition (FGR'02),* 381-386.

Granström, B., House, D. (2005). Audiovisual representation of prosody in expressive speech communication. *Speech Communication* 46, 473-484.

Hadar, U., Steiner, T. J., Grant, E. C., and Rose, F. C. (1983). Head movement correlates of juncture and stress at sentence level. *Language and Speech* 26, 117–129.

Hagler, D.J. Jr., Riecke L., Sereno M.I. (2007). Parietal and superior frontal visuospatial maps activated by pointing and saccades. *NeuroImage* 35(4), 1562-1577.

Hewes G.W. (1981). Pointing and language. In: T. Myers, J. Laver, and J. Anderson (eds.) *The cognitive representation of speech,* 263-269. Amsterdam: North-Holland.

Hickok, G. & Poeppel, D. (2001). Towards a functional neuroanatomy of speech perception. *Trends In Cognitive Sciences* 4(4), 131-138.

Higginbotham, D. (1992). Reference and control. In: R.K. Larson, S. Iatridou, U. Lahiri, and J. Higginbotham (eds.). *Control and grammar,* 79-108, Dordrecht: Kluwer.

Hornby, P.A. & Hass, W.A. (1970). Use of contrastive stress by preschool children. *Journal of Speech and Hearing Research* 13, 395-399.

Iacoboni, M., Woods, R.P, Brass, M., Bekkering, H., Mazziotta, J.C., and Rizzolatti, G. (1999). Cortical mechanisms of human imitation. *Science* 286, 2526-2528.

Iacoboni, M., Koski, L.M., Brass, M., Bekkering, H., Woods, R.P., Dubeau M.-C., Mazziotta J, C., and Rizzolatti, G. (2001). Reafferent copies of imitated actions in the right superior temporal cortex. *Proceedings of the National Acadamy of Sciences USA*, 98(24), 13995-13999.

Jackendoff, R. (2002). *Foundations of Language - Brain, Meaning, Grammar, Evolution*. Oxford University Press.

Jisa, H. & Kern, S. (1998). Relative clauses in French children's narrative texts. *Journal of Child Language* 25, 623-652.

de Jong, K., Beckman, M. E., and Fletcher J. (1991). The articulatory kinematics of final lengthening. *Journal of the Acoustical Society of America* 89, 369-382.

Jun, S.-A. & Fougeron, C. (2000). A Phonological Model of French Intonation. In: A. Botinis (ed.) *Intonation: Analysis, modelling and technology*, 209-242, Dordrecht: Kluwer Academic Publishers.

Just, M.A., Carpenter, P.A., Keller, T.A., Eddy, W.F., and Thulborn K.R. (1996). Brain activation modulated by sentence comprehension. *Science* 274, 114-116.

Kendon, A. (1996). An Agenda for Gesture Studies. *Semiotic Review of Books* 7(3), 8-12.

Kendon, A. (2004). *Gesture: Visible Action as Utterance*. Cambridge: Cambridge University Press.

Kertzman, C., Schwarz, U., Zeffiro, T. A., and Hallett, M. (1997). The role of posterior parietal cortex in visually guided reaching movements in humans. *Experimental Brain Research* 114(1), 170-183.

Kidd, E. & Bavin, E.L. (2002). English-speaking children's comprehension of relative clauses: Evidence for general-cognitive and language-specific constraints on development. *Journal of Psycholinguistic Research* 31, 599–617.

Kita, S. (2003). *Pointing: where language, culture, and cognition meet*. Mahwah, NJ: Lawrence Erlbaum Associates Publishers.

Klima, E.S. & Bellugi, U. (1988). *The signs of language*. Harvard University Press.

Konopscynsky, G. (1986). *Du prélangage au langage : acquisition de la structuration prosodique*. PhD thesis, University of Strasbourg.

Krahmer, E,. Ruttkay, Z., Swerts, M., and Wesselink, W. (2002). Pitch, Eyebrows and the Perception of Focus. *Proceedings of Speech Prosody 2002*, 443-446.

Lacquaniti, F., Perani, D., Guigon, E., Bettinardi, V., Carrozzo, M., Grassi, F., Rossetti, Y., and Fazio, F. (1997). Visuomotor transformations for reaching to memorized targets: a PET study. *Neuroimage* 5(2), 129-146.

Leavens, D.A., Hopkins, W.D., and Bard, K.A. (2005). Understanding the Point of Chimpanzee Pointing. Epigenesis and Ecological Validity. *Current Directions in Psychological Science* 14, 185-189.

Liberman, A.M. (1982). On Finding that Speech Is Special. *American Psychologist* 37, 2, 148-167.

Lœvenbruck, H. (1996). *Pistes pour le contrôle d'un robot parlant capable de réduction vocalique.* Unpublished Doctoral Dissertation in Cognitive Sciences, INPG, Grenoble (France).

Lœvenbruck, H. (1999). An investigation of articulatory correlates of the Accentual Phrase in French. *Proceedings of the XIVth International Congress of Phonetic Sciences* 1, San Francisco (USA), 667-670.

Lœvenbruck, H., Baciu, M., Segebarth, C., and Abry, C. (2005). The left inferior frontal gyrus under focus: an fMRI study of the production of deixis via syntactic extraction and prosodic focus. *Journal of Neurolinguistics* 18, 237-258.

Lœvenbruck, H., Vilain, C., Carota, F., Baciu, M., Abry, C., Lamalle, L., Pichat, C., and Segebarth, C. (2007). Cerebral correlates of multimodal pointing: An fmri study of prosodic focus, syntactic extraction, digital- and ocular- pointing. *Proceedings of the XVIth International Congress of Phonetic Sciences*, Saarbrücken (Germany).

Magne, C., Astesano, C., Lacheret-Dujour, A, Morel, M., Alter, K., and Besson, M. (2005). On-Line processing of "pop-out" words in Spoken French dialogues. *Journal of Cognitive Neurosciences* 17(5), 740-756.

Macwhinney, B. & Ple'h, C. (1988). The processing of restrictive relative clauses in Hungarian. *Cognition* 29, 95–141.

Mayer, J., Wildgruber, D., Riecker, A., Dogil, G., Ackermann, H., and Grodd, W. (2002). Prosody production and comprehension: converging evidence from fMRI studies. *Proceedings of Speech Prosody 2002*, Aix-en-Provence (France), 487-490.

McNeill, D. (1992). *Hand and Mind*. Chicago: University of Chicago Press.

Mckee, C., Mcdaniel, D., and Snedeker, J. (1998). Relatives children say. *Journal of Psycholinguistic Research* 27, 573–96.

Ménard, L., Lœvenbruck, H., and Savariaux, C. (2006). Articulatory and acoustic correlates of contrastive focus in French: a developmental study,. In: J. Harrington & M. Tabain (eds) *Speech Production: Models, Phonetic Processes and Techniques*, 227-251, New York: Psychology Press.

Morford, M. & Goldin-Meadow, S. (1992). Comprehension and production of gesture in combination with speech in one-word speakers. *Journal of Child Language* 19(3), 559-580.

Munhall, K.G., Jones, J. A., Callan, D. E., Kuratate, T., and Vatikiotis-Bateson, E. (2004). Visual Prosody and Speech Intelligibility – Head Movement Improves Auditory Speech Perception. *Psychological Science* 15(2), 133-137.

Nelson, W.L. (1983). Physical principles for economies of skilled movements. *Biological Cybernetics* 46(2), 135-147.

Oldfield, R.C. (1971). The assessment and analysis of handedness: the Edinburgh Inventory. *Neuropsychologia* 9(97), 113.

Pollick, A.S. & de Waal, F.B.M. (2007). Ape gestures and language evolution. *Proceedings of the National Academy of Sciences* 104(19), 8184-8189.

Povinelli, D.J. & Davis, D.R. (1994). Differences between chimpanzees (Pan troglodytes) and humans (Homo sapiens) in the resting state of the index finger: Implications for pointing. *Journal of Comparative Psychology* 108, 134–139.

Povinelli, D.J., Bering, J.M., & Giambrone, S. (2003). Chimpanzee 'pointing': Another error of the argument by analogy? In: S. Kita (ed.) *Pointing: Where language culture and cognition meet*, 35-68, Lawrence Erlbaum Associates.

Rizzolatti, G., Fogassi, L., and Gallese, V. (1997). Parietal cortex: from sight to action. *Curr. Opin. Neurobiol*, 7(4), 562-567.

Rolfe, L. (1996). Theoretical stages in the prehistory of grammar. In: A. Lock & C.R. Peters (eds.) *Handbook of human symbolic evolution*, 776-792. Oxford: Clarendon.

Rossi, M. (1999). La focalisation. In *L'intonation, le système du français: description et modélisation*, 116-128, Ophrys.

Séguinot, A. (1976). L'accent d'insistance en français standard. *Studia Phonetica* 12, 1-58.

Sheldon, A. (1974). The role of parallel function in the acquisition of relative clauses in English. *Journal of Verbal Learning and Verbal Behavior* 13, 272–81.

Simon, O., Mangin, J.F., Cohen, L., Le Bihan, D. & Dehaene, S. (2002). Topographical layout of hand, eye, calculation, and language-related areas in the human parietal lobe. *Neuron* 33, 475–487.

Tabain, M. (2003). Effects of prosodic boundary on /aC/ sequences: Articulatory results. *Journal of the Acoustical Society of America*, 113(5), 2834-2849.

Tavakolian, S. (1981). The conjoined clause analysis of relative clauses. In: S. Tavakolian (ed.) *Language acquisition and linguistic theory*, 167–187, Cambridge (MA): MIT Press.

Tomasello, M., Carpenter, M., and Liszkowski, U. (2007). A new look at infant pointing. *Journal of Child Language* 34, 1-20.

Tong, Y., Gandour, J., Talavage, T., Wong, D., Dzemidzic, M., Xu, Y., Li, X., and Lowe, M. (2005). Neural circuitry underlying sentence-level linguistic prosody. *NeuroImage* 28, 417-428.

Touati, P. (1987). Structures prosodiques du suédois et du français. *Lund Working Papers* 21, Lund University Press.

Tour, de la, G. (1635). *Le Tricheur à l'as de carreau (The cheat with the ace of diamonds).* Musée du Louvre, Paris (France).

Vallar, G., Guariglia, C., Nico, D., and Pizzamiglio, L. (1997). Motor deficits and optokinetic stimulation in patients with left hemineglect. *Neurology* 49(5), 1364-1370.

Volterra, V., Caselli, M.C., Capirci, O., and Pizzuto, E. (2005). Gesture and the emergence and development of language. In: M. Tomasello & D. Slobin (eds.) *Beyond Nature-Nurture. Essays in Honor of Elizabeth Bates.* 3-40, Mahwah, NJ: Lawrence Erlbaum Associates.

Wechsler, S. & Wayan, A. (1998). Syntactic ergativity in Balinese: an argument structure based theory. *Natural Language and Linguistic Theory* 16, 387-441.

Wildgruber, D., Hertrich, I., Riecker, A., Erb, M., Anders, S., Grodd, W., and Ackerman, H. (2004). Distinct Frontal Regions Subserve Evaluation of Linguistic and Emotional Aspects of Speech Intonation. *Cerebral Cortex* 14(12), 1384-1389.

Wilkins, D. (2003). Why pointing with the index finger is not a universal (in sociocultural and semiotic terms). In S. Kita (ed.) *Pointing: where language, culture, and cognition meet*. 171-216, Mahwah, NJ: Lawrence Erlbaum Associates Publishers.

Wurmbrand, S. (2001). *Infinitives: restructuring and clause structure*. Berlin: Mouton de Gruyter.

APPENDICES

A.1. Methods for the EMA Study

Recordings

Simultaneous acoustic and articulatory recordings were collected using EMA (Carstens AG100), for a female native speaker of French. Five pellets were glued midsagittally to the apex, middle and dorsum of the tongue, and to the lower and upper incisors. The EMA data were sampled at 500 Hz, the acoustic data at 16000 Hz. The data were corrected for rotation, low-pass filtered and normalized by the reference pellet to correct for head movements. Velocity and acceleration traces were obtained using a finite difference method.

Corpus

The corpus consisted of several read sentences, containing 4-syllable target words, which constituted an Accentual Phrase. Position of the target word in the sentence was varied (initial, central, final), as in the example below for which the target word is "l'illuminée" (the crank):

'L'illuminée a allumé néanmoins le monument.' (Initial).

The crank has nevertheless lighted the monument.

'Il a humilié l'illuminée en l'éloignant.' (Central).

He humiliated the crank by moving her away.

'L'aumonier a néanmoins éloigné l'illuminée.' (Final).

The chaplain has nevertheless moved the crank away.

The corpus was designed so that analyses were made easier. To facilitate F0 tracking, only sonorants were used, and to obtain clear tongue movements, syllables containing vowels /i/ and /a/, which correspond to large tongue displacements in the horizontal and vertical dimensions, were selected. Several target words were pronounced. Results are presented for the target word: *"l'anomala"* (/la-no-ma-la/, beetle), which entails clear tongue movements on the initial and final syllables. As described in Jun & Fougeron (2000), in the contrastive focus rendition, initial and final syllables are potential spots for the F0 peak to occur.

The sentences were pronounced under two conditions: a neutral (broad focus) condition and a contrastive focus condition. Three speaking rates were produced: slow, normal, fast. Contrastive emphasis or focus was elicited on the target word as follows. Before each recording, a sentence was played to the subject, where the target word had been replaced by a wrong 4-syllable word. The subjects had to correct the sentence, placing contrastive focus on the target word.

Articulatory data analysis

Among the 8 traces (horizontal and vertical positions of the tongue -apex, -middle and -dorsum and of the lower incisor), the vertical position of the tongue-middle showed the most variation. It was thus chosen as the representative articulator. For each syllable, the tongue-middle vertical position at the time the vowel was fully reached, the peak velocity of the movement from the consonant to the vowel, and the duration of the syllable were measured, using hand-labelled events. The spectrogram of the acoustic signal, as well as velocity and acceleration traces, were used to mark these events. As shown in figure 2 for [**la**-no-ma-la], the beginning and end of the syllable were marked using the spectrogram (and listening to the signal) and provided the duration of the syllable. The tongue-middle minimum vertical position for /a/ was measured using zero-crossing of the velocity trace. The peak velocity was measured using zero-crossing of the acceleration trace.

A.2. METHODS FOR THE OPTOTRAK STUDY

For more details the reader can refer to Dohen et al. (2006).

Corpus

The corpus used for this study consisted of 13 subject-verb-object (SVO) structured sentences with CV syllables and, whenever possible, sonorants. Below is an example of one of the sentences used:
Lou ramena Manu. *Lou gave a lift back to Manu.*

Recordings

Four focus conditions were elicited: subject-, verb- and object-focus (narrow focus) and a neutral version (broad focus). In order to trigger contrastive focus, the speakers had to perform a correction task. They heard a prompt in which two speakers were talking and they were then asked to correct a phrase (S, V or O) which had been mispronounced. Two repetitions of each utterance were recorded.
The Optotrak system consists of three infrared (IR) cameras used to track the motion of infrared emitting diodes (IREDs) which in this case were glued to the speaker's face. The 3D coordinates of each IRED were automatically detected. For this experiment, we used two Optotraks in order to compensate for missing data. A total of 24 IREDs were glued to the speakers' faces. An additional 4 IREDs were attached to a head rig and were used to correct for head motion. IRED positions were sampled at 60 Hz and low-pass filtered. The acoustic signals were recorded simultaneously and sampled at 22 kHz.

Acoustic validation

The data recorded were first acoustically validated i.e. it was checked check whether focus had actually been produced acoustically. For all the speakers, we checked that the focused utterances displayed a typical focused intonation and that focus was well perceived auditorily (informal auditory perception tests).

Articulatory measurements

In our previous studies (see *a.*), two articulatory features had been analyzed, namely inter-lip area and protrusion. These parameters best represented the high segmental variability of speech and were the most relevant parameters to isolate supra-segmental originating variations. However, it is not possible to compute inter-lip area accurately from Optotrak data. This is why, in this study, we separately analyzed lip opening (difference between the vertical coordinates of the upper and lower middle lip markers) and lip spreading (difference between the horizontal coordinates of the two lip corner markers). Jaw vertical movements were analyzed using the chin marker. Upper lip protrusion was computed as well.

Facial movements

Based on other studies of the facial movements accompanying speech and more specifically prosody, we decided to limit our study to the head and eyebrow movements. Cavé et al. (1996) showed that eyebrow movements accompanying prosody were mainly raising movements. Therefore we decided to study the raising of both the left and the right eyebrows (middle eyebrow markers). As for head movements, the three rotations and translations were available. Since Munhall et al. (2004) and Graf et al. (2002) had found that the main movements related to prosody were nods, we analyzed the rotation of the rigid body around the horizontal axis.

Data shaping

In order to be able to isolate and compare supra-segmental variations for different segmental constituents, we used a normalization technique. After normalization, a value of 1 corresponds to no variation of the considered parameter compared to the neutral version, a value above 1 corresponds to an increase and a value below 1 to a decrease. For both articulatory and facial movement parameters, we analyzed the inter- and intra-utterance contrasts related to focus (inter: comparison of a phrase in its focused and neutral versions; intra: comparison of a focused phrase with the other phrases of the same utterance).

A.3. METHODS FOR THE FMRI PRODUCTION STUDY

Stimuli

Each sentence was presented for 3 seconds at the beginning of the corresponding condition. Then a fixation mark, alternating every 3 seconds between a '+' and a 'x' sign, appeared in the middle of the screen. This alternation aimed at triggering the silent (covert speech) repetition (14 times per condition) of the sentence presented.

Subjects' performance

Before entering into the magnet, the subjects were trained to execute the tasks, first in overt mode, then in covert mode. In addition, pre- and post-scan audio recordings were carried out to estimate the subjects' task performance during the fMRI scan. Subjects were prompted by exactly the same script as during the scans. They produced each of the sentences 4 times. For the post-scan recording, the instruction was to reproduce in overt speech the intonation patterns mentally produced during the scans. Overall, the subjects' performance, as measured by the audio recordings before and after the scans, indicated that their production varied neither in rhythm nor in intonation between recordings.

fMRI paradigm

Three functional scans were performed. A block paradigm was used. A scan comprised 8 epochs (two repetitions of each condition) of 42 seconds each. The order of presentation of the four conditions was varied across scans and across subjects.

Functional MR imaging was performed on a 1.5T imager (Philips NT) with echo-planar (EPI) acquisition. Twenty-five adjacent, axial, slices (5mm thickness each) were imaged 10 times during each epoch. The imaging volume was oriented parallel to the bi-commissural plane. An EPI MR pulse sequence was used. The MR parameters were: TR = 3700ms, TE = 45ms, pulse angle = 90°, acquisition matrix = 64x64, reconstruction matrix = 128x128, field-of-view = 256x256mm^2. Between the first and second functional scans, a high-resolution 3D anatomical scan was acquired.

fMRI data processing

Data analysis was performed using the SPM-99 software (Wellcome Department of Cognitive Neurology, London). First, motion correction was applied. All images within a functional scan were realigned by means of a rigid body transformation. Then, the anatomical volume was spatially normalized into a reference space using the Montreal Neurological Institute template. The normalization parameters were subsequently applied to the set of functional images. Finally, to conform to the assumption in SPM that the data are normally distributed, the functional images were spatially smoothed.

Contrasts between conditions were determined voxelwise using the General Linear Model. Statistical significance threshold for individual voxels was established at $p = 0.001$. Clusters of activated voxels were then identified, based on the intensity of the individual responses and the spatial extent of the clusters. Finally, a significance threshold of $p = 0.05$ (corrected for multiple comparisons) was applied for identification of the activated clusters.

A.4. Methods for the fMRI perception study

Subjects

Twelve healthy right handed volunteers (Edinburgh Inventory; Oldfield 1971), native speakers of French (4 women and 8 men), with normal or corrected-to-normal vision and normal neurological history were examined. The study was approved by the ATR Human Subject Review and subjects gave informed written consent for experimental procedures.

Stimuli

The stimuli consisted of sentences spoken by a native French speaker (women). 24 were pronounced in normal speech and 6 in whispered speech. The structure of the sentences was: subject (two-syllable first name) - two-syllable action verb - object (two-syllable noun preceded by a one-syllable singular determiner). All syllables were CV syllables (sonorant consonants). An example of one of the sentences used is given below:

Nico mangea le bonbon. *Nico ate the candy.*

The audiovisual stimuli were recorded at ex-ICP (now Speech & Cognition Department – GIPSA-lab) in a sound attenuated room. Two focus conditions were recorded for each sentence: no-focus (neutral) and focus on the subject. A question/answer procedure was used to elicit prosodic focus as naturally as possible. After the recordings, audio data was normalized regarding intensity. Video clips were re-centred for the head of the speaker to be in the middle of the image. Three types of stimuli were designed: audio only (A), visual only (V) and audiovisual (AV). The AV stimuli (avi) were directly extracted from the recordings. Both audio and video streams were then isolated to design the A (wav) and V (avi) stimuli. The duration of all the stimuli was 3s.

During the functional MRI sessions, whenever no video stimulus was displayed on the screen (A only condition and Null Events), the subjects saw a mid-centred black cross that they were asked to fixate (fixation cross).

Procedures

The subjects were told that they would see and/or hear a sentence extracted from a dialogue of the following type:

A: Nico mangea le bonbon. *Nico ate the candy.*

B: Sarah mangea le bonbon ? *Sarah ate the candy?*

A: NICO mangea le bonbon. *NICO ate the candy.*

Two situations were possible: 1. B did not understand who performed the action (as in the example above) and A corrected him (focus case); 2. B understood well but was unsure and repeated the sentence in a question mode and A simply repeated the correct sentence in a neutral mode (no focus case). The subjects were asked to identify the situation: A corrected B or not. They were therefore indirectly asked to identify focus cases.

The stimuli (video and/or audio) were presented to the subjects inside the MR scanner using Neurobehavioural Systems' Presentation software. Audio was presented via MR-compatible headphones (Hitachi Advanced Systems' ceramic transducer headphones). Video was presented through a projector located outside the MR room and a mirror positioned inside the head coil just above the subject's eyes. The subjects responded via a MR-compatible two-button response box placed in their right hand. They were told beforehand that they had to provide an answer even if they were not sure and that they should respond only once the stimulus was finished (fixation cross back).

Prior to the experiment, subjects were trained with the experimental task. Once inside the MR-scanner, the subjects could train using the response box and audio volume was adjusted.

fMRI paradigm

The fMRI procedure consisted of an event-related pseudo-random design. Four functional scans were acquired: two for normal speech and two for whispered speech. Each functional scan consisted of 12 sentences in six conditions: AV+focus, AV+no focus, A+focus, A+no focus, V+focus and V+no focus (72 stimuli). For normal speech, one functional scan used the first 12 sentences available in all conditions and the second the last 12 sentences. For whispered speech, the two sessions both consisted of the same 6 sentences replicated twice for all conditions. A total of 14 null events (NE, fixation cross) were added to the 72 stimuli to vary intertrial interval times. Trials were presented as events lasting 5.1s: stimulus (3s) + response delay (2.1s). NE also lasted 5.1s. The trial sequences were presented following a pseudo-random order. Total duration of a scan was approximately 7 min (5.1s × 86 trials).

fMRI data collection and processing

Blood Oxygenation Level-Dependent (BOLD) contrast was measured over the whole brain using a Shimadzu-Marconi Magnex Eclipse 1.5 Tesla Power Drive 250 imager at the ATR Brain Activity Imaging Center. T2*-weighted images were acquired using a gradient echo-planar sequence (repetition time: 2000ms; echo time: 48ms; flip angle: 80°; 5 initial dummy scans). A total of 20 axial sequential slices with a 3×3×6 mm voxel resolution were acquired. They covered the cortex and cerebellum. A high-resolution 3D anatomical MR scan of the volume examined functionally was acquired after the four functional MR scans (191 slice RF-FAST sequence: repetition time: 12ms; echo time: 4.5ms; flip angle: 20°; voxel size: 1x1x1 mm).

Functional data analysis was performed using the SPM2 software (Statistical Parametric Mapping-Wellcome Department of Cognitive Neurology, London, UK) running on a PC under MATLAB (Mathworks, Sherbon, USA). All the functional images were pre-processed as follows. Movement artifact was corrected for by realigning the images. Differences in acquisition time between slices were accounted for and images were spatially normalized to a standard space. Finally, the images were smoothed using a 6×6 ×14 Gaussian kernel.

The haemodynamic response to the onset of each event was modeled using a delayed haemodynamic response function (HRF). Contrasts were determined voxelwise using a General Linear Model. Statistical significance threshold for individual voxels was established at $p<.01$ uncorrected. Clusters of activated voxels were then identified, based on the intensity of the individual responses and the spatial extent of the clusters (10 voxels). A random effect analysis was then conducted for the group of 12 subjects.

A.5. Methods for the multimodal fMRI study

fMRI paradigm

A pseudorandom, event-related fMRI paradigm was employed. Four functional scans were acquired, one for each type of pointing. Each functional scan included a sequence of the following five conditions: Preparation of the control task (Pc), Preparation + Execution of the control task (PEc), Preparation of the pointing task (Pp), Preparation + Execution of the pointing task (PEp) and a null event (NE, black fixation cross). The five conditions were alternated between scans and between subjects. 24 repetitions of each condition were presented. Trials were presented as events lasting 4.5 s. The duration of the PEp and PEc conditions was of 0.5 s for the initial fixation cross + 2 s for the preparation phase + 2 s for the execution phase. The Pp and Pc conditions consisted of 0.5 s for the fixation cross + 4 s for the preparation phase. NE condition also lasted 4.5 s. The trial sequences were presented in a pseudo-random optimized order. Total duration of a scan was approximately 9 min (4.5 s × 5 conditions × 24 trials).

Apparatus

Three types of behavioural responses were recorded: vocal production, eye movement and index finger movement. Verbal responses were recorded using an fMRI-compatible microphone. To minimize the amount of noise recorded, the microphone was positioned out of the scanner, at one extremity of a wave guide consisting of a soft plastic tube. The other extremity of the tube was connected with a mask placed over the subjects' mouth. This apparatus reinforced the signal-to-noise ratio. Eye position was monitored using an ASL 504 eye-tracker (Applied Science Laboratories, Bedford, MA) coupled with the scanner. Right index finger responses were recorded using a digital camera placed out of the fMRI room, behind the window.

fMRI data acquisition and processing

A whole-body 3 Tesla MRI imager (Bruker) with gradient echo acquisition was used to measure blood oxygenation level-dependent contrast over the whole brain (repetition time: 2.5s; echo time: 30 ms; field of view: 216 x 216 mm, acquisition matrix: 72x72; reconstruction matrix: 128 x 128; 7 dummy scans). Forty-one 3.5 mm axial interleaved slices were imaged parallel to the bi-commissural plane, encompassing the whole brain and the cerebellum. A high-resolution 3D anatomical scan was obtained. Anatomical images were acquired using a sagittal MPRAGE sequence (inversion time: 900ms, volume: 176 x 224 x 256 mm; resolution: 1.375 x 1.750 x 1.33 mm; acquisition matrix: 128 x 128 x 192; reconstruction matrix: 256 x 128 x 128). A B0 fieldmap was acquired twice. Functional data analysis was performed using SPM2 software (Wellcome Department of Cognitive Neurology, London). Functional data were realigned to correct for head motion using a rigid body transformation. A spatial normalisation was applied. The functional images were spatially smoothed.

To examine cerebral activation during the crucial part of the trials (after the preparation phase), the haemodynamic response to the onset of each event was modelled with a delayed haemodynamic response function, empirically shifted to onset 3.5 s later. Contrasts between conditions were determined voxelwise using the General Linear Model. To perform a random effect analysis, the contrast images (pointing vs control) were calculated for each subject individually and were then entered into a one-sample t test with a significance threshold of $p<.005$ uncorrected.

Behavioural results

Monitoring the subjects' utterances included word accuracy and correct prosodic contour productions. Word recognition was possible in the audio signals from all subjects but 2. F0 examination was possible on 9 out of 16 subjects. In the other cases, technical problems with the microphone or the mask drastically degraded the signal. Word accuracy and F0 patterns were correct in all available prosodic and syntactic conditions (and their controls). Eye-tracking data were analyzed with the eye-tracker software. Horizontal positions of the eyes were checked using a Matlab script. Subjects behaved according to the instructions. An overview of the video data on finger movements shows that all the subjects performed adequately.

10

How special is speech?

RUDOLPH SOCK
BÉATRICE VAXELAIRE

Abstract: The main thrust of this work is to show, from experimental evidence, *how* and *to what extent* speech may be considered as being special. A major rationale for stating that speech is special is that the kinematics of speech is different from usual biological movements, as are the configurations or postures adopted by the vocal tract during the production of real words. Underlying such differences in behaviour between speech and other biological movements are the following *constraints,* which are either *speech-specific* or more *salient* in speech as a motor behaviour: 1) there is a constant necessity to *preserve the identity* of a given linguistic category; 2) it is vital to *maintain phonetic and phonological contrasts* even when the speech task becomes difficult, as in fast speech conditions; 3) emerging articulatory and acoustic patterns that are linguistically relevant must be *viable, in motor terms, guided by linguistic constraints.*

1. INTRODUCTION

The title of this chapter inevitably evokes 'The motor theory of speech perception' advocated by Liberman and Mattingly (1985). This is wilful, albeit the various points that will be discussed here are mainly based on production data. We shall, however, endeavour to show relations that may exist between articulatory-acoustic patterns and linguistic constraints.

If we do believe that speech as a human behaviour is special, to some extent, compared with other biological motor activities, it is much more convincing to base our arguments on observable articulatory and kinematic data. This has the convenience of avoiding strong claims that are not always possible to verify experimentally. Although supporting data will be presented and discussed in this chapter, it should be kept in mind that our intention here is rather to bring up theoretical issues than to go into the details of experimental designs and statistical results.

To adequately show how special speech may be, we suggest to distinguish between speech acts that convey meaning from so-called speech acts that may, in certain laboratory conditions be useful, but are meaningless. The latter are judiciously referred to as speech acts because they emanate from the speech production system, without necessarily being constrained by any phonological system. One example of a meaningless speech act is producing sustained vowels.

Varying speech rate will be used across most of the experiments reported here, as a natural means of perturbing the production-perception system. This paradigm has the advantage of helping to observe the flexibility of the speech motor system, and thus evaluating the robustness of emerging articulatory-acoustic patterns. We shall also see later how articulatory and acoustic modifications, induced by increasing speaking rate, may not only help to distinguish between speech motor behaviour and other non semiotic biological movements, but also to understand some aspects of sound change.

We shall, first of all, briefly recall 'The motor theory of speech perception' and explain our stance regarding this theory.

Then we shall present a series of experimental evidence to support our claim that speech is special, and to what extent it could be so. A good amount of results reported here is based on investigations that we have carried out on several vowel quantity languages. However, data from related works will also be presented and commented.

1.1. Recalling the Motor Theory of Speech Perception

It is important to recall, first of all, that Liberman and Mattingly's revised motor theory (1985) is more about perception. However, they later addressed this issue within a speech production framework, providing methodological landmarks in order to examine this problem (Liberman & Mattingly, 1988).

The *first claim* of the theory is that the objects of speech perception are the intended phonetic gestures of the speaker. These intended phonetic gestures are presumably represented in the brain as invariant motor commands. They solicit specific articulatory movements which are linguistically relevant configurations of the vocal tract. These gestural commands are the physical reality underlying traditional phonetic notions such as 'tongue fronting', 'lip spreading' and 'jaw lowering'. They provide the rationale for phonetic categories. According to Liberman and Mattingly (1985), they are the elementary events of speech production and perception, and phonetic segments are merely groups of one or more of such elementary events.

In their terms, to perceive an utterance is to perceive a specific pattern of intended gestures. The choice of the expression 'intended gestures' is deliberate for various reasons: due to coarticulation, the gestures are not directly manifested in the acoustic signal or in the observable articulatory movements. However, a description of invariant gestures of some kind is inevitable, according to the proponents of the theory, in their particular theory and in *any* [their emphasis] theory of speech production (Liberman & Mattingly, 1985, p. 3).

The *second claim* of the theory, resulting from the first is that if speech perception and speech production share the same set of invariants, then they must be closely linked. It is argued that the link is not a learned association (during speech production and speech perception) but rather an innately specified one which requires only epigenetic development to activate it. Further, perception of the gestures are said to occur in a specialised mode, significantly different from the auditory mode. This specialised mode would also be responsible for the production of phonetic structures and part of the larger specialisation for language. In such a perspective, speech perception is not to be explained by principles that apply to perception of sounds in general, but must rather be considered as a specialisation for phonetic gestures. Incorporating a biologically based link between perception and production, this specialisation prevents listeners from hearing the signal as an ordinary sound, but enables them to use the systematic, yet special, relation between signal and gesture to perceive the gesture. The relation is systematic because it results from lawful dependencies among gestures, articulatory movements, vocal-tract shapes, and signal. It is special because it occurs only in speech.

1.2. DIVERTING FROM THE THEORY: A SENSORY-MOTOR PERSPECTIVE

The main thrust of this work is not to confirm or infirm these two major claims of the motor theory. Rather, as was mentioned earlier, we intend to show, from experimental evidence, how and to what extent speech may be considered as being special. Nonetheless it is necessary to make some preliminary clarifications as to our stance regarding the motor theory of speech perception.

We follow the proponents of the theory to say that there are principled dependencies among gestures, articulatory movements, vocal-tract shapes, and the acoustic signal. This systematic relation indeed makes speech special, as it has not been shown to exist in other biological non human 'communicating' systems. For all these reasons, the data presented here is an attempt to examine such relationships, in a sensory-motor perspective.

However, we do not think that a description of *invariant gestures* is inevitable in any theory of speech production. It is now commonplace in speech production and perception research to search for *spatial and/or temporal regularities* rather than absolute or relative invariance in articulatory, acoustic and perceptual data. The pinpointing of such regularities in speech data has contributed significantly to understanding production and perception mechanisms, and to refining models.

Saying that a sensory-motor link is not a learned association but rather an *innately specified* one is a *too powerful* statement to be ascertained experimentally. The same is true of the concept of a specialised mode that would be responsible for the production of phonetic structures and part of the larger specialisation for language (but see Hoonhorst et al., chapter 1, whose works will be discussed later).

As stated earlier, Liberman & Mattingly (1988) did indeed furnish arguments to support the idea of speech being special from the *speech production* point of view.

"Speech movements are, for the most part, peculiar to speech; they have no obvious nonspeech functions. The peculiarity of phonetic gestures is further demonstrated in consequence of the fact that, in most cases, a gesture involves more than one articulator. [...] Cooperation between the articulators is also required in such nonphonetic gestures as swallowing, but the particular cooperative patterns of movement observed in speech are apparently unique, even though there may be nonspeech analogues for one or another of the components of such a pattern. A further indication of the specialness of speech production is that certain of the limited and eccentric set of gestures executed by the tongue tip are paralleled by gestures executed by other major articulators. Thus stops and fricatives can be produced not only by the tongue tip but also by the tongue blade, the tongue body, the lips and the larynx, even though these various articulators are anatomically and physiologically very different from one another [...] Our final argument for the specialness of speech production depends on the fact of gestural overlap. Thus in the syllable [du], the tongue-tip closure gesture for [d] overlaps the lip-rounding and tongue-body-backing gestures for [u]. Even more remarkably, two gestures made by the same articulator may overlap. [...] As we have already suggested, it is gestural overlap, making possible relatively high rates of information transmission, that gives speech its adaptive value as a communication system. But if the strategy of overlapping gestures to gain speed is not to defeat itself, the gestures can hardly be allowed to overlap haphazardly. [...] the gestures are apparently phased so to provide the maximum amount of overlap consistent with the preservation of the acoustic information that specifies either of the gestures [...]. Thus, to borrow Fujimura's (1981) metaphor, the gestural timing patterns of consonants and consonant clusters are iceberg floating on a vocalic sea. Like the individual gestures themselves, these complex temporal patterns are peculiar to speech and could serve no other ecological purpose. We would conclude, then, that speech production is specialized, just as speech perception is. But if this is so, we would argue further that these two processes are not two systems, but, rather, modes of one and the same system."

The latter arguments are, we believe, more convincing as they could be addressed with more reliable empirical backup.

Following this Liberman & Mattingly (1988) perspective, we shall try to show in this chapter that the major rationale for stating that speech is special is that the kinematics of speech is different from usual biological movements; as are the configurations or postures adopted by the vocal tract during the production of real words. Underlying such differences in behaviour between speech and other biological movements are the following constraints, which are either speech-specific or *more salient* in speech among the other motor behaviours:

1) There is a constant necessity to *preserve the identity* of a given linguistic category (this point is not unique to speech but motor constraints are more imposing in speech production compared with handwriting production, for example).

2) It is vital to *maintain phonetic and phonological contrasts* even when the speech task becomes difficult, as in fast speech conditions.

3) Emerging articulatory and acoustic patterns that are linguistically relevant must be *viable, in motor terms, guided by linguistic constraints.*

Above, we have emphasised the notion of *more salient constraints,* because certain motor activities that convey 'linguistic' information (hand writing, sign-language, etc.) could indeed be 'semantically' constrained. We will argue, however, that contrary to speech, which is a precociously acquired sensory-motor behaviour, general motor activities which carry 'linguistic' information and learned relatively tardily *are less constrained.*

The novelty of the discussion of the 'speech is special matter' in this chapter, we believe, is the attempt to rationalise our production data (articulator kinematics and vocal tract postures) in terms of preservation of phonological identity, of phonological contrasts and also of viability constraints.

Let us now turn to experimental data which support our aforementioned claims.

2. EXPERIMENTAL EVIDENCE

2.1. QUANTITY CONTRASTS AND TIMING PATTERNS

Having presented the main motives for stating that speech is a special biological motor behaviour, we will discuss data from vowel quantity languages from an articulatory-acoustic point of view.

Only acoustic data were obtained for some languages. However, conclusions drawn here are based on kinematic and acoustic data that were collected simultaneously for certain languages, using an electromagnetic system (EMMA). They were then analysed within the articulatory and corresponding acoustic domains, called cycles (see below), thus enabling us to establish robust articulatory-acoustic timing regularities. The behaviour of such regularities was further examined in a sensory-motor perspective, with constant reference to linguistic constraints.

The syllabic structures of vowel quantity languages attested in the literature are usually of two types: in one category of languages, that we have called the *simple contrast* category (Sock, 1999), short vowels contrast with long vowels, i.e. VC vs VVC. In another category of languages, called the *complementary distribution* category (Elert, 1964), when the vowel is long, it is followed by a short consonant, and when the vowel is short, it is followed by a long consonant, i.e. VVC vs VCC.

Together with some of our colleagues and students, we have examined the syllabic structures of various vowel quantity languages and classified them within these two categories. Thus German (Elchinger, 1998; Grosshans, 2002), Alsatian (Witz, 1998), Danish (Herzfeld, 1998), Twi (Adu Manyah & Sock, 2002) and Gambian Wolof (Sock, 1983; 1999) would belong to the *simple contrast* group.

Swedish (Sock & Löfqvist, 1995; Sock & Vaxelaire, 2001) and Senegalese Wolof (Becerra Castellano, 1996; Martins, 1996; Camara, 1997) would figure among languages of the *complementary distribution* category.

As for dialectal variations of Arabic, quantity contrasts may rely on the two types of contrastive syllabic configurations. Kuwaiti Arabic (Delattre et al., 1990), Moroccan Arabic (Rhardisse et al., 1990) and Tunisian Arabic (Boussaffa et al., 1991; Jomaa 1991) may thus be classified among the two groups, the *simple contrast* group and the *complementary distribution* one, depending on quantity contrast cognates.

2.2. MEASUREMENT PROCEDURES FOR ACOUSTIC AND MOVEMENT DATA

Based on articulatory and acoustic events in the velocity and audio signals respectively, one interval (among several possible intervals) was identified in the movement of each articulator, and another interval (among several other intervals) was also measured in the acoustic waveform, for all repetitions. Movement and acoustic durations, within the relevant intervals, were then determined by specific articulatory and acoustic timing relations respectively (e.g., Abry et al., 1985). Figure 1 is a representative example of the acoustic signal and the position curve for the vertical displacement of the tongue body (Sock, 1999), for one of the words extracted from the corpus: /fatam/.

The acoustic *Vowel-to-Vowel* duration, measured in the Vowel-Consonant (VC) domain, is defined in the audio signal as the interval from onset of a clear formant structure for the first vowel (V1on) to onset of the same formant structure for the subsequent vowel (V2on). This *Vowel-to-Vowel* duration thus includes the consonant closure of the medial consonant. A *Vowel* interval is determined within the *Vowel-to-Vowel* span, as the steady-state portion between onset of a clear formant structure of the first vowel (V1on) and offset of the formant structure, due to closure (V1of) of the following consonant /t/.

The *Peak-to-Peak Velocity* interval, measured in the VC domain, for the lower lip, the jaw and the tongue body, is defined in the position signal, with the help of the velocity curve, as the duration between successive negative peaks, associated with lowering movements in the production of the vowels. This interval goes from the first negative peak, for the production of the first vowel (Pv1), to the second negative peak (Pv2), associated with the production of the second vowel, which is always /a/.

An articulatory measure, referred to as *Vowel* duration in the position signal, is determined for each articulator, within the *Peak-to-Peak Velocity* duration, as the interval between the first negative peak (Pv1) and peak velocity (Pc1), in the raising movement associated with the production of the medial apical consonant /t/.

It should be mentioned that the acoustic Vowel-to-Vowel interval and the articulatory Peak-to-Peak Velocity span, both specified in the VC domain, had proven useful in portraying quantity contrasts for various languages examined in previous studies (Delattre et al., 1990). Moreover, the kinematic Peak-to-Peak Velocity interval seems to coincide best, in terms of timing characteristics, with the acoustic Vowel-to-Vowel duration, compared with other intervals (such as movement onsets) that could also be defined on a position signal.

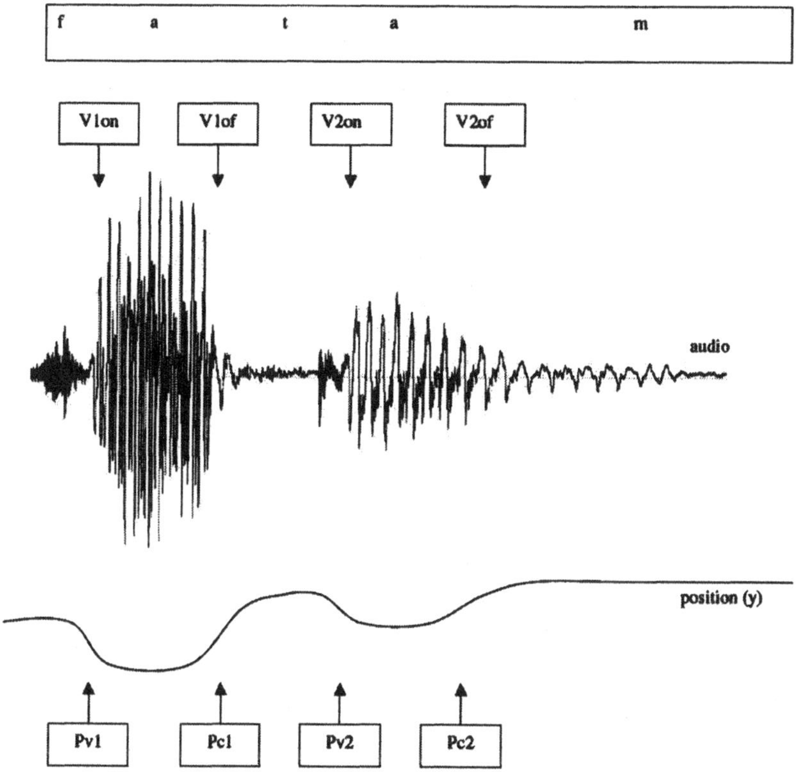

Figure 1: A representative signal of the audio for the Wolof word /fatam/ and the position signal of the tongue-body (adapted from Sock, 1999). In the audio signal, 'V1on' corresponds to the onset of a clear formant structure of the first vowel and 'V1of' to the offset of the formant structure of this vowel, due to the closure of the following consonant /t/. Likewise, 'V2on' corresponds to the onset of a clear formant structure of the second vowel, which is always /a/, and 'V2of' to the offset of the formant structure of this second vowel, due to the closure of the following consonant /m/. In the position signal 'Pv1' is the first negative peak in the production of the first vowel and Pv2 is the second negative peak, associated with the production of the second vowel. Pc1 is the first positive peak associated with the production of the medial consonant /t/ and Pc2 corresponds to the second positive peak associated with the production of the final consonant /m/.

Results obtained for several quantity languages, and reported in Sock (1999), have shown that articulator movements are efficient in portraying quantity contrasts, for both vowels and consonants, only when the peak velocity of the movement of the articulator is attained, and not at its onset.

Please keep in mind that the discussion of the results that follow systematically refers to kinematic and acoustic phasing patterns. This is so because the cycles retained have allowed unveiling *structurally similar* patterns in the articulatory and acoustic domains.

2.3. LINGUISTIC AND PHYSICAL CONSTRAINTS AND THE COMPLEMENTARY DISTRIBUTION CATEGORY

Our data systematically show that *relative stability* of vocalic phasing patterns is the preferential manoeuvre deployed in order to obtain and preserve quantity contrasts in languages which belong to the *complementary distribution* category. It is posited that, in this case, the relative stability observed is essentially determined by linguistic constraints. Thus intra-class relative stability serves to ensure the linguistic contrast in a given speech rate condition. Inter-class stability is the strategy used to preserve vowel quantity contrasts in all speech rate conditions. Such results allow stating that maintaining phasing patterns relatively stable is principally a phonological constraint: only trajectories that are *viable* for the phonological contrast are borrowed.

Apart from this strategy, which consists in maintaining phases relatively stable, are there other trajectories that phonetic classes could follow while remaining within viability limits of the phonological contrast (see Figure 2)?

Long vowels could increase their vocalic phases in both rate conditions. Such a behaviour has been observed in very rare cases; however, the increase was quite insignificant. This is so, because the proportion of the vowel phase may not be increased beyond certain limits without provoking remarkable consequences on the nature of the complementary consonantal phase in the Vowel-Consonant domain.

Indeed, in a voiceless stop context, a too pronounced increase in the vowel phase would, of course, imply significant reduction of the proportion of the consonant, eventually provoking voicing of the latter.
In a voiced stop context, any remarkable augmentation of the vowel phase will have the same shortening effect on the complementary consonantal phase. In such a case, a remarkably reduced voiced consonant could end up being too short, becoming a *flapped* consonant. Consequently, from a perspective of voicing preservation – whether phonologically relevant or phonetically realised – choosing to increase the proportion of the vowel phase in the Vowel-Consonant domain does not correspond to a viable trajectory.
Another option would be to reduce the proportion of the vowel phase of the long vowels. This implies a drift towards the short vowels, which is absolutely an unwanted strategy, if one accepts that a fundamental *raison d'être* of phonological productions is to preserve distinctions in all speech conditions. It happens at times, for the complementary distribution languages, that long vowels are constrained to slightly reduce the proportion of their vowel phases when speech rate is increased: the reduction, however, is always small and statistically not significant. The best solution for this category of long vowels is thus to maintain the proportion of their vocalic phasing patterns relatively stable: it is generally such a timing behaviour that is adopted.
As regards short vowels, no increase of the proportion of the vocalic phase is observed in general; this avoids collision with their longer counterparts. However, when such behaviour is observed, it is only in cases where phase differences between the two phonological categories are sufficiently large in order to tolerate eventual vowel phase lengthening in the short category.
Another consequence of increase of the vocalic phase of short vowels would be a reduction of the proportion of the complementary consonantal phase in the Vowel-Consonant domain. Let us recall that vowel quantity contrast for the complementary distribution class is always reinforced by a difference in consonantal phase.

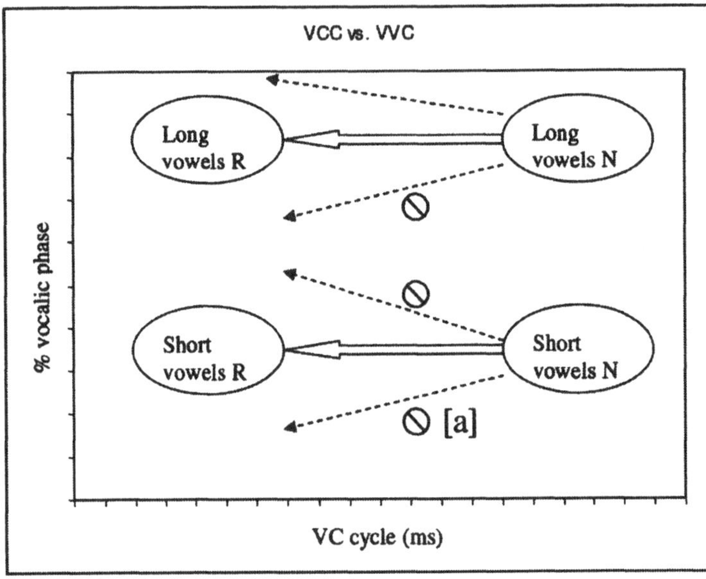

Figure 2: A schemata, adapted from Sock (1999) showing the percentage of the vocalic phase (and opening movement phase) in the Vowel-Consonant (VC) cycle. Short vowels belong to the VCC category and long vowels to the VVC one. The letters 'N' and 'R' refer respectively to normal and rapid or fast speech rates. Unfilled arrows indicate preferred trajectories, broken-line arrows correspond to possible trajectories, which may also be detrimental to preservation of quantity contrasts or to the identity of the vowel, and the symbol '⃠' indicates a proscribed reduction of the phonologically short vowel [a].

It is thus clear that kinematic pathways followed under increased speaking rate (and the corresponding acoustic patterns) are not dictated by usual motor control principles. When biological tasks, like pointing or grasping, are sped up, absolute and relative durations in executing the task are most usually compressed. It could indeed be considered surprising for a given vowel phase to maintain its proportion within its cycle relatively stable, let alone increase it in fast speech. Such behaviours may only become clear when linguistic constraints are taken into account, as has been done above.

2.4. LINGUISTIC AND PHYSICAL CONSTRAINTS AND THE SIMPLE CONTRAST CATEGORY

Concerning quantity contrasts for languages belonging to the *simple contrast* category, *variability* is the most frequent strategy adopted in order to maintain linguistic contrasts. Differences between phonological categories rely on both vocalic phases and vocalic cycles, in normal and fast speaking conditions. Intra-class variability is sufficiently low, such that linguistic entities remain distinct. Intra-class variability serves to maintain or even enhance quantity contrasts, when speaking rate is increased. The goal, here also, is to avoid trajectories that may be borrowed by vowels that belong to the other degree of quantity. The result is obtained by either an increase or a reduction of the vowel phase proportion in the VC cycle.

Thus, when long vowels reduce the proportion of their vowel phase under the effect of speech rate, the shorter counterparts also do likewise. Correlatively, when short vowels can no longer reduce the proportion of their vowel phase – for reasons related to preservation of their linguistic identity – it is the longer counterparts that are constrained to increase theirs. Here again, it is the linguistic viability of trajectories that is the most determining factor. Now, let us take a closer look at permitted trajectories in this VC domain (see Figure 3).

Long vowels may reduce the proportion of their vowel phase when speech rate is increased, while avoiding a too pronounced compression, which may provoke collision with their shorter counterparts. The amount of reduction of long vowels thus directly depends on that of short vowels and vice versa, if the general behaviour observed is vowel phase reduction in fast speech.

Reduction of long vowels will have, as may be foreseen, consequences on the proportion of the consonantal phase in the VC domain, i.e. increase in the proportion of this consonantal phase. However, such consequences will not provoke modifications in the voiced vs voiceless phonological stop distinction (if this distinction is relevant at all in the quantity language studied).

Long vowels may also increase their vocalic phase in fast speech; it is indeed the behaviour usually observed in cases where the duration of short vowels resist reduction. This strategy has the effect of enhancing the linguistic contrast. It should be noted that this vowel phase increase remains sufficiently small so as to avoid having major effects on the proportion of the consonant. Nevertheless, the immediate consequences on the consonant do not seem to be of particular concern here, since this consonantal phase does not contribute to reinforcement of quantity contrasts (as is the case in the *complementary distribution* category; see below). Under the effect of increased speaking rate, short vowels reduce their vowel phase, if the intrinsic nature of the vowel calls for it. Thus the short vowel /a/, intrinsically long, is in some cases incompressible beyond certain limits. If, however, a short vowel may not resist compression imposed by a very fast speaking rate, it is the consonantal context which seems to largely ensure the identity of the vowel, transformed into an ultra-short vowel. The consonantal context catering for an ultra-reduced vowel's identity, will be even more efficient, the higher the articulatory proximity between the vowel and the consonant. One finding (Sock, 1983; 1999) could illustrate this phenomenon: the Gambian Wolof word /futam/ ('his blister') becomes at times /f*tam/, but is still perceived /futam/ in fast speech.

If indeed the timing of such short vowels may largely depend on the consonantal context for their identity, that of the long vowels are generally more constrained in their trajectories when speech rate is increased. A certain *threshold* and *critical* value of the vowel phase for long vowels has to emerge, and any drift of this vowel phase, when speaking rate increases, has to be adequately negotiated.

Here also, determining factors that seem to condition speech motor behaviours (and the corresponding acoustic patterns) are to be found in the linguistic domain.

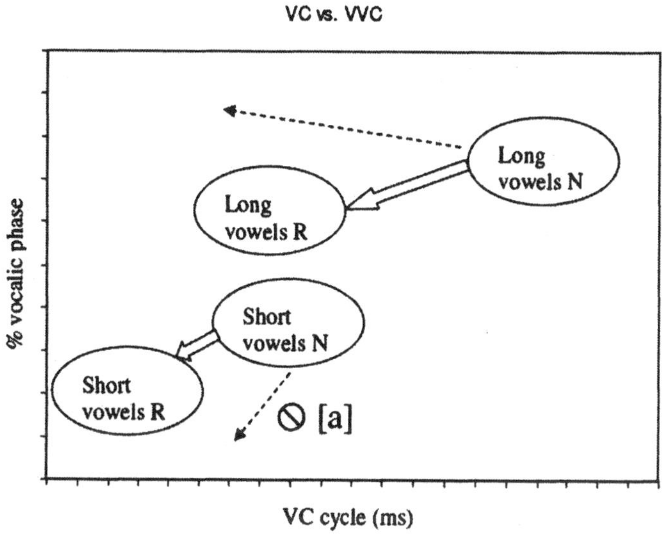

Figure 3: A schemata showing the percentage of the vocalic phase (and opening movement phase) in the Vowel-Consonant (VC) cycle. Unfilled arrows indicate preferred trajectories, broken-line arrows correspond to possible trajectories, which may also be detrimental to preservation of quantity contrasts or to the identity of the vowel, and the symbol '⊘' indicates a proscribed reduction of the phonologically short vowel [a].

2.5. SPEECH RATE AND THE DRIFT OF COMPLEX SYLLABIC STRUCTURES

The tendency for complex structures of the type VVCC, VCC and VVC to drift towards a simple VC structure when speaking rate increases, i.e. when the speech task becomes more 'difficult', could help in distinguishing, to a certain extent, speech motor behaviour from general biological motor ones.

The effect of the drift on phonological distinctions depends on the nature of phasing patterns in the different kinematic and acoustic cycles.

As regards vowel quantity contrasts, increasing speech rate provokes compression of cycle durations with either:

1) A *convergence tendency* of contrasting syllabic structures in the VC zone in fast speech (or the abovementioned trend for complex structures to drift towards a simple VC structure): this has been observed for some languages (some variants of Arabic and Gambian Wolof) that belong to the *simple contrast* category (VC vs VVC) that we have labelled relatively fragile quantity languages or

2) A more or less parallel drift of contrasting syllabic structures without, however, merging of phonological classes: it is the case for languages (some variants of Arabic and Swedish) that belong to the *complementary distribution* category (VCC vs VVC) that we have called more robust quantity languages.

From data on consonantal quantity contrasts (Christmann, 1998 for Italian; Chardi, 2004 for Kabyle; Bouarourou, 2006 for Tarifit Berber) it has been shown that increasing speech rate also provokes compression of cycle durations. In the consonantal cycle, contrastive structures have distinct consonantal phasing patterns in normal speech, and a drift of classes towards the single consonant zone in fast speech occurs without collision of phonological classes. This is the case for geminates in Arabic with contrasts of the type VC vs VCC and VVC vs VVCC. The scenario is thus similar to that of syllabic structures that rely on the complementary distribution of quantity, such as in Arabic and in Swedish.

In summary, our data on trajectories borrowed by vocalic and consonantal phonological classes, due to increase in speech rate, reveal two major articulatory-acoustic strategies:

1) in the simple contrast category, a drift of contrasting classes towards the simplest syllabic structure, with a tendency for convergence;

2) in the complementary distribution category and in the case of geminates, a drift of contrasting classes towards the zone of the simplest structure while resisting to any convergence. In the latter case, it is parallel paths that are adopted by contrasting classes.

Let us take the liberty of making a slight detour into *structural drifts* in relation to *phonetic changes*. Such changes are usually due, *among other factors*, to speaking rate conditions (McCarthy, 1986; Browman & Goldstein, 1986). To illustrate this phenomenon, we would like to cite an example of rationalisation of the evolution of certain consonantal categories, which was adequately re-interpreted in motor terms by Kelso et al. (1986). They judiciously recalled that Stetson (1928) was the real precursor in the matter. Let us remind the paradigm. The task that Stetson had asked his subjects was to repeat, while *accelerating* speech rate, CVC syllables in order to produce a continuum, beginning with double abutted consonants, then going on to geminates to singletons, (CV**C**+**C**VC => CV**CC**VC => CV**C**VC). The idea behind this experiment was to demonstrate the fact that current modifications, provoked by speech rate, were the main causes of permanent historical linguistic changes (see e.g. *'abbam'* in Latin which gave *'abe'* in Ancient French, or *'addubare'* which gave *'adouber'* in French, etc.). It was in this perspective that Kelso et al. (1986) took up another experiment by Stetson analysed within the conceptual framework of *phase transitions*. Preferential in-phase relations between vowels and consonants could explain the universality of CV syllables compared with VC ones (see also Wioland, 1985 for a study on a more frequent occurrence of CV syllables in French). The fact that /ip+ip => ipip.../ ends up in /pipi/ but never the contrary, seems to coincide fairly well with an experiment on the control of finger movements. The index fingers that were, at movement onset, in phase opposition (i.e. anti-symmetrically in flexion and in extension), switched on 'inevitably' towards an in-phase mode when the task was sped up (Tuller & Kelso, 1990).

On this point about modifications of phase relations, Tuller & Kelso (1990) finally presented speech data which, in general, did not highlight expected phase transitions (except for one phonetician subject). In fact, several problems cropped up while subjects tried to carry out the basic task:

1) The first problem related to suppressing the juncture /ip#ip => ipip/.

2) The second had to do with absence of a real vocalic gesture, from vowel to vowel (since within this paradigm, one is dealing with the same vowel).

3) Finally, and most importantly, having to control two consonantal gestures, lip closing and glottal opening, creates an idiosyncratic phenomenon in English: subjects end up producing aspirated /p^{h}i/, which is a phase opposition.

Regardless of all these obstacles, it must be admitted that this phase dynamics approach seems promising, even if the problem of conceptual transfer in terms relevant to speech has not yet been completely solved.

It is, however, crucial here, talking about simplification processes and about the problem of conceptual transfer of motor control paradigms to the area of speech production, to reaffirm the major claim in this chapter: the production of linguistic gestures (that have acoustic and perceptual dimensions) do *not follow* the same organisational principles as those generally attested in human motor control studies. Indeed, our investigations in speech motor control indicate that trajectories adopted by various phonological categories, when speaking rate is increased, are largely constrained by demands of the linguistic type (phonology and, in a broader sense, semantics). More specifically, quantity phasing patterns that are preferentially adopted, when speaking rate is sped up, are not the most stereotyped ones. Such is, however, the case in other human motor control behaviours, which follow general principles of movement control economy.

We have seen that some complex syllabic entities maintain their initial phasing patterns relatively stable, thus resisting any simplification process towards a simpler zone, because of preservation of quantity contrasts. Such is the case in VCC vs VVC contrasts.

Other complex patterns of quantity contrasts – VVCC, VCC, VVC – do not usually merge with the simplest VC category. However, in vowel quantity languages where the linguistic contrast is regarded as being fragile, ultimate convergence of categories implies neutralisation of the contrast, at least in the temporal domains observed. The simplification process would thus contribute to the disappearance of quantity contrasts in such languages. It therefore seems clear why linguistic systems – which essentially are systems based on contrastive relations – tend to resist such evolutionary processes, contrary to most non-semiotic human motor control behaviours.

It could be argued, however, that some non-semiotic human behaviours such as walking and running may adopt motor characteristics similar to those found in speech. Indeed, Shapiro and colleagues (1981), and also Hildebrand (1985) reported variations in cycle durations as a function of walking and running speed. Regardless of these changes in cycle durations provoked by variations in speed, differences between the two motoric activities are preserved by maintained differences in their phasing patterns.

In an earlier study (Abry et al., 1990), a comparison between speech timing patterns and those observed in locomotion, indeed served to pinpoint similarities between these two motor activities. However, such a comparison may not go beyond factors such as control strategies related to limb anatomy, biomechanics and dynamics, mechanical interactions between 'articulators'... (see Fuchs & Perrier, 2005, for a discussion on the far from straightforward interpretation of speech kinematics in terms of underlying speech motor control). The phasing patterns in speech are specific in that *in addition* to the physical properties they share with locomotion, such patterns are constrained by linguistic factors. We have endeavoured to uncover these linguistic factors in our quantity studies reported above, and have also tried to show to what extent they weigh on the physical properties of speech movements.

Motor activities devoted to 'linguistic' communication do, in general, show speech-like characteristics. Thus looking at the simultaneity of the two limb movements in sign-language production for brain damaged signers, Tyrone (2007) observed the following:

"*Simultaneity is affected in a variety of ways in atypical signers with aphasia or with movement disorders* [...] *Some aspects of simultaneity do not seem to be inherently linguistic in nature* [...] *By contrast, there are aspects of simultaneity that are fundamentally linguistic in nature, as evident from the fact that they are preserved in individuals with articulatory disorders but not in those with aphasia.*" (p. 330)

These results indeed show that, as is the case in speech production, inter-articulator timing in sign-language is strongly constrained by linguistic factors. Tyrone (2007) judiciously raises the idea of carrying out research particularly on the characteristics of sign articulation, so that the properties of the language that result from motor control can be teased apart from those that are linguistic and arbitrary in nature. The question that naturally crops up is the relationship between signing and mouthing during typical and atypical sign production. We wonder if it is not mouthing, i.e. a speech component, which conveys linguistic constraints to signing? This issue needs to be looked into.

Looking at the literature on monkey calls, Ghazanfar et al. (2007), for example, have shown that rhesus monkeys use formant variability in 'coo' calls to assess the age-related body-size differences of conspecifics. This finding may suggest that the acoustic variability of the rhesus monkeys' calls could be constrained by communication purposes, ensuring the right perception of the calls and allowing the distinction between communication-related and subject-related information.

It is likely, as suggested by Ghazanfar and Logothetis (2003), and Ghazanfar et al. (2007) that the existence of multimodal perception in an animal's communication signals may correspond to an evolutionary predecessor of humans' capability to make the multimodal associations essential for speech perception. It is also likely that the link between rhesus monkey perception and human perception is direct since they are closely related species. Nonetheless, as mentioned by Ghazanfar et al. (2007), in human speech perception, indexical cues (or the above-mentioned capacity to extract important information related to the physical characteristics of the speaker from formants) are *coupled with phonetic cues*. 'Coo' and 'threat' calls are the most frequently produced calls in the rhesus monkey repertoire, both in the wild and in captivity. As Ghazanfar et al. (2007) tell us, coo calls are *long*, tonal signals and are produced in an affiliative context, threat calls, by *contrast*, are noisy, pulsatile calls of *short* duration and are produced during agonistic encounters. Coo calls are associated with a small mouth opening and protruding lips, whereas threat calls are accompanied with a large mouth opening and no lip protrusion. It is quite tempting to see in these animal sensory-motor behaviours speech-like acts. It is, however, a far cry from, for example, long and short vowels in quantity languages. Long and short vowels in such languages are usually produced across a broad range of sounds, and arranged in complex contrasting phonological systems. This is a few, among other aspects, that are unique to speech, compared with vocalisations of nonhuman primates.

2.6. QUANTITY CONTRASTS AND CONSTRAINED VELOCITY PROFILES

Examining velocity profiles may also reveal speech-specific patterns, furnishing complementary information on gestural control and on the formation of trajectories in the production of quantity contrasts. A study carried out by Abry et al. (1993) on the search for correlates of quantity contrasts in the temporal domain, and similar to ours (Sock et al., 2006), allows comparing jaw phasing patterns with velocity profiles (see Figure 4).

The figure shows velocity profiles for the jaw elevation gesture, i.e. the consonantal closing gesture which goes from onset of jaw raising, in order to produce the consonant, to onset of jaw lowering to produce the subsequent vowel (CCO or Consonantal Cycle Onset – VCO or Vocalic Cycle Onset). The acceleration phase (CCO – MCV or Maximum Consonantal Velocity), corresponding to the interval between onset of jaw lowering and peak velocity of this elevation gesture, is given as a percentage of the global closure gesture. The authors retained this closure gesture because, according to them, it is within this phase (and not in the lowering phase) that differences in velocity profile symmetries/asymmetries were better correlated with phasing patterns of quantity contrasts, VCC vs VVC. It could indeed be seen in Figure 4 that at a normal speaking rate, VCC velocity profiles of all speakers are skewed to the left, whereas those of the VVC category are rather symmetrical. According to the authors, the fact that VCC velocity profiles are skewed to the left, thus tending to present a plateau on the right, may directly be related to the production of the geminate consonant /zz/, which follows the short vowels. The production of this geminate consonant would recruit the jaw in order to reinforce the tongue blade gesture.

Abry et al. (1993) note, however, that the fact that for the VVC category, both slow and fast closing gestures may be clearly symmetrical is an observation contrary to results attested in the literature on motor control, be it in speech (Nelson et al., 1984; Kelso et al., 1985; Ostry & Flanagan, 1989) or in mastication. It is worthwhile signalling that a study by Adams et al. (1993) recalls that the *tendency* to produce bell-shaped velocity profiles in fast speech is a generalized behaviour, whereas in slow speech, profiles are more chaotic.

Certain speakers who lose their quantity contrasts in fast speech (presumably relayed by correlates of quality), thus adopting relatively symmetrical profiles, is in line with general principles of gestural economy in motor control.

Such findings correspond to tendencies found in some of our results, thus depicting a drift of complex structures (VVC, VCC, VVCC...)

towards a VC convergence zone, when speech rate is increased. This behaviour corresponds to a simplification process of phasing patterns and a tendency for bell-shaped velocity profiles, to the detriment of preservation of robust phonological distinctions. Again, simplification processes have only been depicted in very few quantity languages, classified as fragile quantity languages.

Thus *some aspects of motor behaviour,* in these particular cases for such languages, are no more special than other biological motor areas, i.e. when linguistic quantity constraints have been relayed by other constraints, like quality, for example.

Indeed, real bell-shaped symmetrical velocity profiles were shown to correspond to an optimal control (see, for example, Nelson, 1983), but only in the case of target directed single movements, and in the absence of any friction or contact with external bodies. This is obviously not the case in jaw elevation gestures associated with the production of geminate alveolar consonants. It could be argued that this is the reason why we do not observe bell-shaped symmetrical velocity profiles in speech. However, tendencies for bell-shaped symmetrical velocity profiles in speech could help in uncovering those aspects that relate more to the physical properties of the production system than to underlying linguistic constraints.

Clear experimental evidence supporting the hypothesis that speech movement control could be different from other orofacial movement control was found by Tremblay et al. (2003). These authors found that the perturbation of jaw opening gestures with velocity-dependent horizontal forces induces, over time, compensations in speech movements, which preserve the articulatory path, while no compensation was observed in non-speech movements. Compensations in speech movements had no measurable or perceptible effect on acoustic output. In other words, they show that somatosensory information by itself is essential to the emergence of speech movements. Their demonstration comprised a dissociation of somatosensory and auditory feedback (in a silent speech condition that explicitly removed auditory feedback) during speech production.

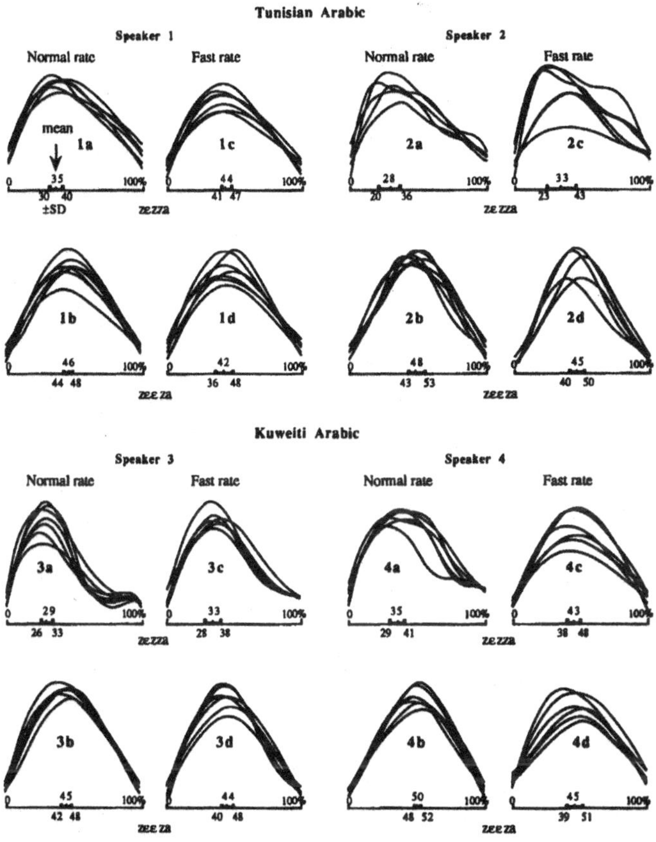

Figure 4: Velocity profiles of the jaw elevation gestures (CCO-VCO) in four subjects, duration normalised. N.B.: amplitude scales were normalised by rounding up values to the higher integer; initial and final values correspond to samples closest to zero+ velocity (Abry et al., 1993).

They posit that the positions of speech articulators and associated somatosensory inputs constitute a goal of speech movements that is wholly separate from the sounds produced. Particularly in line with our major claim in this chapter is the finding that speech movements are readjusted, to reassemble regular articulatory speech patterns, following a perturbation, whereas no compensatory readjustment is found for non-speech movements, thus pointing to the specificity of speech gestures.

In this realm of research works, another interesting study suggesting a possible specificity of speech movement control was proposed by Tremblay et al. in 2008. The question they addressed is a dominant hypothesis in motor control studies, i.e. the idea that the brain controls movement based on a neural representation of limb dynamics. Thus, if speech learning results in a generalisable dynamics representation, then, at least, learning should transfer when similar movements are couched in phonetically different utterances. Using a velocity-dependent perturbation paradigm, similar to that in the Tremblay et al. (2003) study, these authors observed that speech learning is highly contextually sensitive and fails to transfer even to utterances that involve very similar movements. Speech learning thus seems to be very local and the specificity of learning is contradictory with any generalization across the whole articulatory space.

2.7. SPEECH MOVEMENTS AND VOCAL TRACT POSTURES THAT CONVEY MEANING

Our X-ray data have allowed us to confirm the existence of a tight coupling between the movement of the larynx and that of the hyoid bone (Vaxelaire & Sock, 1997). The displacement of the hyoid bone is diagonal in nature, with an elevation movement accompanied by a backward translation. This backward translation thus corresponds to the horizontal component of the hyoid bone movement. High correlations have been found (Vaxelaire & Sock, 1997) between the vertical displacement of the larynx and the horizontal component of the diagonal movement of the hyoid bone. Figures 5 and 6 show larynx (and hyoid bone) trajectories across VCV sequences, where V1 is always the high vowel /u/ and V2 the low vowel /a/. In Figure 5, in normal speech (left graph), it can be seen that the position of the larynx for Speaker MM (female) is 18 mm on average during vocal tract configurations corresponding to the production of the vowel /u/ (frames 863 to 867); this larynx position attains an average value of 24 mm in vocal tract configurations relative to the production of the vowel /a/ (frames 871 to 876). When speaking rate increases (right graph), the initial position of the larynx to produce vowel /u/ (frames 544 to 546) is now at 23 mm on average (we will take up this point again below); it will attain a 29 mm value in the vowel /a/ configurations (frames 550 to 555).

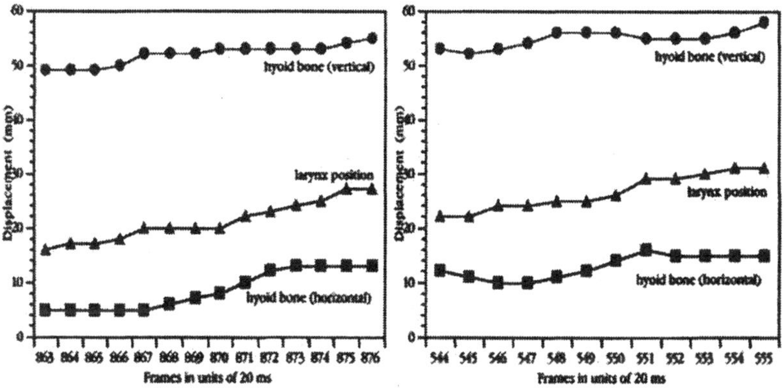

Figure 5: Larynx (vertical displacement) and hyoid bone (vertical and horizontal displacements) for an /uta/ sequence in normal speech (left) and fast speech (right); speaker MM (female). The y-axis shows displacement of these structures (mm) and the x-axis indicates time, in frames of 20 ms (Vaxelaire & Sock, 1997).

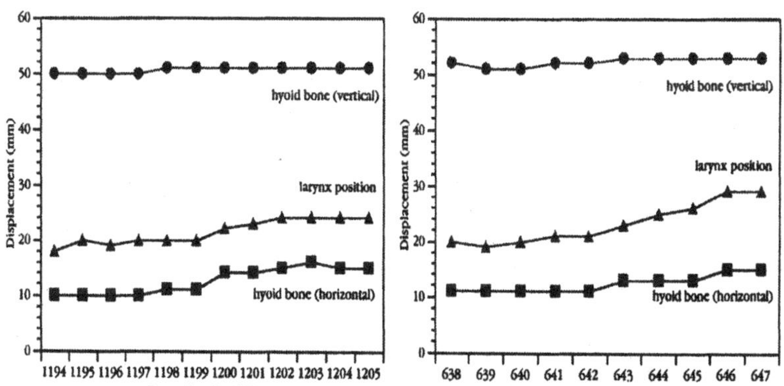

Figure 6: Larynx (vertical displacement) and hyoid bone (vertical and horizontal displacements) for an /uka/ sequence i+n normal speech (left) and fast speech (right); speaker MM (female). The y- axis shows displacement of these structures (mm) and the x-axis indicates time, in frames of 20 ms (Vaxelaire & Sock, 1997).

Notice, incidentally, that displacement amplitude of the larynx, from configurations related to the production of the high vowel to those of the low vowel is similar in both speech rate conditions: it is of 6 mm on average. When we compare Figures 5 and 6, two facts can be observed:
1) a similarity between larynx and hyoid bone trajectories across VCV sequences;
2) a structural resemblance of trajectories, despite differences in the consonantal context /t/ or /k/, and speakers.
This robust correlation between the two structures, regardless of segmental (vocalic or consonantal) and prosodic contexts (speech rates, male voice, female voice, high pitch, low pitch, etc.), have authorised us to consider these two entities as a single functional unit as from now on.
It has been found that the position of the larynx is systematically lower for so-called closed vowels compared with their open counterparts. Such a finding corroborates results obtained by Bothorel (1975) for a dialect of Breton spoken in Argol. Our data reveal that for sequences like /upa/ (in the sentence "Nous pâlissons." and /apu/ (in the sentence "Il a pourri.") – sequences for which production of the consonant does not require active intervention of the tongue – the tongue body moves in a direction opposite to that of the larynx-hyoid bone couple. While the tongue body adopts a constantly descending trajectory during production of /upa/ sequences, the larynx-hyoid bone unit, on the contrary, continues its elevation movement. Figure 7 shows these trajectories of the larynx (coupled with the hyoid bone) and the tongue body across an /upa/ sequence, in normal (on the left) and fast (on the right) speech rates. This gestural pattern is symmetrical opposite to that observed for the production of an /apu/ sequence. In both cases, the result for an /u/ configuration is a maximal distance between the tongue body and the larynx-hyoid bone couple. For the /a/ configuration, this distance between the tongue body and the larynx-hyoid bone couple is minimal. The scenario is the same in fast speech, and when the vowel /u/ is replaced by the vowel /y/ (Vaxelaire, in preparation).

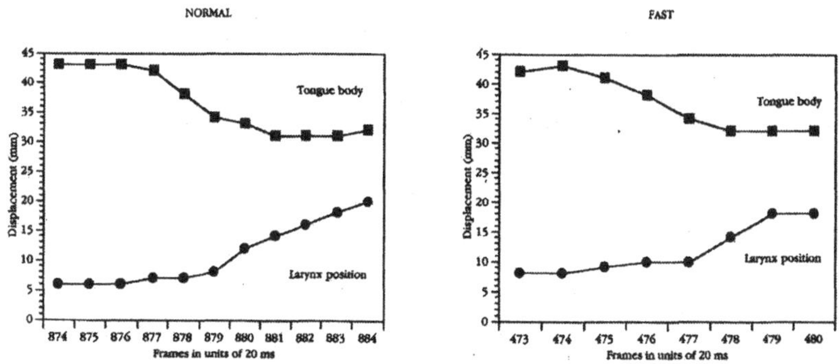

Figure 7: A frame-by-frame analysis of an /upa/ sequence in normal (left) and fast (right) speech rates. It can be seen in the figure that relative timing of the gestures of the tongue body and of the larynx are similar in the two speech rate conditions (Vaxelaire & Sock, 1997).

Since the movement of the set larynx-hyoid bone is inversely correlated with the vertical displacement of the tongue body, and consequently, with vowel aperture, our data systematically reject the tongue-pull hypothesis. More precisely, we are making reference here to a version of this hypothesis which claims a strong relation between tongue body raising, the hyoid bone and the rigid structures of the larynx. There would thus be a high and positive correlation between displacement of these three structures, where the vertical displacement of the tongue body would cause vertical displacement of the larynx-hyoid bone couple and, thereby, reduction of vowel constriction diameter. This hypothesis that was first advocated by Ladefoged (1964), then Lehiste (1970), also tried to establish a correlation between these raising gestures and variations in F0: the tongue, while rising to produce the most closed vowels, would pull the hyoid bone and the larynx upwards, thus provoking tension in the vocal folds and, consequently, F0 elevation. However, data attested in the literature do not confirm this hypothesis. Later, the different proponents of the hypothesis had either simply to reject it (Ladefoged et al., 1972) or to revise it claiming its relevance in *singing* or in the production of *sustained vowels,* and admitting its invalidity in speech production (Ohala & Eukel, 1978). The behaviour of these three structures has been explained by contraction of specific

muscles: the geniohyoid, the anterior belly of the digastric and the mylohyoid (see Perkell, 1969 for an explanation).
The point that is being made here is simply that since speech acts like singing and producing sustained vowels do not convey meaning, gestural control for the larynx and the hyoid bone, for instance, differ from control strategies observed during speech.

2.8. SOME PERCEPTION STUDIES AND THE SPEECH-SPECIFIC ISSUE

Animal, baby and adult comparative studies have served to find out how much speech characteristics are one manifestation of a general sensory-motor behaviour and to what extent some characteristics may be speech-specific. It should be mentioned that most works carried out in these areas do not support the Motor Theory of Speech Perception (see Hawkins, 1999, for an extensive review). However, findings do not give clear-cut answers either to the speech-specific problem.
A key-question that arises in the domain of categorical perception is the following: are perceptual magnet effects (or when a well-formed prototypical sound perceptually attracts similar sounds towards itself) and perceptual constancy (or the categorisation of acoustically very different stimuli into classes based on phonemic contrasts of adults) specific to babies and adults or could they also be found in animals?
Iverson and Kuhl (1995), for example, have shown that in addition to being able to discriminate *between* phonetic categories, 6-month-old babies show evidence of structure *within* phonetic categories, at least for vowels, in that the perceptual space is compressed near the phonetic prototype. This is evidence of the perceptual magnet effect. However, it has also been demonstrated that animals do have magnet effects and that the magnet effect seems to require linguistic experience to develop.
For example, Kuhl and Miller (1975) tested chinchillas' discrimination between /Ca/ syllables containing alveolar stops that varied across a VOT continuum (0 ms, heard as English /d/ at one end, and +80 ms, heard as English /t/, at the other). There were two different responses, and the task was to choose which response to make for each stimulus of the acoustic series. It was thus possible to estimate where the perceptual

boundary between /da/ and /ta/ lay for these birds. After a training period, the chinchillas' response function was remarkably close to that of a group of adult native speakers of English to the same stimuli: the boundary values (50% crossover points) were 33 ms for chinchillas and 35 ms for the humans.

Findings comparing the perceptual capacities of animals and babies do not say to what extent speech perception may be based on special processes rather than general auditory ones, for which animals' perception of speech is of interest. What we know for sure is that, while the baby gradually develops its phonologically relevant capacities in the surrounding speech environment, animals never acquire language in the final analysis!

Neurophysiological studies could help in positing that phonological perception may have developed from basic auditory mechanisms that humans share with animals. Hoonhorst et al. (in this book) hypothesised that if the N100 morphology was the neurophysiological correlate of basic acoustic characteristics implied in voicing perception, then they should observe a double-peak response according to the acoustic universal boundaries. They use the expression 'acoustic universal boundaries' to refer to the initial -30 ms and +30 ms VOT values that define the voicing continuum, acoustic boundaries to which animals and infants less than 6 months old are sensitive to. This would be so, even though the phonological boundary that French-speaking subjects are sensitive to does not coincide with any of these universal boundaries. The phonological boundary would thus represent a higher mode of perception. Their results indeed show that for French-speaking subjects, there is still a clear evoked-potential correlate of the acoustic boundaries. The trace takes the form of a double-on N100 wave appearing when VOT values exceed both positive and negative universal boundaries, thus corroborating Hoonhorst and colleagues' hypothesis that there remains an N100 trace of the basic neurophysiological mechanism on which phonological percepts are developed. Moreover, they indicate that regardless of the region in the VOT continuum exploited by productions of a particular language, the voiced-voiceless contrast is associated with the single vs double-on responses. According to the authors, contrast between long-lead vs short-lag voicing distributions in French is echoed with a differential double vs single-on peaks of N100.

Knowing how modifications of the basic acoustic boundaries influence phonological percepts would indeed help in pinpointing speech-specific mechanisms.

3. CONCLUSIONS

Speech is indeed special, compared with general human and non human behaviours. This statement is in line with Liberman and Mattingly (1988). We have thus made it clear from the beginning that our arguments would rely mainly on production data. Accordingly, we have argued that the processes that underlie speech production motor mechanisms are predominantly governed by linguistic constraints. This does not at all exclude physical constraints related to the production-perception system. The latter, however, do not have the upper hand when the speech production system is in its normal control regime. When pushed to its limits (in accelerated speech for example), linguistic constraints may either prevail over physical constraints and condition the motor behaviour of the production system or, in some rare cases, succumb to the adverse context, and tendencies for stereotyped motor behaviour would then appear.

We have seen that timing patterns of quantity contrasts under fast speech adopt strategies that ultimately serve to preserve phonological entities and also keep them distinct. The different behaviours observed could not be explained in purely motor terms. Syllable types, involved in quantity contrasts, also determine pathways that phonological classes would follow when speech rate is varied. It is on this basis that we have been able to distinguish between languages that belong to the simple contrast category from those that could be classified among the complementary distribution category. In all cases, maintaining quantitative distinctiveness, whatever the category, seems to condition speech motor behaviour.

This is also true for velocity profiles which show speech-specific shapes, explainable however from a phonological perspective. When speech velocity profiles become stereotyped, they appear to obey general motor control principles. Such behaviours allow evaluating the fragility of a phonological distinction in a specific language, and eventually offer insights into sound change phenomena.

Speech-like acts that do not convey meaning differ, to some extent, from real speech acts in motor behaviour. Caution should therefore be taken when paradigms like, for example, production of sustained vowels are retained in order to study laryngeal behaviour. We know from our data that trajectories followed by the larynx and the hyoid bone during speech production are speech-specific.

Other semiotic motor activities, like handwriting, and signing, are also subject to linguistics constraints. Nevertheless, linguistic constraints imposed on such activities are less severe.

We may now want to answer the question: How special is speech? Speech shares many organisational principles with other biological movements. However, the higher the linguistic and the phonological constraints, the more specialised speech motor control strategies become.

ACKNOWLEDGMENTS

The authors are very grateful to Susanne Fuchs, Pascal Perrier and one anonymous reviewer for their insightful comments on an earlier draft of this chapter. We would also like to particularly thank Susanne and Pascal for providing us with relevant bibliographical references. Acknowledgment is also due to Fabrice Hirsch for some of the data collection, and to Kofi Adu Manyah for proof-reading. Some of the findings reported in this chapter were partly funded by an Agence Nationale de la Recherche contract (ANR – DOCVACIM, 2008 – 2011) and a Maison Inter-universitaire des Sciences de l'Homme d'Alsace contract (MISHA – ACM, 2005 – 2008).

REFERENCES

Abry, C., Autesserre, D., Barrera, C., Benoît, C., Boë, L.-J., Caelen J., Caelen-Haumont, G., Rossi, M., Sock, R., and Vigouroux, N. (1985). Propositions pour la segmentation et l'étiquetage des sons du français. *14èmes JEP du GCP du GALF*, 156-163.

Abry, C., Orliaguet, J.-P., and Sock, R. (1990). Patterns of speech phasing. Their robustness in the production of a timed linguistic task: single *vs* double (abutted) consonants in French. *European Bulletin of Cognitive Psychology* 10(3), 269-288.

Abry, C., Bailly, G., Boë, L.-J., Jomaa, M., Laboissière, R., Lallouache, T., Perrier, P., Savariaux, C., and Sock, R. (1993). Contrôle du Mouvement et Cognition en Parole et en Écriture. *Rapport Final du Groupe Représentations Cognitives et Motrices (Pôle régional Rhônes-Alpes de Sciences Cognitives).*

Abry, C.; Boe, L.-J., Cheik Rohou, M. (1995). Facteurs de variation et stabilité de la quantité vocalique en franco-provençal de Saint-Pierre-de Soucy (Savoie): Situation typologique. In : J.-F. BONNOT (ed.) *Parole Régionales, Normes, Variétés Linguistiques et contexte Social,* 38, 289-316, Strasbourg: Presses Universitaires de Strasbourg (Collection:Maison des Sciences de l'Homme de Strasbourg).

Adu Manyah, K., Sock, R. 2002. La quantité vocalique en twi. Considérations phonologiques et étude acoustique préliminaire. *Travaux de l'Institut de Phonétique de Strabourg – TIPS* 31, 1-10.

Becerra Castellano, M.J. (1996). Le statut du /A/ en wolof du Sénégal. Observations phonologiques et étude acoustique. *Mémoire de Maîtrise de Phonétique, UFR PLISE,* Institut de Phonétique de Strasbourg.

Bothorel, A. (1975). Positions et mouvements de l'os hyoïde dans la chaîne parlée. *Travaux de l'Institut de Phonétique de Strasbourg* 7, 80-132.

Bouarourou, F. (2006). Etude de la gémination en tarifit. *Projet de Recherche de Phonétique, UFR PLISE,* Institut de Phonétique de Strasbourg.

Boussaffa, F., Jomaa, M., Sock, R. (1991). Les contraintes temporelles des types consonantiques sur le timing mandibulaire de la quantité en arabe tunisien. *XIIth International Congress of Phonetic Sciences,* Aix-en-Provence (France), 306-309.

Browman, C.P. & Goldstein L. (1986). Towards an articulatory phonology. *Phonology Yearbook* 3, 219-252.

Camara, M. (1997). L'organisation temporelle de l'opposition de quantité en wolof du Sénégal. *Mémoire de Maîtrise de Phonétique,* Institut de Phonétique de Strasbourg.

Chardi, D. (2004). Etude de la quantité et de la qualité consonantiques des constrictives du kabyle. *Mémoire de Maîtrise de Sciences du Langage, UFR PLISE,* Institut de Phonétique de Strasbourg.

Christmann, A. (1998). La résistivité de la gémination en italien. *Mémoire de Maîtrise de Phonétique,* Institut de Phonétique de Strasbourg.

Delattre, C., Jomaa, M., Al-Dossari, A., Worley, C., and Sock, R. (1990). Comparaison articulatori-acoustiques des structures temporelles en arabe et en français ou peut-on séparer les classes dans les VC ? *XVIIIèmes JEP du GCP de la SFA.* Montréal, 113-117.

Elchinger, P. (1998). La résistivité de l'opposition de quantité vocalique en allemand. *Mémoire de Maîtrise de Phonétique,* Institut de Phonétique de Strasbourg.

Elert, C.-C. (1964). *Phonologic studies of quantity in Swedish.* Stockholm-Göteborg-Uppsala: Almqvist & Wiksell.

Fuchs, S. & Perrier, P. (2005). On the complex nature of speech kinematics. *ZAS Papers in Linguistics* 42, 137–165.

Gaitenby, J.H. (1965). The elastic word. *Haskins Laboratories, Status Report, Speech Research* 2, 1-12.

Ghazanfar A.A. & Logothetis, N.K. (2003). Facial expressions linked to monkey calls. *Nature* 423, 937–938.

Ghazanfar, A.A., Turesson, H.K., Maier, J.X., and Dinther, van R. (2007). Vocal tract resonances as indexical cues in Rhesus monkeys. *Current Biology* 17, 425–430.

Grosshans, C. (2002). L'étude de l'opposition vocalique tendue/lâche en allemand. Une approche acoustique et cinématique. *Mémoire de Maîtrise de Phonétique – Lettres Modernes,* Institut de Phonétique de Strasbourg/Université Ludwig-Maximilians de Munich.

Hawkins, S. (1999). Auditory capacities and phonological development: animal, baby, and foreign listeners. In: J.M. Pickett *The Acoustics of Speech Communication: Fundamentals, Speech Perception Theory, and Technology.* 183–197, Needham Heights (MA): Allyn and Bacon,.

Hawkins, S. (1999). Looking for invariant correlates of linguistic units: Two classical theories of speech perception. In: J.M. Pickett *The Acoustics of Speech Communication: Fundamentals, Speech Perception Theory, and Technology,* 198–231, Needham Heights (MA): Allyn and Bacon.

Hawkins, S. (1999). Re-evaluating assumptions about speech perception: Interactive and integrative theories. In: J.M. Pickett *The Acoustics of Speech Communication: Fundamentals, Speech Perception Theory, and Technology,* 232–288, Needham Heights (MA): Allyn and Bacon.

Herzfeld, J. (1998). La résistivité de l'opposition de quantité vocalique en danois. *Mémoire de Maîtrise de Phonétique.* Institut de Phonétique de Strasbourg.

Hildebrand, M. (1985). Walking and running. In: M. Hildebrand, D.M. Bramble, K.F. Liem and D.B. Wake (eds.) *Functional Vertebrate Morphology,* Cambridge (MA): The Belknap Press of Harvard University Press.

Hoonhorst, I., Colin, C., Markessis, E., Radeau, M., Deltenre, P., and Serniclaes, W. (2008). N100 component: an electrophysiological cue of voicing perception, 5-34. In S. Fuchs, H. Loevenbruck, D. Pape & Perrier, P. (eds.) *Some aspects of speech and the brain.* Peter Lang Verlag: Berlin

Iverson, P., Kuhl, P.K. (1995). Mapping the perceptual magnet effect for speech using signal detection theory and multidimensional scaling. *Journal of the Acoustical Society of America* 99, 1130–1140.

Jomaa, M. (1991). *Organisation temporelle acoustique et articulatoire de la quantité en arabe tunisien : comparaisons avec l'arabe standard et l'arabe koweïtien.* Thèse de Doctorat en Sciences du Langage, Institut de la Communication Parlée, Université Stendhal - Grenoble III (France).

Jomaa, M., Abry, C. (1988). La résistivité de la quantité vocalique aux variations de la vitesse d'élocution : le cas de l'arabe tunisien. *17èmes Journées d'Etudes sur la Parole du Groupe Communication Parlée organisées par la S.F.A.*, Nancy, 231-236.

Kelso, J.A.S. & Scholz, J. (1985). Cooperative phenomena in biological motion. In: H. HAKEN (ed.) *Complex Systems: Operational Approaches in Neurobiology, Physical Systems, and Computers*, 124- 149, Berlin: Springer.

Kelso, J.A.S., Saltzman, E.L., and Tuller, B. (1986). The dynamical perspective on speech production: Data and theory. *Journal of Phonetics* 14, 29-59.

Kuhl, P.K. & Miller, J.D. (1975). Speech perception by the chinchilla: Voiced-voiceless distinction in alveolar plosive consonants. *Science* 190, 69–72.

Ladefoged, P. (1964). *A phonetic study of West African Languages. An auditory-instrumental survey*. Cambridge (MA): Cambridge University Press.

Ladefoged, P., Declerk, J., Lindau, M., and Papçun, G. (1972). An auditory-motor theory of speech production. *University of California Los Angeles Working Papers in Phonetics* 22, 48-75.

Lehiste, Ilse. (1970). *Suprasegmentals*. Cambridge (MA): MIT Press.

Liberman, A.M. & Mattingly. I.G. (1985). The motor theory of speech perception revised. *Cognition* 21, 1-36.

Liberman, A. & Mattingly, I.G. (1988). Specialized perceiving systems for speech and other biologically significant sounds. In: G.M. Edelman, W.E. Gail, and W.M. Cowan (eds.) *Auditory Function*, 775-793, John Wiley & Sons.

Martins, P. (1996). Organisation temporelle de la gémination en wolof. Différences dialectales et effets de la vitesse d'élocution. *Mémoire de Maîtrise de Phonétique*, Institut de Phonétique de Strasbourg.

McCARTHY, J.J. (1986). OCP effects: gemination and anti-gemination. *Linguistic Inquiry* 17, 207-263.

Nelson, W.L. (1983). Physical principles for economies of skilled movements. *Biological Cybernetics* 46, 135-147.

Nelson, W.L., Perkell, J.P., Westbury, J.R. (1984). Mandible movements during increasingly rapid articulation of single syllables: preliminary observations. *Journal of the Acoustical Society of America* 75, 945-951.

Ohala, J. & Eukel, B. (1978). Explaining the intrinsic pitch of vowels. *Report of the Phonology Laboratory*, Berkerley, 118-125.

Ostry, D.J. & Flanagan, J.R. (1989). Human jaw movement in mastication and speech. *Archives of Oral Biology* 34, 685-693.

Perkell, J. (1969). *Physiology of speech production: results and implications of a quantitative cineradiographic study*, Cambridge (MA) and London (England): MIT Press.

Rhardisse, N., Sock, R., Abry, C. (1990). "L'Efficacité des cycles acoustiques dans la distinction des quantité vocalique et consonantique". *XVIIIèmes JEP du GCP de la SFA*. Montréal, 108-112.

Shapiro, D.C., Zernicke, R.F. Gregor, R.J., and Diestel, J.D. (1981). Evidence for generalized motor programs using gait pattern analysis. *Journal of Motor Behavior* 13, 33-47.

Sock, R. 1983. *L'organisation temporelle de l'opposition de quantité vocalique en wolof de Gambie. Sa résistivité aux conditions de durée segmentales et suprasegmentales.* Thèse de Doctorat de Troisième Cycle, Institut de Phonétique de Grenoble, Université de Grenoble III, (France).

Sock, R. (1999). *Organisation temporelle en production de la parole. Emergence de catégories sensori-motrices phonétiques.* Villeneuve d'Ascq Cedex (France): Presses Universitaires du Septentrion.

Sock, R., Löfqvist, A. (1995). Quantity Contrasts in Swedish. Kinematic and Acoustic Patterns. *XIIIth International Congress of Phonetic Sciences*, 580-583.

Sock, R., Vaxelaire, B. (2001). Réflexions sur le timing de la quantité. *Travaux de l'Institut de Phonétique de Strasbourg TIPS* 31, 89-126.

Sock, R., Vaxelaire, B., Roy J.P, Hirsch, F., and Hecker, V. (2006). Temporal and spatial correlates of quantity contrasts in Wolof, In J. Harrington & M. Tabain (eds.): *Speech Production – Models, Phonetic Processes and Techniques*, 253-274, New York: Psychology Press.

Stetson, R.H. (1928). Motor phonetics. A study of speech movements in action. *Archives Néerlandaises de Phonétique Expérimentale* 3 (Reedition 1987: J.A.S. KELSO & K.G. MUNHALL (eds.), 1-216, Boston: Little, Brown and Company.

Tremblay, S., Shiller, D.M., and Ostry, D.J. (2003). Somatosensory basis of speech production. *Nature* 423, 866-869.

Tremblay, S., Houle, G., and Ostry, D.J. (2008). Specificity of speech motor learning. *The Journal of Neuroscience* 28(10), 2426–2434.

Tuller, B. & Kelso J.A.S. (1990). Phase transitions in speech production and their perceptual consequences. In: M. Jeannerod (Ed.) *Attention and Performance XIII: Motor representations and control*, 429-452, Hillsdale (New Jersey): Erlbaum.

Tyrone, M.E. (2007). Simultaneity in atypical signers. Implications for the structure of signed language. In: M. Vermeerbergen,L. Leeson & O. Crasborn (eds.) *Simultaneity in Signed Languages, Form and Function*, 317-335, John Benjamin Publishing Company.

Vaxelaire, B. (1995a). Single vs Double (Abutted) Consonants across Speech Rate. X-Ray and Acoustic Data for French. *XIIIe Congrès International des Sciences Phonétiques (ICPhS)* 1, Stockholm, 384-387.

Vaxelaire, B. (1995b). Geometric and temporal constraints in the production of French consonantal sequences. X-ray and acoustic data. *Eurospeech 1995* 2, 1285-1288.

Vaxelaire, B. & SOCK, R. (1997). Laryngeal movements and speech rate. An X-ray investigation. *Eurospeech 1997* 2, Rhodes, 1039-1042.

Warren, M.R. & Gregory, R.L. (1958). An auditory analogue of the visual reversible figure. *American Journal of Psychology* 71, 612–613.

Wioland, F. (1985). Les structures syllabiques du français. Fréquence et distribution des phonèmes consonantiques. Contraintes idiomatiques dans les séquences consonantiques. *Slatkine-Champion*, Genève, Paris.

Witz, S. (1998). Quantité vocalique en alsacien : une variante dialectale du Bas-Rhin. *Mémoire de Maîtrise de Phonétique*, Institut de Phonétique de Strasbourg.

11

Pre-lexical speech processing in the brain

GEORG MEYER
SOPHIE WUERGER
ELVIRA PEREZ

Abstract: The many computational steps involved in translating heard or seen speech into meaning are well documented by a wealth of linguistic research and theories. Recent developments in brain imaging have helped to identify regions of the brain involved in speech perception and production and have given new impetus to the development of theoretical models of pre-lexical speech perception.
We review some of the major theories with an emphasis on the predictions the models would make for speech processing in the brain and consider existing models that are based on imaging studies. We present example fMRI and EEG data to highlight some of the methodological issues that have to be considered in drawing conclusions from neuroimaging data and evaluate the extent to which neuroimaging can differentiate between the theoretical pre-lexical speech processing models that have been proposed.

1. PRE-LEXICAL SPEECH PERCEPTION

Speech is not a sequence of discrete tokens but a sequence of overlapping segments that are shaped by the speaker's vocal tract and that reflect not only the current, but also past and future segments. This co-articulation makes a direct mapping from acoustic properties to phonetic categories difficult and also means that there are no clearly defined segment boundaries between the elements of speech. Further variability of the acoustic signal is introduced by speaker characteristics, such as sex, size and age and speaking rate or the environment (review: Miller and Eimas, 1995). There is also no stable and unique mapping between individual acoustic features and phonetic categories, but phonetic segments are specified by multiple properties (e.g. Lisker, 1986) which take on different importance depending on the phonetic and environmental context (trading relations, e.g. Repp, 1982).

In spite of all this, there is convincing evidence that we perceive a restricted set of sub-lexical units. The challenge therefore is to explain how listeners translate the highly variable and context dependent acoustic signal into an invariant representation.

There are two fundamental approaches. The most common view is that perception requires normalization: the acoustic signal is first mapped into an abstract, invariant representation which is then used for lexical access. Exactly what this representation is - distinctive features (e.g. Jakobson and Halle, 1956; or Chomsky and Halle, 1968), phonemes (e.g. McClelland & Elman, 1986), syllables (e.g. Diehl and Kluender, 1989) or something else is subject to a lively debate. An opposing view is that speech is directly mapped into a lexical representation. This could be achieved by accessing stored traces of all acoustical manifestations of speech (e.g. Goldinger, 1998) or via direct perception of linguistically significant actions of the vocal tract that occur during speech (e.g. Fowler, 2003).

For the discussion we will split the theories into two rough classes, depending on whether they postulate intermediate representations or direct access. If intermediate representations are used to provide lexical access, then this should be visible in neuroimaging and lesion studies. Within both classes there are theories that argue that the objects of perception are articulatory or motor based and others that argue for an auditory basis of speech perception. This distinction should also be clearly visible in imaging studies since auditory representations are localised in the superior temporal lobe while motor representations are found in the frontal lobe.

Neuroimaging has led to a number of models that link anatomical structures to speech perception and production.

1.1. LEXICAL ACCESS VIA INTERMEDIATE REPRESENTATIONS

There is behavioural evidence for a range of sub-lexical representations (e.g. McQueen & Cutler, 1997), that may even be used interchangeably depending on the processing task at hand (Pisoni & Luce, 1987). Intermediate representations have consequently been proposed as the basis for many models. We will review a number of influential models and discuss their implication for neuroimaging data.

The **Search Model** (Forster, 1976) assumes the use of syllables in a sequential search through lists or stacks of candidates that are ordered in terms of word frequency. Parallel and distributed computations that are compatible with the neural system are proposed by the **Cohort Model** (Marslen-Wilson & Tyler, 1980) where candidate words are de-selected from a list of initial matches as acoustical, syntactical or contextual information is evaluated. The **TRACE Model** (McClelland & Elman, 1986) explains lexical access in terms of a hierarchical network of interactive nodes that each code specific features in the input stream.

The TRACE and Cohort model generate an invariant representation by explicitly taking context into account.

An alternative proposal is that the acoustic signal contains sufficient invariant features to enable a direct mapping from signal to phoneme (e.g. Stevens, 2002; Stevens and Blumstein, 1981; Kewley-Port, 1983; Sussman et al., 1991). The **Lexical Access From Features** (LAFF) theory posits that invariant features are recognized at acoustic landmarks that are characterized by maxima or minima of spectral change. Sets of features would uniquely specify phonetic segments. The assumed underlying representation of this model are acoustic features. The model predicts that speech perception is based on intermediate, speech specific acoustically derived representations and does not need a close interaction with memory subsystems.

The **Fuzzy Logic Model of Speech Perception** (FLMP) developed by Massaro (1989) is a data-driven rather than a theory-driven model that uses fuzzy logic as its mathematical foundation. Matching received data to idealised prototypes in memory is an important aspect of the theory, but Massaro makes no claims about the nature of the representation, except that it has to be compatible with the sensory representation. In contrast to other models of pre-lexical speech processing this model

predicts human performance for auditory and visual speech by postulating early integration. Behavioural data (e.g. Summerfield, 1979; Schwartz et al., 2004) are consistent with this view, which requires intermediate representations.
Cohort, TRACE, LAFF and FLMP invoke parallel interactive invariant sub-lexical representations that are evaluated in a graded fashion to explain speech recognition. While they make no claim that speech is separate from other perceptual mechanisms all models postulate specialised representations that code prototypical feature representations for lexical access. Imaging and lesions studies should be able to provide evidence for these intermediate representations and show differences in activation for speech and non-speech stimuli.
Liberman and colleagues (1967), based on the finding that perceptual categories appeared to be much more closely associated with articulatory than auditory patterns, proposed the **Motor Theory of Speech Perception**. Initially they proposed that articulatory gestures are the object of speech perception. Invariance is achieved by virtue of an articulatory representation that negates the variability of the acoustic signal introduced by, for instance, co-articulation. The strong claim of a direct motor representation was weakened in later descriptions of the theory to a more abstract claim of a representation based on the intended gesture of the speaker (Liberman and Mattingly, 1985). This means that the theory no longer assumes direct access to motor patterns for speech perception. A central claim of motor theory, however, is that speech perception is 'special' and separate from other auditory perception and that the speaker's intended gesture is the intermediate and invariant representation that links acoustics to lexical entries. An anatomically separate area that is active for speech, but not for other sounds would be strong support for this theory.

1.2. DIRECT LEXICAL ACCESS

One of the arguments for postulating a stepwise recoding of acoustic information to lexical entries is the evidence for perceived categories in the perceptual units that make up speech (e.g. McQueen & Cutler, 1997), but there is no theoretical reason why there should not be a direct mapping from acoustics to lexical entries. The categorical perception of sub-lexical units could be explained by complementary processes that operate in addition to the direct lexical access as for non-speech categorisation.

The fundamental claim of **Exemplar Theory** is that we learn phonetic and linguistic categories by storing labelled exemplars. These exemplars are information-rich so that speaker characteristics or contextual information is retained. Variability is dealt with by accessing a rich set of context and speaker specific exemplars (review: Goldinger, 1998). Exemplar theory makes a number of predictions for imaging and lesion data: there is no need for invariant intermediate representations, so that lexical access is a 'one-shot' operation that draws on auditory signal representations and is intricately tied to memory access. Recognising speech is no different from recognising other sounds so that shared processing might be expected.

Klatt's (1979) **Lexical Access from Spectra** (LAFS) model is much more precisely specified than exemplar theory but shares many of the fundamental assumptions. He proposes that lexical access is mediated directly via a set of canonical spectral diphone sequence templates. As such it deals with co-articulation not by looking for invariance in the acoustics but by coding all possible instantiations of phonetic sequences making up the listener's language.

The **Direct Realist Theory (DRT)**, drawing on ideas by Gibson (1966), has been proposed by Fowler and colleagues (review: Fowler, 2003). The fundamental claim is that perception is direct, that is without intervening representation or processing stages. This also means that DRT should not be considered as an explanation for lexical access, since this would again imply a lexical representation. The objects of perception, in contrast to Exemplar Theory or LAFS, are vocal tract movements that are mediated via the auditory and visual modality. Within the direct perception framework there is no specialised (speech) representation. Fowler and Rosenblum (1991, p 743) argue that "there is no need to look inside the perceiver to explain how the percept acquires its motor character". While the statement did not refer to neuroimaging, the model suggest a close link between articulation and perception and therefore activity in motor areas during speech perception.

1.3. THE ACTIVE/PASSIVE CONTROVERSY

Another way to distinguish models of perception is to classify them into active or passive perception models (MacKay, 1968). Many of the models of speech perception can be considered 'passive' models because identification is a signal-driven filtering operation where the best fitting explanation for the observed data is selected from a range of available candidates. Whether this selection process is based on spectra (LAFS), acoustic features (LAFF), prototypes that are selected from lists (Search model) or combined using fuzzy logic (FLMP) does not change the fundamental approach. The passive approach is an attractive model because it is ideally suited for implementation by a population of parallel signal detectors in neural architectures. Simple exemplar-based models (e.g., Jacoby, 1983) or stimulus-response associating models (e.g., Shiffrin & Schneider, 1977), however, cannot account for some aspects of perceptual learning or the action imitation necessary for language acquisition which requires close integration of perception and production systems.

Active perception uses 'analysis by synthesis'. For speech perception this would mean that we relate auditory patterns to internally generated speech pattern hypotheses. The mirror neuron system (review: Rizzolatti et al., 2001; Buccino et al., 2001), a neural system that is active during the execution as well as the observation of motor action is an obvious candidate. It provides the neural hardware to relate observed gestures (speech or other motor activity) to the observer's own motor plans that would be used to generate this movement. Skipper et al. (2006) draw on the mirror neuron system to propose an active model that consists of a forward and an inverse component to explain audio-visual speech perception. The forward half of the model predicts the acoustic consequence of motor commands while the inverse part converts observed visual and auditory signals into motor patterns. The interplay of the two systems is at the heart of audiovisual speech perception. Active perception models are consistent with motor theories of speech perception because hypothesis generation requires (motor) action synthesis. While active models trivially explain the action/perception link and provide an explanation for language acquisition, they are slow, because successive hypotheses have to be evaluated, and metabolically expensive, because of the putative simultaneous involvement of production and perception systems in speech perception.

Skipper's model is motivated by findings from neuroimaging and therefore fits well with other models that explain speech processing in terms of the underlying neuroanatomy.

2. NEUROANATOMICAL MODELS OF SPEECH PERCEPTION

The **dual stream model of speech perception**, proposed by Hickok and Poeppel (2007) is based on functional neuroimaging data and is necessarily more concerned with the anatomical structures that underlie speech perception and production than the signal representations used. The model consists of two functionally separate processing streams that share common input. The dorsal superior temporal gyri (STG, Figure 1) bilaterally are responsible for spectrotemporal analysis while medial and posterior sections of the superior temporal sulci (STS), also bilaterally, provide a phonological network. At this stage speech processing diverges into a ventral stream that is concerned with speech recognition and a dorsal stream that is primarily involved in speech production.

The ventral stream consists of a lexical interface in the posterior section of the middle temporal gyri and inferior temporal sulci (MTG, ITS) bilaterally. The degree of lateralisation in these structures is controversial; Hickok and Poeppel concede a 'left bias'. Speech perception is completed by a combinatorial network in the anterior section of the MTG and ITS.

The dorsal stream, according to the model, is left lateralised and consists of a sensori-motor interface located in the left Sylvian fissure at the border between temporal and parietal cortex (Spt, Figure 1). Broca's area and a premotor cortical area dorsal to it provide the articulatory network.

The processing of pre-lexical speech, according to this model, is limited to the ventral stream while articulation would activate the dorsal stream.

The areas relevant for speech perception are labelled on an 'inflated brain' (Figure 1). The representation overcomes the problems inherent in rendering activity in the sulci (grooves) of the brain where the cortex is folded inward by modelling the effect of 'inflating' the cortical sheet so that both gyri (ridges) (lighter shade of grey) and sulci (darker shades of grey) are visible.

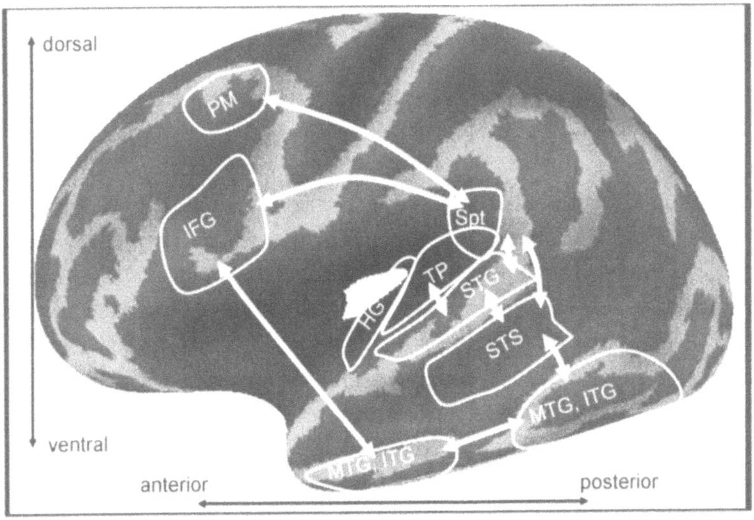

Figure 1: Schematic diagram of the dual stream model proposed by Hickok and Poeppel (2007). Spectrotemporal analysis is carried out in the superior temporal areas (Heschl's Gyrus - HG/ planum temporale - TP/ superior temporal gyrus - STG) while the superior temporal sulcus (STS) contains a phonological network. The diagram only shows the left hemisphere but processing up to this stage is bilateral. After this stage processing diverges into a dorsal path that is concerned with speech production and a ventral pathway that is concerned with speech recognition. The ventral pathway consists of a lexical interface in the posterior parts of the middle and inferior temporal gyrus (MTG and ITG) (with a weak left bias) and a combinatorial network predominantly in left anterior MTG and ITG. Speech production draws on a left dominant network consisting of a sensorimotor interface at the border of the parietal and temporal lobes (Spt) and an articulatory network in the posterior inferior frontal gyrus (IFG) anterior insula and premotor cortex (PM).

Hickok and Poeppel's dual stream model treats the dorsal STG as a general auditory analysis stage. Warren et al. (2006) argue for a processing hierarchy within the STG where general source attributes are analysed in the posterior superior temporal lobe, abstraction occurs in the posterior superior temporal sulcus, and further analysis occurs in the anterior superior temporal sulcus and higher order cortices in the middle and anterior temporal lobe. The same group (Warren et al., 2005), drawing on human imaging as well as animal models, argues that the role of the posterior superior temporal plane (STP) is to disambiguate auditory signals arriving from the primary auditory cortex using stored templates to generate sequences of auditory patterns, which, in turn are the basis of constrained motor representations that are computed in the dorsal pathway. This auditory motor transformation is the primary purpose of the dorsal auditory pathway and applies to auditory localisation as much as to auditory pattern classification, be it speech or other actions. Information is transferred bidirectionally between auditory and motor regions to account for imaging data showing activation of the dorsal stream during speech perception. Warren and co-workers argue that the posteromedial planum temporale (PT) may also be involved in self monitoring of speech and in the generation of articulatory representations that have been implicated in the perception of distorted speech (Davis and Johnstrude, 2003).

While auditory input is without doubt the primary source of information, visual cues, lipreading, can also be used to receive speech signals. There is clear evidence for direct visual input into speech perception (McGurk and MacDonald, 1976). Early fMRI studies (Calvert et al., 1997) suggested an involvement of auditory cortex in silent lipreading. This would support theoretical models arguing that auditory and visual information is integrated at or before phonetic classification (Summerfield, 1992). More recent work (e.g. Paulesu et al., 2003) failed to replicate this finding but identifies frontal areas as being involved in phonetic categorisation of visible speech. Paulesu et al. (2003) argue for very early processing of visual cues in visual areas that are also associated with motion extraction (MT) and object recognition (LOC). They implicate the left anterior IFG (BA 45) and left ITS in lexical processing. The most posterior bank within the STS (BA 22) is commonly found to be activated by auditory as well as visual speech stimuli (e.g. Calvert and Lewis, 2003; Wise et al., 2001).

Skipper and co-workers (2005; 2006; 2007) consider auditory, visual and audio-visual speech perception and invoke the mirror neuron system as

a key aspect in an active perception paradigm. They suggest that lip movements and speech sounds are translated into a hypothesis that is represented in the posterior parts of the STS. This is consistent with imaging data from speech (e.g. Poeppel and Hickok, 2007) and lip-reading (e.g. Calvert and Lewis, 2003). They argue that the posterior part of the pars opercularis (posterior section of Broca's area in the IFG, BA 44) is responsible for specifying this hypothesis in terms of motor goals, which could then be turned into actions via premotor (PM / BA 6) and motor cortical areas. It is clear that the proposed model draws on the same circuitry that is identified by Poeppel and Hickok (2007) as being responsible for speech generation.
It is clear that there is broad consensus about the brain areas involved in speech perception although there is still a lively debate about their detailed function.

3. LOCALISING PRE-LEXICAL SPEECH PROCESSING IN THE BRAIN

A first step in looking at the nature of pre-lexical speech processing is to examine the neural correlates of the classification and discrimination of nonsense syllables. These signals require a full phonemic analysis, but do not rely on syntactic or semantic analysis. We will show a series of fMRI imaging data of our own to highlight some of the methodological approaches and issues involved in isolating speech-specific processing centres. Our experiment compared responses to auditory, visual and audiovisual instances of speech (VCV syllables with the vowels /a,i,u/ and consonants /b,d,g/), biological body motion (e.g. steps, drinking, rowing, using a broom or saw, playing tennis or snooker) and meaningless matched stimuli because body motion and speech consistently activate similar areas in the brain. The auditory signals were high quality recorded natural stimuli while the visual stimuli consisted of motion signals defined by 13 points, defining the lip shape or body joints, which causes a compelling percept of biological body motion or lip movement. The meaningless visual signals consisted of a mixture of local motion vectors extracted from an example of lip and body motion with randomised starting points, so that they had the same luminance,

spatial extent, and local motion parameters as the lip and body motion signals. The auditory meaningless signal consisted of a spectrally reversed speech signal (Blesser, 1972) that was envelope modulated with a body motion signal.
A group of 11 subjects was presented with the signals in a block design consisting of 16 seconds stimulus presentation followed by 16 seconds rest. Subjects were asked to press a button whenever they saw the same signal twice in direct succession. The stimulus conditions enable us to directly compare the activations for speech, body motion and meaningless signals and to isolate modality specific processing.

3.1. CHANGES IN BRAIN ACTIVITY DURING SPEECH PERCEPTION

Figure 2 shows statistical parametric maps (Frackowiak et al., 2004) showing the average activation in response to perceive spoken, visual and audio-visual VCV nonsense syllables against the rest condition where no signal was presented. The t-values are projected onto an 'inflated brain' to show activity in the gyri (ligher shade of grey) as well as in the sulci (darker shade). The top row shows the left hemisphere while the bottom row shows the right hemisphere. The activation pattern was thresholded to only show voxels at $t > 2.0$ ($p < 0.02$) in clusters with significance levels of $p < 0.001$. The experimental data matches the dual stream model well. Auditory presentation alone leads to bilateral activation of the superior temporal gyrus (BA 42) and the upper bank of the posterior STS (BA 22) (Hickok and Poeppel, 2007).
For visual presentation of the same speech signals, the activation pattern is very different. We find bilateral activation in occipital lobe areas MT+ and lateral occipital complex (LOC). The superior parietal cortex (BA 7) shows bilateral activation while activation in the inferior parietal lobule (IPL) is limited to the left hemisphere. Three areas in the frontal cortex show bilateral activation: the medial frontal gyrus (BA6), the inferior/middle frontal gyrus (BA 44/45 – Broca's area) and the anterior insula (IN). Activation in these areas is consistent with previous results (review: Calvert and Lewis, 2003; Skipper et al., 2005). The only area that is significantly co-activated for unimodal auditory and visual speech is the most posterior bank of BA 22.

Audio-visual activation leads (right hand column in Figure 2) to an activation pattern that is largely a compound of the two unimodal patterns. There is relatively less activity in frontal areas and more in temporal sites. The pattern of activity mirrors data from Skipper et al. (2005) where subjects passively listened to stories rather than actively matching VCV syllables. Skipper also observed that activity in the auditory condition was confined to the ventral stream. They argue that in typical listening conditions the production system may only be weakly or transiently activated such that activity is not visible in fMRI studies with their associated poor temporal resolution. This finding is inconsistent with previously reported activity in motor areas in a passive 'listening to monosyllables' task (Wilson et al., 2004). This may be due to thresholding (see section 3.2) or task differences.

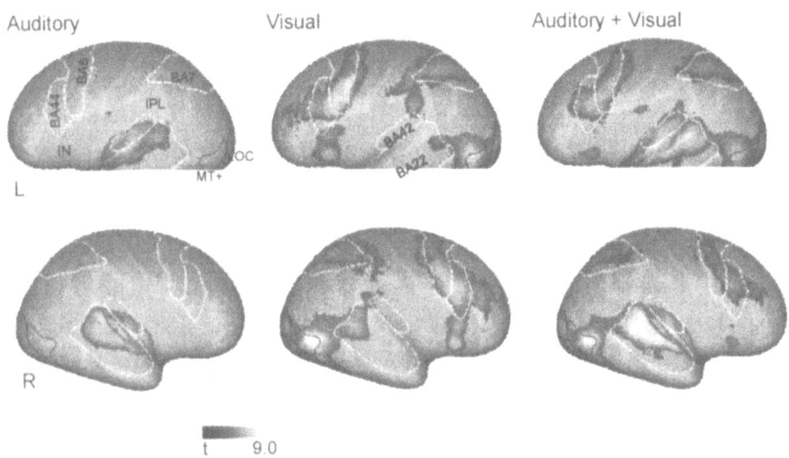

Figure 2: Inflated brains showing average activation in a /VCV/ syllable recognition relative to rest. Activation patterns are presented for three conditions: auditory alone (left), visual alone, and audiovisual presentation (right). The top row shows the left hemisphere while the bottom row shows the right hemisphere. Auditory presentation leads to bilateral activation in Brodmann areas (BA) 42 (superior temporal plane), BA 22 (superior temporal sulcus). Visual speech causes increases in BOLD response in areas BA44 (Broca's area) and BA6 (premotor cortex) the anterior insula (IN), the superior parietal cortex (BA 7) as well as visual areas MT+ and lateral occipital complex (LOC).

A first conclusion from the imaging data is that a large network of brain areas, distributed over both hemispheres, is used to process pre-lexical speech. The activation is entirely consistent with models that assume a hierarchy of processing steps or the parallel extraction of low level features that are required to produce an invariant representation at the lexical interface.

The data shown in Figure 2 also highlight some of the limits and problems associated with this approach. The primary auditory cortex (PAC), located in area BA 41, which is located just anterior to BA 42 (e.g. Morosan, 2001) does not show significantly increased activation in the speech condition. This does not mean that PAC was not active during the speech perception task, but simply that it was not significantly more active than during the control condition where the noisy MRI scanner was running while the subjects were resting. Not seeing activity does therefore not necessarily mean that no signals are processed.

Seeing activity in response to speech signals, on the other hand, does not mean that the observed activity is speech *specific*. Many of the areas activated by speech signals are activated by a host of other auditory and visual stimuli. The visual areas MT+ and LOC, for instance are implicated in general visual motion processing, the primary and secondary auditory cortex are active in all auditory tasks.

A fundamental challenge, therefore, is to isolate speech specific processing.

3.2. ISOLATING SPEECH SPECIFIC ACTIVATION

The most obvious way to isolate speech specific responses from non-speech responses is to compute differences in activation for a speech task and a matched non-speech task. While this strategy sounds simple in principle it is surprisingly difficult to achieve in practice.

The human speech processing system is designed to tolerate large and highly unnatural manipulations of the speech signal (Whalen and Liberman, 1987), such as locally time reversed speech (Saberi and Perrott, 1999) or sine-wave speech where sine-waves replace formant peaks (Remez, 1981). This means that it is extraordinarily difficult to produce non-speech signals that are statistically matched to speech signals but are not perceived as speech.

The analysis of imaging data, whether it is fMRI or EEG data, always involves some degree of thresholding by defining significance levels for responses. This means that small stimulus differences or task modify-cations can have a profound effect on the outcome because they may cause the response to be just above or below the significance level. Differential activation in speech and non-speech conditions may there-fore not reflect any processing, but simply stimulus differences. These potential confounds are unavoidable in any area of research and tolerable where factual activation differences are reported. One should be aware of the limitations, however, before accepting activation differences in response to different stimuli as proof for any of the theoretical frameworks explaining speech perception (e.g. Benson et al., 2001; Whalen et al., 2006).

One control signal that has been used in the past is spectrally reversed speech (e.g. Narain et al., 2003; Obleser et al., 2007). The speech spectrum is reversed and filtered such that formant positions are mirror images of natural speech but the long term spectrum and overall levels closely match speech data. Both groups report a stronger response in the left anterolateral superior temporal cortex (BA 22) for speech than for spectrally reversed speech.

Figure 3 shows contrasts between the three auditory conditions to illustrate the effect of choosing the appropriate contrast. The significance levels are set deliberately low to show all activated clusters containing voxels at significant levels of $p < 0.001$ ($t > 3.09$). No constraints were set to define the minimum of significant voxels in a cluster or a maximum cluster probability.

The comparison of natural speech with a meaningless signal shows activation in anterolateral areas of BA 22 as expected but also low level activation in BA 43 which is concerned with sensorimotor representation of the mouth and taste reception and a large cluster in BA 39, an association cortical area in the angular gyrus that has been linked to language (e.g. Obleser et al., 2007b), as well as visual motion perception (Vaina et al., 2001) (Figure 3, top left). When natural speech is contrasted with meaningful non-speech signals (bottom, Figure 3) BA 39 shows no activation. Taken at face value the two contrasts would lead to very different conclusions about the involvement of area BA 39 in speech perception.

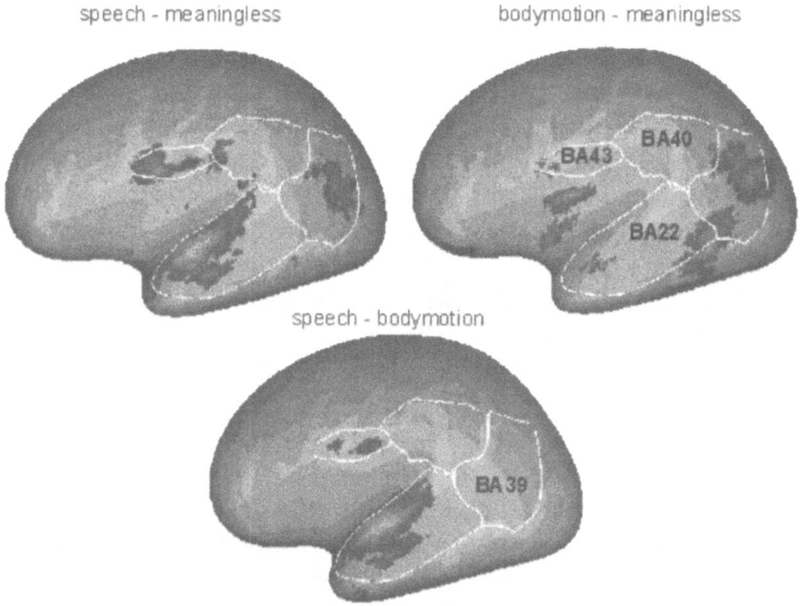

Figure 3: Inflated brains showing average activation contrasting the three auditory signal types: speech, meaningless items and body motion. Speech stimuli cause significantly higher activation in BA22 for both contrasts, but both speech and body motion cause activation in BA 39 relative to meaningless speech. When speech is contrasted with body motion no activity is visible in BA39.

Neither area BA 39 nor BA 43 are linked to pre-lexical speech processing and neither shows significant activations if conservative acceptance levels (family wise error correction - FWE) for clusters were used: the cluster in BA 22 for the speech-meaningless condition is highly significant ($p_{FWE} < 0.001$ at cluster level) while neither the activation in BA 39 ($p_{FWE} = 0.53$) nor in BA 43 ($p_{FWE} = 0.47$) is significant.
The point that significant activation in response to speech stimuli may not mean speech specificity, however, is critical. It is made eloquently by Price et al. (2005). The authors systematically compare foci of activation for speech stimuli when contrasted with matched control stimuli, such as

reversed speech, noise and other sounds with those seen for similar non-speech tasks. They show that brain areas in STG/STS that are typically considered to be speech selective also activate for a range of clearly defined non-speech sounds, such as melodies, meaningful sounds, pitch chroma or written sentences. They conclude that speech and other auditory processing tasks share the same substrates rather than occupying specialised cortical structures. In our data the superior temporal plane (BA 42) shows increased activity relative to rest for speech stimuli but no significant differential activity when compared to the two non-speech conditions. This is consistent with shared processing of speech and (some) non-speech signals in this area. The highly significant selective activation within BA 22 we observed might not be seen if the control stimuli were chosen differently. Price and co-workers show that a range of non-speech stimuli activate the same areas as speech signals. The stimuli, however, all contain features that are important for speech perception: pitch or melody recognition are necessary for the extraction of intonation contours, written text recognition will activate shared lexical and higher representations. Finding differential activity that is linked to specific features supports models that postulate intermediate representations rather than direct access.

It may be argued that finding shared processing areas is evidence against speech specific processing and the motor theory. Functional specialisation, however, does not require spatial separation. It is entirely possible that populations of highly stimulus-specific local processing networks, some specialised for speech and some for non-speech processing, could co-habit the same space and it would not be surprising to find local specificity for similar tasks as Price et al. (2005) demonstrated.

3.3. ISOLATING MODALITY INDEPENDENT ACTIVATION

One of the characteristics of speech perception is that the phonological representation is not directly linked to the physical stimulus and may therefore be driven by both visual and auditory stimulation. Wise et al. (2001) analysed four PET imaging experiments and suggested that the role of the left superior temporal sulcus is the transient representation of phonetic sequences, whether heard or internally generated. This area then would be the final destination of any pre-lexical processing. In our comparison of auditory and visual conditions we identified this area (bilaterally) as being activated by unimodal visual and unimodal auditory speech signals. This can be formally shown by computing those areas that are significantly activated by unimodal auditory and unimodal visual stimulation (conjunction analysis). Figure 4 shows the results for the speech, body motion and scrambled data.

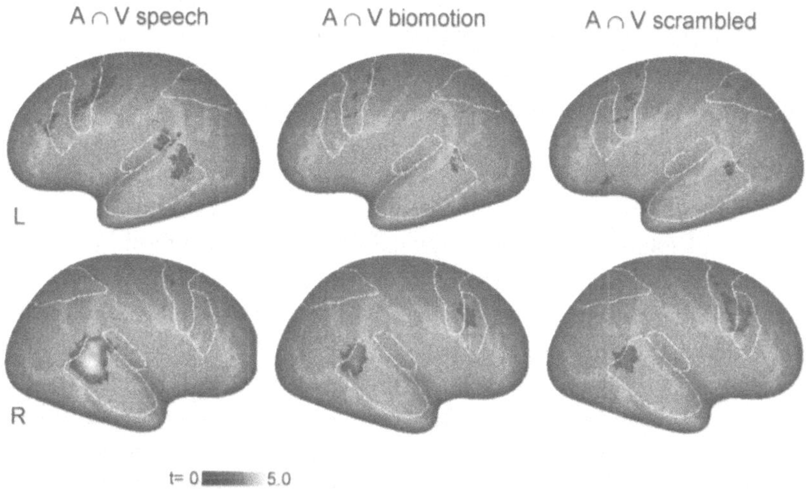

Figure 4: Conjunction analysis showing areas where voxels for both auditory *and* visual conditions cause activations greater than the threshold significance threshold (p = 0.001) for individual voxels. Three conditions were tested: speech, body motion and scrambled motion. All three conditions cause increased activation in the posterior STS (BA 22) bilaterally. The difference in activation was consistently greater in the right hemisphere and stronger for speech stimuli than for biological and scrambled motion signals.

We see bilateral activation of the posterior STS with more activation on the right, activation in the posterior section of BA42 in the speech condition as well as left lateralised activation in BA 44 / 45 (Broca's area) and premotor cortex (BA 6). These results fit previous work on auditory pre-lexical speech processing (review Hickok and Poeppel, 2007) and lipreading (Calvert et al., 1997; Paulesu et al., 2003) well. Note that the relatively higher activation on the right BA 22 is a direct consequence of the greater right hand side area of activation for visual stimuli (Figure 2). If we compare the activation in the speech conditions with those for non-speech, however, it is clear that the same areas that are activated by speech signals are, albeit at a lower level, also activated during non-speech perception.

The conclusion from the conjunction analysis, therefore, is that it is plausible to think of the posterior STS as an area that provides the interface between pre-lexical analysis and further processing stages. It is, however also clear that the region appears to be involved in providing a modality independent interface for other visual and auditory signals.

We also see left lateralised low level activation of dorsal stream areas (BA 44/45 and BA 6) in the speech condition while activity in these areas is right lateralised in the body motion and scrambled conditions.

Davis and Johnsrude (2003) presented listeners with stimuli of systematically varying intelligibility and correlated the BOLD response with intelligibility. Different stimulus pre-processing was employed to enable them to distinguish differences that were due to stimulus differences from those that were due to intelligibility differences. They found that activity in the superior and middle temporal gyri, the left hippocampus and the left inferior frontal gyrus (Broca's area) was correlated to intelligibility but not acoustic form. Callan et al. (2004) and Wilson and Iacoboni (2006) showed increased motor area and superior temporal activation when listeners were presented with non-native speech signal compared to stimulation with native speech sounds. Zekfeld et al. (2006) extended this work and argue that two distinct systems operate in speech comprehension, a bottom-up system that predominantly uses the bilateral temporal areas and a supplementary top-down system that draws on Broca's area. They conclude that speech comprehension does not draw on a single system, or even a single strategy. Instead we can dynamically switch from a passive, bottom-up, strategy for highly intelligible signals to a generative, top-down, system that draws in centres involved in speech production.

Our auditory signals were difficult to interpret in the scanner environment so that an involvement of top-down, generative processes for speech recognition is plausible. The proposal that two fundamentally different systems interactively process the data using efficient passive recognition system for previously seen, 'easy' signals and an active system drawing on motor representation for ambiguous signals and in language acquisition would explain the imaging data. It would also bridge some of the divide between the theoretical models and the experimental data that they are founded on.

The imaging data on pre-lexical processing presented here can be summarised as follows: Pre-lexical auditory speech processing appears to draw predominantly on sites in the left *and* right temporal lobe (BA 42 and 22). The upper portion of BA22 bilaterally is selectively activated by speech sounds, whether contrasted with rest or matched non-speech sounds. It therefore appears a likely site of pre-lexical processing.

The posterior section of STS is strongly activated bilaterally for unimodal visual *and* unimodal auditory speech which suggests that it might be a memory interface (Wise et al., 2001).

We tested our subjects with speech, but also body motion and statistically matched meaningless stimuli and found that co-activation for the different stimulus types is the norm rather than the exception. In fact we are not aware of conclusive evidence for cortical area that reacts exclusively to pre-lexical speech. Models that postulate speech specific processing cannot, however, be rejected, because local non-overlapping speech and non-speech specific processing networks may co-habit within the same spaces. We feel that the DRT model with its assumption of physical vocal tract variations as the basis for speech perception would be more plausible if there was significant activation in motor cortical or inferior-frontal areas that are implicated in speech production.

4. SQUARING IMAGING AND LESION DATA

Imaging data for speech perception tasks consistently show *bilateral* activation of the auditory related cortical areas in the posterior sections of the superior temporal lobe. This is in stark contrast to early lesion work that found impairments in speech perception with lesions in the *left* superior temporal lobe (Wernicke's area, Wernicke, 1874/1977; Luria 1970), the *left* inferior parietal lobe (Caplan et al., 1995) or the *left* inferior frontal cortex (Fiez et al., 1995). Indeed, the Wernicke-Lichtheim-Geschwind Model (WLG, Geschwind, 1965a,b) based on works by Broca, Wernicke and Lichtheim captures a striking difference between patients who have anterior damage and those who have posterior lesions. Anterior damage causes non-fluent speech characterized by articulation difficulties, while posterior damage affects speech perception while speech remains fluent and rapidly articulated although marked by phonological, grammatical, and semantic errors (e.g. Caplan, 1987). It is notable that anterior lesions affect production but spare perception while posterior lesions tend to affect perception as well as production. This suggests a close coupling between perception and production which is a key feature of all motor focussed theories, but the dissociation suggests a functional link from perception to production rather than vice versa and is consistent with a putative motor interface in area Spt/ pPT as suggested by the neuroanatomical models.

The highly lateralised sensitivity to lesions is reflected in statistical analyses of lesion data (e.g. Hier et al., 1994) as well as fMRI data (Springer et al., 1999). It is also consistent with perceptual data, which suggests that the right ear (predominantly processed in the left hemisphere) has a consistent advantage in processing speech signals (right ear advantage, e.g. Shankweiler and Studdard-Kennedy, 1967).

Poeppel and Hickok (2004) attempt to reconcile the lesion and imaging data by arguing for a more differentiated look at the lesion data, anatomical models and imaging data. Hickock and Poeppel (2000; 2007) propose a model that consists of two left-dominant processing streams for lexical representations that share common *bilateral* pre-lexical processing stages. Speech recognition would obviously have to draw on the left lateralised and the bilateral components.

Most models of speech perception, consistently with imaging data, propose a hierarchy of processing levels as the basis for lexical access. If intermediate representations are computed in distinct areas of the brain then selective deficits should be seen in lesion studies.

Verbal auditory agnosia or 'pure word deafness' (PWD) is a rare deficit where patients have difficulties identifying spoken words, but have normal audiometry, identify non-speech sounds and are able to repeat spoken words. The ability to comprehend written text shows that a semantic representation remains intact. This is the basis of the argument for a dissociation between phonological and semantic representation

(Kohn and Friedman, 1986). Poeppel (2001) links PWD to bilateral lesions in the posterior superior temporal areas. A clear dissociation between phonological and semantic processing would provide evidence that pre-lexical speech perception uses separable intermediate representations, whether they are articulatory or acoustically derived.

If this idealised type of PWD was typical or widely spread, the existence of a specialised pre-lexical speech representation would be uncontroversial. In reality there is considerable debate that is fuelled by the rarity of the condition and the difficulty to dissociate speech and non-speech perception experimentally. Riley and Cogan (2007) review the current literature and highlight the fact that much of the non-speech control stimuli discussed in the literature fail to capture the spectro-temporal characteristics of speech and that the majority of PWD cases are characterised by a generalised difficulty in integrating spectro-temporal information. This suggests damage to generalised feature extraction or integration mechanisms rather than damage to speech specific representations. They do, however, highlight the fact that a small number of cases are consistent with a model that proposes speech specific feature representations and also present reverse dissociations where patients failed to recognise environmental sounds but had unimpaired speech perception (Eustache et al., 1990; Godefroy et al., 1995; Lambert et al., 1989) and patients that failed to recognise music but not speech or environmental sounds (Griffiths et al., 1997).

Saygin et al. (2003) systematically tested verbal and non-verbal auditory processing in a group of 30 left hemisphere damaged patients in an identification task and found very highly correlated deficits in both tasks. The verbal and non-verbal tasks were carefully matched in a prior experiment with healthy volunteers. The authors conclude that verbal and non-verbal processing use shared neural resources. Lesion analysis implicated posterior sections of the middle and superior temporal gyri and inferior parietal lobe in both verbal and non-verbal processing deficits. These results, the fMRI data, and the scarcity of the pure PWD reports suggest that while there may well be speech specific pre-lexical representations that are affected by lesions to posterior superior temporal areas, there is good reason to believe that a shared neural system is responsible for processing speech and other sounds.

Selective deficits that impair phonetic categorisation, for instance vowel or consonant identification as opposed to word recognition, but spare the perception of non-speech stimuli would provide evidence for a separate phonetic representation such as postulated by the TRACE model (McClelland and Elman, 1986). Martin (2003) reviews the literature and comes to the conclusion that there is currently no evidence for a separate *phonetic* representation in the lesion data.

Lesion data support the view that pre-lexical analysis of speech is multi-modal. Campbell et al. (1990) found that patients with acquired cortical deafness benefit from lipreading provided higher order lexical representations are still intact. Conversely patients with lesions impairing the phonological lexicon cannot compensate through lip-reading. This finding is consistent with models that propose pre-lexical integration of auditory and visual cues.

5. SPATIO-TEMPORAL CORRELATES OF SPEECH AND NON-SPEECH PERCEPTION

If speech and non-speech signals are processed separately then one might not only expect a different spatial activation pattern but also differences in the fine time course of activation. Electroencephalography (EEG) or Magnetoencephalography (MEG) enable recordings of electrical activity in the brain with very high temporal resolution and are therefore good tools to study temporal correlates of speech processing.

We will describe data from an experiment that was specifically designed to address the question whether attention to speech or non-speech components within the *same* signal modulates the evoked response. This approach overcomes an important problem of imaging studies that use different stimuli as speech and control stimuli. Skipper et al. (2005) suggested that the lack of dorsal activation in audio-only speech perception might be due to a transient activation of the dorsal stream that may not be visible in fMRI data.

The stimuli in our experiment were vowel-nasal syllables that have been shown to change their perceived identity when a 20 ms frequency modulated sine (chirp) is presented at the position of the second formant (F2) transition (Harding and Meyer, 2003). The chirp simultaneously changes the perceived identity of the nasal and is heard as a separate sound. The signal therefore belongs to the class of duplex signals that are considered as evidence for the presence of separate processing of speech and non-speech sounds (Liberman and Mattingly, 1985): the addition of the chirp changes the identity of the perceived nasal, which means that it is processed by a putative speech processing subsystem, and simultaneously is heard as a whistle which means that it also maintains a separate identity as a non-speech signal.

The duplex stimulus used by Liberman and co-workers consisted of a plosive-vowel syllable where one formant transition (F2 of the consonant) was presented in one ear and the remainder of the stimulus in the other. This dichotic presentation is problematic in EEG studies that aim to quantify response lateralisation because lateralised presentation may confound the resulting data.

Our stimuli were presented diotically and therefore avoid some of the possible confounds of dichotic stimulation while still eliciting a clear duplex effect.

Data was recorded in blocks where 10 subjects had to either report the presence of a non-speech component (chirp) or identify the nasal (/m/ or /n/) for the same stimuli. The task was designed to elicit the same manual responses in both target conditions and to be roughly equally difficult to ensure that manual responses and task difficulty would not confound the results. The EEG was recorded in a dense electrode array (Electrical Geodesics Inc. 129 channel system) to enable source localisation. Further details of the stimulus presentation and EEG signal analysis are given in Perez et al. (in press).

EEG data is usually presented as evoked responses, that is the voltage recorded at a particular electrode is averaged over many (typically more than 100) stimulus presentations for each subject. If dense electrode arrays are used, then activity in adjacent electrode areas can be further averaged to reduce noise in the recordings (Figure 5). All frontal and lateral electrode assemblies show large ERPs that are typical for auditory stimulation but only the three assemblies located over the fronto-lateral areas of the left hemisphere show significant differences between speech and non-speech conditions between approximately 120 and 250 ms after stimulus onset. This time window is consistent with phonological processing (review: Pulvermüller & Shtyrow, 2006). Statistical analysis shows significant differences in amplitude in the N1 and P2 components of the evoked potentials in the left temporal, parietal and frontal areas when the 'attend speech' and 'attend chirp' condition are compared. This is consistent with models proposing lateralised selective processing of speech sounds in these areas.

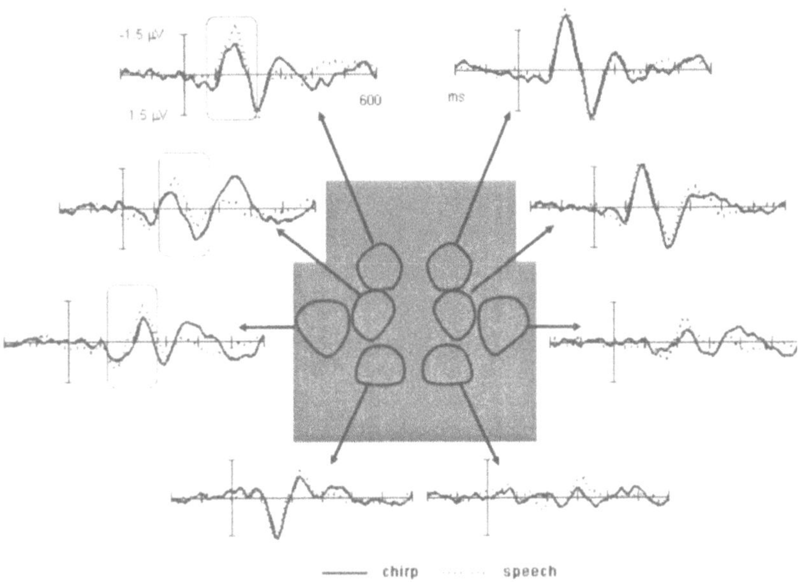

Figure 5: Grand mean waveforms for both conditions. In the non-speech condition (solid line) listeners are attending to the chirp, while in the speech condition (dashed line) they are attending to the speech signal. Vertical lines mark the onset of the stimuli. There are significant differences in the amplitude of the N1/P2 components in left temporal, parietal and frontal electrode arrays, as highlighted by the rectangles superimposed on the ERP traces. Further significant differences are found after around 300 ms post signal onset.

The data may also help to bridge the divide between functional imaging and lesion data. It is consistent with the lesion data because it shows a difference in the evoked potentials in left lateralised locations in a time window that has been linked to phonological processing. Activity, on the other hand, is clearly visible in both hemifields and therefore matches fMRI data for pre-lexical processing that shows bilateral activation. A

key trade-off between EEG and fMRI data is temporal versus spatial resolution. The EEG data shows differences in a narrow time window, 120 – 250 ms after the signal onset. BOLD responses, measured by fMRI, have very broad impulse responses (FWHM = 5.0 s; Glover, 1998) so that short events are unlikely to be resolved. A possible explanation, therefore, might be that speech specific differences are temporally sufficiently constrained and masked by non-speech specific bilateral activation to not cause measurable differences in the fMRI signals.
The ERPs recorded in EEG experiments show the voltage distribution on the scalp. One way to link ERPs to anatomical structures generating them is to model the observed voltage distribution on the scalp using equivalent dipole sources in the cortex (e.g. Scherg and von Cramon, 1985). The modelling is highly underconstrained because the same voltage distributions on the scalp can be produced by a number of dipole configurations. Typical auditory responses, for instance, can be explained by a single generator located centrally or a pair of symmetrical generators located in the auditory cortical areas. Both the location and orientation determine the observed scalp distribution so that a range of positions with appropriate orientations give similar results (review: Michel et al., 2004). The precise position of a fitted dipole or fine comparisons of fitted dipole positions across multiple conditions that explain (noisy) EEG data should therefore be treated with suspicion. A more conservative approach is to ask whether two voltage topologies, one for the speech condition, one for the non-speech condition, can be explained by the same dipoles. If very different neural assemblies are active during the two conditions, then one might expect to see that the solution for one condition cannot explain the data observed for the other. We took this approach with the speech/non-speech EEG data by initially fitting a pair of dipoles to the combined data for both conditions and then comparing the goodness of fit for separate conditions (we used BESA, MEGIS Software GmbH, Munich). We found that the same pair of dipoles (labelled 1 and 2 in Figure 6) well explains the initial ca. 300 ms of both conditions, provided a slightly different activation pattern (more negative activation to the left dipole in the speech condition) is assumed. A third dipole, located in the left anterior cingulate cortex, was required to model a negative deflection over left fronto-lateral sites in response to the non-speech condition (ca. 300-400 ms. after stimulus onset).

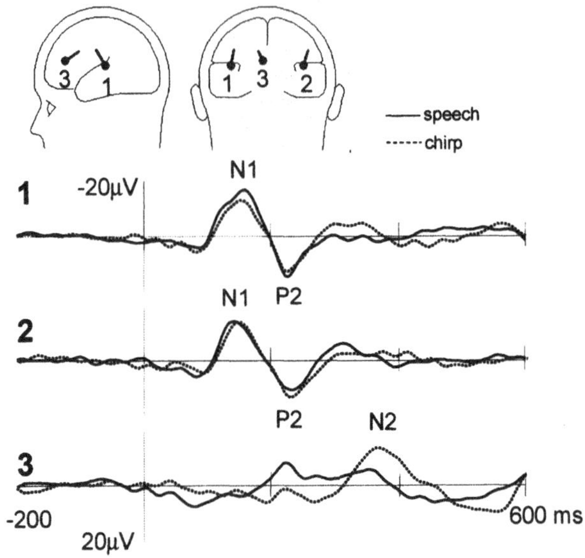

Figure 6: Results of the dipole source analysis of the ERP data. The graph shows the locations of the three dipole and associated generator patterns that account for the observed scalp activations in the two conditions. In the time range 120-250 ms the response is dominated by activation in the auditory cortex (dipoles 1 and 2). Activity between 280 and 380 ms is accounted for by a third dipole located in the left anterior cingulate cortex.

The dipole modelling, in summary, suggests that the observed difference between the speech and the non-speech condition in the time window consistent with phonological processing can be explained by differential activation of the same brain areas. This finding is entirely consistent with the fMRI data described in section 3. The EEG data locates pre-lexical processing in superior temporal areas with a bias towards the left hemisphere. We observe strong, shared auditory evoked responses bilaterally for both conditions which presumably explain bilateral fMRI activation.

6. CONCLUSION

The aim of this chapter was to evaluate theoretical approaches that explain pre-lexical speech processing in the light of recent imaging data. The data on auditory and visual speech perception suggest distributed and largely separate processing networks for the two modalities that are shared with processing for other, related, signals. This is consistent with multi-stage models of speech processing assuming that a hierarchy of representations is extracted to explain behavioural data.

Passive listening causes dominant activation in superior temporal areas bilaterally. Left hemisphere speech specific modulation of the response, not dipole localisation shifts, are seen in EEG data. This is consistent with models of speech perception that assume the parallel processing of speech and non-speech data in overlapping areas. Passive listening does not cause extensive activation in areas typically associated with articulation. We see clear evidence for activity in motor-related areas for visual speech processing. This suggests that motor-representations are not the primary representation for pre-lexical speech processing.

Unimodally presented auditory *and* visual syllables activate the posterior edge of BA 22. This suggests that this area processes abstract, modality independent representations and is consistent with the idea that this area is providing the interface between pre-lexical and higher order processing. We found bilateral activity – with generally more significant activation in the right hemisphere. The area does not appear to be speech specific.

We found significant overlap in the areas activated by speech, body motion and meaningless signals and we have no evidence for areas exclusively devoted to speech processing although the differential activation for the three conditions is compatible with a model that assumes co-localised stimulus specific networks.

The ventral pathway in our data, consistently with Hickok and Poeppel (2007) and Skipper's (2005; 2007) data and model, is the primary processing pathway for spoken speech. As soon as lip movements are visible, either alone or in combination with auditory signals, high levels of activity are seen in the dorsal pathway. If we accept the suggestion that the dorsal pathway is part of a generative active perception network, which presumably codes motor patterns, and is invoked for unintelligible speech (Zekfeld et al., 2006), then this raises a number of questions. It is clear how the dorsal system would be invoked by visual speech, but not why it strongly responds to audiovisual speech, which is, if anything, more intelligible than auditory-alone speech. A possible explanation might be that the invocation of the dorsal stream is optional for (poor intelligibility) speech, but compulsory for visual speech.

The notion that there might be an (articulatory) gesture based system that is invoked when necessary to complement the primary ventral pattern matching system, is attractive from an ecological perspective. It would mean that we rely on an efficient, passive primary speech perception system that uses an auditory representation, but is complemented by an active secondary system that is expensive in terms of metabolism and processing time. A compulsory involvement of the dorsal stream (whenever visual input is present – whether it aids intelligibility or not) might explain the imaging data as well the McGurk effect, which a purely auditory processing strategy for highly intelligible speech cannot explain.

The data presented and reviewed here raise a number of issues that models of speech perception should take into account. While there is no evidence for the extraction of speech specific features, there is clear evidence that multiple processing sites activate, which presumably have specific functions. There is also clear evidence for audio-visual interactions at a pre-lexical stages from lesion data. This makes models that propose a direct transformation of spectral information into a lexical representation (e.g. Klatt, 1979) less plausible than models that propose intermediate representations.

The imaging is consistent with the lesion data in supporting a distinction between speech production and perception. Spoken speech activates primarily auditory areas. This, in our view, makes DRT (Fowler, 1996) less likely because we would have expected to see dominant activity in motor cortical areas or Broca's area where articulatory gestures are processed in speech production. It is not possible to dismiss the theory because one could postulate duplicate articulatory representations in areas linked to production and perception.

The same argument can be applied to the original motor theory of speech perception (Liberman et al., 1967), because it postulated that speech is perceived by reference to the motor patterns so that perception and production should draw on the same circuitry. The revised motor theory of speech perception proposes that it is the 'intended gesture' rather than the physical realisation that is the object of speech perception. This means that the involvement of areas concerned with the physical realisation of motor activity is no longer required for speech perception. Whalen et al. (2006) use differential activity in the primary auditory cortex for speech and non-speech sounds of different complexity to argue for a specialised speech processing system. This would be consistent with the revised motor theory of speech perception but it would, of course, also be consistent with any other theory that posits an intermediate representation, such as general auditory accounts. This highlights one of the limitations of brain imaging methods: while brain imaging may provide evidence for specialised processing centres or distributed representations, it is unable to distinguish the underlying representations or algorithms. Even if one could identify a processing centre that specifically codes an intermediate representation for speech sounds, there is no way to distinguish potential articulatory from auditory *internal* representations. We expect the debate whether speech is special and what the underlying representations are to go on for a good while yet.

REFERENCES

Benson, R., Whalen, D.H., Richardson, M., Swainson, B., Clark, V., and Lai, S. (2001). Parametrically dissociating speech and nonspeech perception in the brain using fMRI. *Brain and Language* 78, 364-396.

Blesser, B. (1972). Speech perception under conditions of spectral transformation. I. Phonetic characteristics. *Journal of Speech and Hearing Research* 15, 5–41.

Buccino, G., Binkofski, F., Fink, G.R., Fadiga, L., Fogassi, L., Gallese, V., Seitz, R. J., Zilles, K., Rizzolatti, G., and Freund, H.J. (2001). Action observation activates premotor and parietal areas in a somatotopic manner: an fMRI study, *European Journal of Neuroscience* 13, 400-404.

Callan, D.E., Jones, J.A. Callan, A.M., and Akahane-Yamada, R. (2004). Phonetic perceptual identification by native- and second-language speakers differentially activates brain regions involved with acoustic phonetic processing and those involved with articulatory-auditory/orosensory internal models. *NeuroImage* 22, 1182-1194.

Calvert, G.A. & Lewis, J.W. (2003). Hemodynamic studies of audiovisual interactions. In: G.A. Calvert, C. Spence, and B.E. Stein (eds.) *The Handbook of Multisensory Processes*, Cambridge (MA): MIT Press.

Calvert, G.A. & Campbell, R. (2003). Reading speech from still and moving faces: The neural substrates of visible speech. *Journal of Cognitive Neuroscience* 15(1), 57-70.

Calvert, G.A., Bullmore, E.T., Brammer, M.J., Campbell, R., Williams, S.C.R., McGuire, P.K., Woodruff, P.W.R., Iversen, S.D., and David A.S. (1997). Activation of Auditory Cortex During Silent Lipreading. *Science* 276, 593–596.

Campbell, R., Garwood, J., Franklin, S., Howard, D., Landis, T., and Regard, M. (1990). Neuropsychological Studies of Auditory Visual Fusion Illusions - 4 Case-Studies and Their Implications. *Neuropsychologia* 28, 787-802.

Caplan, D. (1987). *Neurolinguistics and Linguistic Aphasiology: An Introduction*. New York: Cambridge University Press.

Caplan, D., Gow, D., and Makris, N. (1995). Analysis of lesions by MRI in stroke patients with acoustic-phonetic processing deficits. *Neurology* 45(2), 293-298.

Chomsky, N. (1991). Linguistics and Cognitive Science: problems and Mysteries. In: A. Kashler (ed.) *The Chomskyan Turn*, 26-53, Cambridge (MA): Blackwell.

Chomsky, N. & Halle, M. (1968). *Sound Pattern of English*. New York: Harper Row.

Davis, M.H. & Johnsrude, I.S. (2003). Hierarchical Processing in Spoken Language Comprehension. *Journal of Neuroscience* 23, 3423-3431.

Diehl, R.L. & Kluender, K.R. (1989). On the Objects of Speech Perception. *Ecological Psychology* 1, 121-144.

Diehl R.L., Lotto, A.J., and Holt, L.L. (2004). Speech Perception. *Annual Revues Psychology* 55, 149-179.

Eulitz, C. & Lahiri, A. (2004). Neurobiological Evidence for Abstract Phonological Representations in the Mental Lexicon during Speech Recognition. *Journal of Cognitive Neuroscience* 16, 577–583.

Eustache, F., Lechevalier, B., Viader, F., and Lambert, J. (1990). Identification and discrimination disorders in auditory perception: a report on two cases. *Neuropsychologia* 28, 257-570.

Fiez, J.A., Raichle, M.E., Miezin, F.M., Petersen, S.E., Tallal, P., and Katz, W.F. (1995). Pet Studies Of Auditory And Phonological Processing: Effects Of Stimulus Characteristics And Task Demands. *Journal Of Cognitive Neuroscience* 7, 357-375

Forster, K.I. (1976). Accessing the mental lexicon. In: R.J. Wales & E. Walker (eds.) *New Approaches to Language Mechanisms*. 257-287, Amsterdam: North-Holland.

Fowler, C.A. (1996). Listeners do hear sounds, not tongues, *Journal of the Acoustical Society of America* 99, 1730-1741.

Fowler, C.A. (2003). Speech as a supramodal or amodal phenomenon. In: G. Calvert, C. Spence, and B.E. Stein (eds.), *The handbook of multisensory processes*, 189-202, Cambridge (MA): MIT press.

Fowler, C.A. & Rosenblum, L.D. (1991). Duplex perception: A comparison of monosyllables and slamming doors. *Journal of Experimental Psychology: Human Perception and Performance* 16, 742-754.

Frackowiak, R.S.J., Friston, K.J., Frith, C.D., Dolan, R.J., Price, C.J., Zeki, S., Ashburner, J.T., and Penny, W.D, (2004). *Human Brain Function*, Academic Press.

Geschwind, N. (1965). Disconnexion syndromes in animals and man I, *Brain* 88, 237-294.

Geschwind, N. (1965). Disconnexion syndromes in animals and man II, *Brain* 88, 585-644.

Gibson, J.J. (1966). *The Senses Considered as Perceptual Systems*. Boston: Houghton Mifflin.

Glover, G.H. (1999). Deconvolution of impulse response in event-related BOLD fMRI1. *NeuroImage* 9, 416-429.

Godefroy, O., Leys, D., Furby, A., De Reuck, J., Daems, C., Rondepierre, P., Debachy, B., Deleume, J.F., and Desaulty, A. (1995). Psychoacoustical Deficits Related to Bilateral Subcortical Hemorrhages. A Case with Apperceptive Auditory Agnosia. *Cortex 31*, 149–159.

Goldinger, S.D. (1996). Words and voices: Episodic traces in spoken word identification and recognition memory. *Journal of Experimental Psychology: Learning, Memory and Cognition* 22, 1166–1183.

Goldinger, S.D. (1998). Echoes of echoes? An episodic theory of lexical access. *Psychological Review* 105, 251–279.

Griffiths, T.D., Rees, A., Witton, C., Cross, P.M., Shakir, R.A., and Green, G.G.R. (1997). Spatial and temporal auditory processing deficits following right hemisphere infarction. A psychophysical study. *Brain* 120, 785-794.

Harding, S. & Meyer, G. (2003). Changes in the perception of synthetic nasal consonants as a result of vowel formant manipulations. *Speech Communication* 39, 173-189.

Hickok, G. and Poeppel, D. (2000). Towards a functional anatomy of speech perception. *Trends in Cognitive Sciences* 4,131-138.

Hickok, G & Poeppel, D. (2007). The cortical organization of speech processing. *Nature Reviews, Neuroscience* 8, 393-402.

Hier, D.B., Yoon, W.B., Mohr, J.P., Price, T.R., and Wolf, P.A. (1994). Gender and aphasia in the Stroke Data Bank. *Brain and Language* 47, 155–167.

Jacoby, L.L. (1983). Perceptual enhancement: Persistent effects of an experience. *Journal of Experimental Psychology: Learning, Memory, and Cognition* 9, 21-38.

Jakobson, R. & Halle, M. (1956). *Fundamentals of Language*. The Hague: Mouton.

Kewley-Port, D. (1983). Time-Varying features as correlates of place of articulation in stop consonants. *Journal of the Acoustical Society of America* 73, 322-335.

Klatt, D.H. (1979). Speech perception: A model of acoustic–phonetic analysis and lexical access. *Journal of Phonetics* 7, 279–312.

Klatt, D.H. (1989). Review of selected models of speech perception. In: W.D. Marslen-Wilson (ed.) *Lexical representation and process*, 169–226, Cambridge(MA): MIT Press.

Kohn, S.E. & Friedman, R.B. (1986). Word-meaning deafness: A phonological-semantic dissociation, *Cognitive Neuropsychology* 3, 291-308.

Lambert, J., Eustache, F., Lechevallier, B., Rossa, Y., and Viader, F. (1989). Auditory agnosia with relative sparing of speech perception. *Cortex* 25, 71 -82.

Liberman, A.M., Cooper, F.S., Shankweiler, D.P., and Studdert-Kennedy, M. (1967). Perception of the speech code. *Psychological Review* 74, 431-461.

Liberman, A.M. & Mattingly, I.G. (1985). The motor theory of speech perception revised, *Cognition* 21, 1-36.

Liberman, A.M. & Whalen, D.H. (2000). On the relation of speech to language *Trends in Cognitive Neuroscience* 4, 187-196.

Lisker, L. (1986). "Voicing" in English: a catalogue of acoustic features signaling /b/ versus /p/ in trochees. *Language and Speech* 29, 3-11.

Luria, A.R. (1970). *Traumatic Aphasia*. The Hague: Mouton.

Mackay, D.M. (1968). The 'active/passive' controversy. *Zeitschrift für Phonetik, Sprachwissenschaft und Kommunikationsforschung* 21, 40-42.

Martin, R.C. (2003). Language processing: Functional organization and neuroanatomical basis. *Annual Reviews Psychol*ogy 54, 55-89.

Marslen-Wilson, W.D. & Tyler, L.K. (1980). The temporal structure of spoken language understanding. *Cognition* 8, 1-71.

Marslen-Wilson, W.D. & Warren, P. (1994). Levels of perceptual representation and process in lexical access: Words, phonemes, and features. *Psychological Review* 101, 653-675.

Massaro, D.W. (1989). Testing between the TRACE Model and the Fuzzy Logical Model of Speech perception. *Cognitive Psychology* 21, 398-421.

McClelland, J.L. & Elman, J.L. (1986). The TRACE model of speech perception. *Cognitive Psychology* 10, 1–86.

McGurk, H. & MacDonald, J. (1976). Hearing lips and seeing voices, *Nature* 264, 746–748.

McQueen, J.M. & Cutler, A. (1997). Cognitive processes in speech perception. In: W.J. Hardcastle and J. Laver (eds.) *The Handbook of Phonetic Sciences*, 566-585, Oxford: Blackwell.

Michel, C.M., Murray, M.M., Lantz, G., Gonzalez, S., Spinelli, L., and Grave de Peralta, R. (2004). EEG Source Imaging, *Clinical Neurophysiology* 115, 2195-2222.

Miller, J.L. & Eimas, P.D. (1995). Speech perception: from signal to word. *Annual Reviews Psychology* 46, 467-492.

Morosan, P., Rademacher, J., Schleicher, A., Amunts, K., Schormann, T., and Zilles, K. (2001). Human primary auditory cortex: cytoarchitectonic subdivisions and mapping into a spatial reference system. *NeuroImage* 13, 684–701.

Narain, C., Scott, S.K., Wise, R.J.S, Rosen, S., Leff, A., Iversen, S.D., and Matthews, P.M. (2003). Defining a Left-lateralized Response Specific to Intelligible Speech Using fMRI, *Cerebral Cortex* 13, 1362–1368.

Obleser, J., Zimmermann, J., Van Mater, J., and Rauschecker, J. (2007a). Multiple stages of auditory speech perception reflected in event related fMRI, *Cerebral Cortex* 17, 2251-2257.

Obleser, J., Wise, R.J.S., Dresner, M.A., and Scott, S.K. (2007b). Functional Integration across Brain Regions Improves Speech Perception under Adverse Listening Conditions. *The Journal of Neuroscience* 27, 2283–2289.

Paulesu, E., Perani, D., Blasi, V., Silani, G., Borghese, N.A., De Giovanni, U., Sensolo, S., and Fazio, F., (2003). A Functional-Anatomical Model for Lipreading, *Journal of Neurophysiology* 90, 2005-2013.

Perez, E., Harrison, N., and Meyer, G.F. (in press). Brain correlates of speech and non-speech: ERPs associated with duplex perception. *Journal of Neurolinguistics*.

Pisoni, D.B., and Luce, P.A. (1987). Acoustic-phonetic representations in word recognition. *Cognition* 25, 21–52.

Poeppel, D., (2001). Pure Word deafness and the bilateral processing of the speech code. *Cognitive Science* 25, 679-693.

Poeppel, D. & Hickok, G. (2004). Towards a new functional anatomy of speech perception, *Cognition* 92, 1-12.

Price, C., Thierry, G., and Griffiths, T., (2005). Speech specific auditory processing: where is it? *Trends in Cognitive Sciences* 9, 271-276.

Pulvermüller, F. & Shtyrow, Y. (2006). Language outside the focus of attention: The mismatch negativity as a tool for studying cognitive processes. *Progress in Neurobiology* 79, 49-71.

Remez, R.E., Rubin, P.E., Pisoni, D.B., and Carrell, T.D. (1981). Speech perception without traditional speech cues. *Science* 212, 947-950.

Repp, B. (1982). Phonetic trading relations and context effects: new experimental evidence foe a speech mode of perception. *Psychological Bulletin* 92, 91-110.

Riley, J.A. & Cogan, G.B. (2007). A two mechanism model of pure word deafness. *University of Maryland Working Papers in Linguistics* 16, 201-221.

Rizzolatti, G., Fogassi, L., and Gallese, V. (2001). Neurophysiological mechanisms underlying the understanding and imitation of action. *Nature Reviews Neuroscience* 2, 661-670.

Saygin, A.P., Dick, F. Wilson, S.W. Dronkers, N.F., and Bates, E. (2003). Neural resources for processing language and environmental sounds: Evidence from aphasia. *Brain* 126, 928-945.

Saberi, K. & Perrott, D.R. (1999). Cognitive restoration of reversed speech *Nature* 398, 760.

Scherg, M. & von Cramon, D. (1985). Two bilateral sources of the late AEP as identified by a spatio-temporal dipole model. *Electroencephalography and Clinical Neurophysiology* 62, 32-44.

Schwartz, J-L., Berthommier, F., and Savariaux, C. (2004). Seeing to hear better: evidence for early audio-visual interactions in speech identification, *Cognition* 93, B69–B78.

Shankweiler, D. & Studdert-Kennedy, M. (1967). Identification of consonants and vowels presented to left and right ears. *Quarterly Journal of Experimental Psychology* 19, 59-63.

Shiffrin, R.M. & Schneider, W. (1977). Controlled and automatic human information processing: II. Perceptual learning, automatic attending, and a general theory. *Psychological Review* 84, 127-190.

Skipper, J.I., Nusbaum, H.C., and Small, S.L. (2005) Listening to talking faces: motor cortical activation during speech perception. *NeuroImage* 25, 76-89.

Skipper, J.I., Nusbaum, H.C., and Small, S.L. (2006). Lending a helping hand to hearing: another motor theory of speech perception. In: M.A. Arbib (ed.) *Action to language via the mirror neuron system*, 250-285, Cambridge(MA): Cambridge University Press.

Skipper, J.I., van Wassenhove, V., Nusbaum, H.C, and Small, S.L. (2007). Hearing lips and seeing voices: How cortical areas supporting speech production mediate audiovisual speech perception. *Cerebral Cortex* 17, 2387-2399.

Springer, J.A., Binder, J.R., Hammeke, T.A., Swanson, S.J., Frost, J.A., Bellgowan, P.S.F., Brewer, C.C., Perry, H.M., Morris, G.L., and Mueller, W.M. (1999).

Language dominance in neurologically normal and epilepsy subjects. *Brain* 122, 2033-2046.

Stevens, K.N. & Blumstein, S.E. (1981). The search for invariant acoustic correlates of phonetic features. In: P.D. Eimas and J.L. Miller (eds.) *Perspectives on the study of speech.* Hillsdale (NJ): Erlbaum.

Stevens, K.N. (2002). Toward a model for lexical access based on acoustic landmarks and distinctive features. *Journal of the Acoustical Society of America* 111, 1872-1891.

Stromswold, K. (2000). The Cognitive Neuroscience of Language Acquisition, In: M.S. Gazzaniga (ed.) *The New Cognitive Neurosciences* (2nd ed)., 909-932, Cambridge (MA): MIT Press.

Summerfield, Q. (1979). Use of visual information for phonetic perception. *Phonetica* 36, 314–331.

Summerfield, Q. (1992). Lipreading and audio-visual speech perception. *Philosophical Transaction of the Royal Society London. Series B: Biological Sciences* 335, 71-78.

Sussman, H.A., McCaffrey H.A., and Mathews, S.A. (1991). An investigation of locus equations as a source of relational invariance for stop place articulation. *Journal of the Acoustical Society of America* 90, 1309-1325.

Tomasello, M. (2003). *Constructing a Language: A Usage-Based Theory of Language Acquisition,* Cambridge (MA): Harvard University Press.

Tuomainen, J., Andersen, T.S., Tiippana, K., and Sams, M. (2005). Audio–visual speech perception is special, *Cognition* 96, B13–B22.

Vaina, L.M., Solomon, J., Chowdhury, S., Sinha, P., and Belliveau, J.W. (2001). Functional neuroanatomy of biological motion perception in humans. *Proceedings of the National Academy of the Sciences USA* 98, 11656–11661.

Warren, J.D., Jennings, A.R., and Griffiths, T.D. (2005). Analysis of the spectral envelope of sounds by the human brain. *NeuroImage* 24, 1052–1057.

Warren, J.D., Scott, S.K., Price, C.J., and Griffiths, T.D. (2006). Human brain mechanisms for the early analysis of voices. *NeuroImage* 31, 1389-1397.

Wernicke, C. (1874/1977) Der aphasische Symptomenkomplex: eine psychologische Studie auf anatomischer Basis. In: G.H. Eggert (1977) *Wernicke's works on aphasia: A sourcebook and review.* 91-145, The Hague: Mouton.

Whalen, D.H. & Liberman, A.M. (1987). Speech perception takes precedence over nonspeech perception, *Science* 237(4811), 169.

Whalen, D.H., Benson, R.R., Richardson, M., Swainson, B. Lai, S., Mencl, W.E. Fulbright, R.K., Constable, R.T., Liberman, A.M., (2006). Differentiation of speech and nonspeech processing within primary auditory cortex, *Journal of the Acoustical Society of America* 119, 575-581.

Wise, R.J.S., Greene, J., Büchel, C., and Scott, S.K. (1999). Brain systems for word perception and articulation. *Lancet* 353,1057-1061.

Wise, R.J.S., Scott, S.K., Blank, C., Mummery, C.J., Murphy, K., and Warburton, E.A. (2001). Separate neural subsystems within 'Wernicke's area'. *Brain* 124, 83–95.

Wilson, S.M., Saygin, A.P., and Iacoboni, M. (2004). Listening to speech activates motor areas involved in speech production, *Nature Neuroscience* 7, 701-702.

Wilson, S.M., Iacoboni, M. (2006). Neural responses to non-native phonemes varying in producibility: Evidence for the sensorimotor nature of speech perception. *NeuroImage* 33, 316-325.

Zekveld, A.A., Heslenfeld, D.J., Festen, J.M., and Schoonhoven, R. (2006). Top-down and bottom-up processes in speech comprehension, *NeuroImage* 32, 1826-1836.

12

The role of syllabification in the lexical segmentation of German and Slovak

ADRIANA HANULÍKOVÁ

Abstract: Two experiments were carried out to examine the syllable affiliation of intervocalic consonant clusters and their effects on speech segmentation in two different languages. In a syllable reversal task, Slovak and German speakers divided bisyllabic non-words that were presented aurally into two parts, starting with the second syllable. Following the maximal onset principle, intervocalic consonants should be maximally assigned to the onset of the following syllable in conformity with language-specific restrictions, e.g., [dʊ.gru], [zʊ.kro:] (dot indicates a syllable boundary). According to German phonology, syllables require branching rhymes (hence, [zʊk.ro:]). In Slovak, both [dʊ.gru] and [dʊg.ru] are possible syllabifications. Experiment 1 showed that German speakers more often closed the first syllable ([zʊk.ro:]), following the requirement for a branching rhyme. In Experiment 2, Slovak speakers showed no clear preference; the first syllable was either closed ([dʊg.ru]) or open ([dʊ.gru]). Correlation analyses on previously conducted word-spotting studies (Hanulíková, in press, 2008) suggest that speech segmentation is unaffected by these syllabification preferences.

1. INTRODUCTION

The syllable is a fundamental unit in phonological theories and plays an important role in many areas of language research, including research into speech production (e.g., Cholin et al., 2004; Schiller et al., 1997), speech comprehension (e.g., Cutler et al., 1983, 1986; Mehler et al., 1981), and language acquisition (e.g., Brière, 1968; Liberman et al., 1974; Sato, 1984). However, despite its importance across fields, the linguistic description of the syllable is rather controversial in terms of both its structure and its necessity as a linguistic unit (for different views, see, e.g., Hooper, 1972; Kahn, 1976; Lebrun, 1966; Pulgram, 1970; Selkirk, 1982; Vennemann, 1988). The least controversial definition might be one that describes a syllable as a unit of organization comprised of a vocalic nucleus that can have one or more consonants preceding or following it (for further discussion, see, e.g., Blevins, 1995; Itô, 1986, 1988; Selkirk, 1982).

The concept of a syllable comes into play in syllabification. Syllabification is the division of words into syllables, and speakers of any language can normally effortlessly determine how many syllables a word has. However, languages differ as to how they combine speech sounds into syllables and syllables into words. These differences result in language-specific assignment of segments to syllable positions. For example, English allows the combination of the three phonemes /n/, /k/, and /i:/ to form a syllable such as /ki:n/. However, the combination of these three phonemes to form the syllable /kni:/ is not permissible because /kn/ is not a possible English onset. As a consequence, the syllabic division of a word such as *technique* is clearly influenced by such combinatorial restrictions. The second syllable of the word *technique*, as most native speakers of English will agree, is /ni:k/ and not /kni:k/. Other languages, however, permit a combination such as /kni:/. For example, the second syllable of the Slovak word *pekný* 'pretty' can be /kni:/. Unlike English speakers, Slovak native speakers may have differing intuitions about the syllable affiliation of the intervocalic consonants in *pekný*, which could be either *pe.kný* or *pek.ný*, because all these syllables and syllable boundary placements are permissible (see also Rubach, 1993).

In addition to language-specific restrictions on syllable structure, some phonological theories also suggest universal principles that influence syllable boundary placements (e.g., Kahn, 1976; Selkirk, 1982; Vennemann, 1988). One proposed universal principle is that the maximal number of consonants possible should be assigned to the onset of the following syllable in conformity with language-specific restrictions (e.g., Pulgram, 1970), hence *pe.kný*. However, these theoretical suggestions about syllabic divisions do not always coincide with human intuitions about syllable boundaries (e.g., Treiman & Danis, 1988; Titone & Connine, 1997).

Thus, native speakers agree less about the identification of syllable edges than they do about the number of syllables in a word. Syllable boundaries are easy to determine in some languages, as indicated by a high degree of agreement among speakers. In other languages, there is a high variability in speakers' responses, which suggests that syllable boundaries are rather ambiguous (e.g., Treiman & Danis, 1988; Content et al., 2000; Frauenfelder & Content, 1999).

The lack of certainty in syllable identification presents challenges for some psycholinguistic theories about spoken-language comprehension that rely on the concept of the syllable. These theories suggest that syllabic units might help answer the well-known question about how humans segment individual words from the stream of speech. In speech-processing research, the role of the syllable as a psychological unit has been the target of debate for over thirty years (e.g., Savin & Bever, 1970; Cutler & Norris, 1988; Goslin & Frauenfelder, 2000; Mehler, 1981; Mehler et al., 1981; Norris & Cutler, 1985). It has been assumed that the syllable plays a universal role in speech segmentation as well as speech comprehension and is used to access words in the mental lexicon (e.g., Mehler, 1981). If boundaries of lexical units coincide with boundaries of syllables, detecting syllable edges would be a useful strategy in speech segmentation and in lexical matching. However, variation and ambiguity in syllable structure are problematic for such speech-processing theories.

Several methods have been developed to investigate the role of syllabic representations as universal perceptual units that mediate between the acoustic signal and the mental lexicon (e.g., Mehler, 1981; Mehler et al., 1981; see also Grosjean & Frauenfelder, 1996; Morais & Kolinsky, 1992, for overviews). One such method is the sequence detection task (see Frauenfelder & Kearns, 1996). In a study by Mehler and colleagues (Mehler et al., 1981), French listeners were found to be faster at detecting the target sequence *ba* in *balance* 'balance' than in *balcon* 'balcony' because *ba* matches the syllabification of *ba.lance* but not of *bal.con*. Similarly, *bal* was detected faster in *bal.con* than in *ba.lance,* due to the syllabification match. Further investigations, however, revealed crucial distinctions between languages, and different methods and materials (words versus non-words) yielded contradictory results (e.g., Cutler et al., 1983, 1986, 1992; Cutler, 1997; Mehler et al., 1990; Frauenfelder & Content, 1999; Zwitserlood et al., 1993). For example, the effect did not replicate when using French nonsense words (Frauenfelder & Content, 1999; Content et al., 2001) nor was it observed in either English or Dutch listeners who were presented with the same French materials (Cutler, 1997; Cutler et al., 1983, 1986).

It has been further shown that English and Dutch speakers treat intervocalic consonants (following lax short vowels) in bisyllabic words such as *palace* or *letter* as ambisyllabic, thus as part of both syllables (e.g., Fallows, 1981; Schiller et al., 1997; Zwitserlood et al., 1993). Moreover, listeners' knowledge about where one syllable ends and the next begins is subject to great variation, which occurs not only between languages, but also within a given language and even within the same speaker (e.g., Content et al., 2000; Content et al., 2001; Frauenfelder & Content, 1999; Rubach, 1993; see also Cutler, 1993, for an overview).

If there is such disagreement about syllabic boundaries among listeners, how can the syllable be used in speech segmentation and as a universal mediating unit for theories about lexical access? Because of the language-specific differences, Norris and Cutler (1985) argued against the syllable as a universal perceptual unit (see also Cutler et al., 2001). They pointed out limits of the sequence detection task and argued that it is crucial to distinguish between segmentation and classification of the speech input. Classification means that some mental categories are assigned to stretches of the speech input. To classify the input into syllables, the input must be segmented at syllable boundaries (e.g., the sequence detection task requires classification). Segmentation, however, means finding the right alignment points for lexical access. Although classification requires segmentation, it is not necessary to classify the input in order to segment it. It has been shown that lexical access begins as soon as a few speech sounds are available; there is no delay until a syllabic representation has been determined (e.g., Marslen-Wilson, 1987; McClelland & Elman, 1986; Norris, 1994).

Further evidence supporting this idea comes from cross-linguistic studies showing that listeners use language-specific rhythm in speech segmentation (e.g., Cutler & Norris, 1988; Otake et al., 1993). For example, Cutler and Norris (1988) showed that English listeners assume that a potential word onset occurs at strong syllables (syllables with a full vowel) and they are more likely to segment continuous speech at strong and not at weak syllables. Therefore, it is unlikely that syllables are universal prelexical units of perception (see Cutler et al., 2001, for an overview), although they might play a role in speech segmentation in some languages (for further discussion, see, e.g., Morais & Kolinsky, 1992; Kolinsky, 1998; Dupoux, 1993; Content et al., 2001). In French, for instance, the syllable onset has been suggested to play such a role in speech segmentation (e.g., Content et al., 2000; Dumay et al., 1999).

In more recent research, Norris and colleagues proposed that syllables nevertheless might have a universal function in speech processing, not as a perceptual unit but as a viable parsing unit (Norris et al., 1997; Norris et al., 2001). This idea has been implemented in the Possible-Word Constraint (PWC), which proposes that the syllable is used as a unit that is evaluated by a listener in terms of viable and unviable lexical parses of continuous speech. A syllable seems to provide such a viable unit across languages while single consonants do not.

Support for the PWC comes from studies using the word-spotting paradigm developed by Cutler & Norris (1988) in which listeners were asked to respond whenever they found an English target word embedded at the beginning or at the end of a nonsense sequence. In Norris et al. (1997), the English word *apple* was embedded in a single-consonant context ***f**apple* or in a CVC syllable context ***vuff**apple* (context in bold in the examples). Neither of the contexts is an existing English word, but ***vuff*** is a possible well-formed word in English. The results showed that if the target word *apple* was preceded by a single consonant, it was recognized more slowly and less accurately than when it was preceded by a nonsense syllable. This result was interpreted as evidence that a single consonant, which itself cannot be an English word, is not a viable residue of the input. According to the PWC, the activation of lexical candidates is reduced in this way. A single consonant is disfavoured as a parsing unit and this affects lexical segmentation. Norris et al. (1997) implemented this principle in the Shortlist model of spoken-word recognition (Norris, 1994) and specified the nature of a viable residue as one containing a vowel.

To test whether the model was indeed universal, Norris et al. (2001) investigated whether or not English listeners would treat any syllable as a possible parsing unit (i.e., as a viable residue), independently of the phonological constraints in English. A word such as *perturb* was therefore presented in three contexts: a tense-vowel CV syllable (e.g., [**dɑ**pətə:b]), a lax-vowel CV syllable (e.g., [**dɛ**pətə:b]) and a single consonant (e.g., [**s**pətə:b]). None of these contexts are existing English words, but [dɑ] could be a word. While there are English words with tense vowels and an open coda (e.g., *car* [kɑ] in British English), there are none with a lax vowel without the coda being closed (e.g., *deck* [dɛk], but not [dɛ]). The PWC predicts that English listeners would treat both syllables ([dɑ] and [dɛ]) alike and spot words in syllabic contexts faster than in single-consonant contexts. Replicating the results from the previous experiment, listeners' detection of the target word was significantly faster and more accurate in both syllable contexts as compared to the consonant context. The crucial result was that there was no difference between the two syllables [dɛ] and [dɑ], although only the latter is a well-formed English syllable. Moreover, there was a significant difference between [dɛ] and [s], both of which are not possible English words.

According to Norris and colleagues, a possible residue does not have to be a phonologically acceptable word (i.e., any syllable will be acceptable); however, it cannot consist of only consonants. Thus, the actual or potential lexical status of words in a specific language is not relevant and the PWC is a universal principle, a claim that has been supported by studies with further languages including Japanese (McQueen et al., 2001), Dutch (McQueen & Cutler, 1998), Sesotho (Cutler et al., 2002), and Cantonese (Yip, 2004). These languages exhibit differing surface constraints on possible syllables and differing phonological processes, as well as differing language-specific cues to word boundaries. For example, possible stand-alone words in Sesotho must consist of minimally two syllables. If the PWC were sensitive to this language-specific constraint on word structure, a monosyllabic sequence should be penalized in segmentation. However, Cutler et al. (2002) showed that the recognition of a word such as *alafa* 'to prescribe' was as fast in a monosyllabic context (***ro**alafa*) as in a bisyllabic one (***pafo**alafa*), but slower in a single-consonant context (***h**alafa*). This finding is in line with the universal PWC. The effect of the PWC was observed in all these languages, and thus the conclusion was drawn that segmenting a word from a vowelless sequence is always harder.

Such a universal role of the syllable in speech processing has, however, been challenged by recent research on Japanese and Slovak (e.g., Cutler et al., submitted; Hanulíková et al., submitted; Hanulíková, in press, 2008). These studies revealed that word recognition can succeed in the context of single consonants, but only when these consonants receive support from the lexicon. Slovak allows single-consonant words such as the preposition *k* 'to' (with two positional allophones [k] and [g]). In two cross-linguistic studies with a very similar design, Hanulíková et al. investigated how segmentation proceeds in Slovak, a language with single-consonant words, as compared to German (Hanulíková, in press, 2008), a language that does not allow single-consonant words. German and Slovak listeners had little difficulty recognizing a target word (e.g., *Rose* 'rose' and *ruka* 'hand') if between this word and a likely word boundary there was a syllabic stretch of speech (e.g., ***suck**rose*, ***dug**ruka*). If this stretch of speech was a single consonant (e.g., ***k**rose*, ***g**ruka*), target words were less easily recognized in German, but this was only true if the single consonant in the Slovak context was not an existing Slovak word (e.g., *t* in ***t**ruka*). The fastest responses were observed in single-consonant contexts that are existing words in Slovak (e.g., the voiced allophone of the preposition *k* 'to' in *gruka*).
On the basis of this finding, Hanulíková et al. (submitted) argued that word segmentation across languages is not uniformly constrained by vowelless sequences. The PWC seems to be a language-specific segmentation principle. Following this proposal, however, the recognition of words in contexts that are acceptable parses (i.e., word-like units) in a given language should be equally easy. This means that both a syllable (e.g., in ***dug**ruka*) and a prepositional context (e.g., in ***g**ruka*) are possible parsing units in Slovak, therefore the word recognition latencies in these contexts should have been comparable. In the Slovak word-spotting experiments, as noted above, faster latencies were observed for target words in single-prepositional contexts (***g**ruka*) than for those in the syllable contexts (***dug**ruka*). Although it was shown that the missing canonical main stress on the targets in the syllable context resulted in slower detection latencies, once this stress information was provided by cross-splicing in a second experiment, participants were still faster in the

prepositional context than in the syllable context.[1] One explanation for these faster response times (RTs) in the prepositional context could be a stronger lexical support for a real word (i.e., the preposition) as opposed to a possible but nonsense word (i.e., the nonsense syllable). However, there might be an alternative explanation, namely, that specific syllabification preferences (for CV.CCV vs CVC.CV) or the assignment of segments to certain syllables might have affected the segmentation and word recognition in the syllabic contexts. This paper is aimed at an examination of this alternative.

If syllables play a role in segmentation in some languages, do they possibly influence segmentation in Slovak or even in German? If the speech input is organized in terms of syllables, a syllable could be evaluated as shorter or longer during processing. This could influence segmentation and word recognition. For example, both *du* and *dug* are well-formed syllables in Slovak and hence viable residues. On hearing the Slovak nonsense word ***dug**ruka*, as mentioned earlier, Slovak listeners could process the first syllable as *du* and segment the signal at *gruka*. Detection latencies would be slower than in cases where participants assign the consonant to the coda of the first syllable (hence, *dug*) because in the latter case, the lexical search would start with the onset of a syllable that coincides with the word onset of the target word *ruka*. The same would be true for German participants. Recognition of the target word *rose* in ***suck**rose* could be facilitated if German listeners put syllable boundaries between /kr/. The present study hence investigates whether syllabification in Slovak and in German plays a role in speech segmentation.

To answer the question of whether listeners' syllabification preferences might have affected speech segmentation in the previous word-spotting experiments, I first examine how German and Slovak listeners syllabify the input into its individual parts and whether participants in each group agree in syllable boundary placements. One experimental technique that has previously been suggested for these purposes is the

1 Note that stress clash could have emerged by cross-splicing the material (although participants reported perceiving main stress on the second syllable of ***dug**ruka*). This manipulation might have provided a cue for the listener. Notwithstanding this, their performance was not faster in this condition than in the single-prepositional context, where no such cue was provided.

syllable reversal task. It was developed by Treiman and Danis (1988) to investigate the affiliation of intervocalic consonants (e.g., to which syllable the consonant /t/ in *letter* belongs). Since then it has been used to investigate language users' internal representation of words and to address syllabification as well as speech segmentation issues in various languages (e.g., Content et al., 2001; Schiller et al., 1997; Berg & Niemi, 2000). In this task, participants hear bisyllabic non-words and real words with instructions to split these words into two parts and then say these two parts in the reverse order. For example, on hearing the word *monkey*, participants are expected to say [ki.mʌŋ]. The available response interval is kept relatively short in order to increase the likelihood of assessing online processing of the assignment of the consonants. A short response window might further help to avoid giving the participant time to reason about the best syllabification procedure. In such a metalinguistic task, listeners are forced to make explicit choices about syllable onsets. It is therefore possible to examine where in the speech signal German and Slovak listeners find likely syllable onsets.

German and Slovak are both languages with relatively complex syllabic structures and with a considerable amount of ambiguity in terms of syllabification. Slovak phonology allows the occurrence of consonant clusters of up to four consonants in onset position (e.g., *pstruh* 'trout'), while German syllables mainly exhibit complex codas with up to five consonants (e.g., *du kämpfst* 'you fight'). More than two consonants in the Slovak syllable coda are rare and occur only in loan words (e.g., [tɛkst] 'text'; see Rubach, 1993). Furthermore, the Slovak coda exhibits fewer possible combinations than German (see Hanulíková, 2003; Hanulíková & Dietrich, in press, for more details). Vowels and laterals (/l/) can form syllabic peaks in both languages. Nasals /n, m/ in German and rhotic /r/ in Slovak can also be syllabic nuclei. The German vowel system can be characterized by vowel quantity and vowel quality. In contrast to German, Slovak exhibits phonemic quantity but not quality distinctions. One language-specific characteristic of syllabic structure in German is that German syllables should not end with a short lax vowel. In Slovak, no such restriction holds.

According to some phonological theories, the maximal onset principle (e.g., Pulgram, 1970; Kahn, 1976; Selkirk, 1982) is a universal mechanism predicting that intervocalic consonants will be maximally assigned to the onset of the following syllable in conformity with language-specific phonotactic restrictions as well as universal preferences (such as the sonority hierarchy; see Clements, 1990; Hooper, 1972; Vennemann, 1988). Previous studies have shown that English listeners indeed follow the maximal onset principle in syllabification (e.g., Titone & Connine, 1997; Treiman & Zukowski, 1990). Accordingly, Slovak participants might divide the nonsense word *dugru* into [dʊ.grʊ], creating a maximal onset that is phonotactically possible and does not violate the universal sonority scale (as obstruents are less sonorous and hence should precede sonorants in syllable onsets). The same principle would apply for the German non-word [zʊ.kro:]. This syllabification, however, would violate a constraint on well-formed German syllables, as will be shown below.

According to language-specific phonological theories, the syllable in German, but not Slovak, requires a branching rhyme (e.g., Lahiri & Koreman, 1988; Ramers, 1992; Vennemann, 1982, 1994; Wiese, 1988, 1996). This means that open syllables with short lax vowels are not permissible and require at least one consonant in the coda[2] (hence, [zʊk.ro:]). For German, there are therefore two conflicting predictions concerning theoretical syllabification (universal versus language specific). One plausible solution is that German native speakers are sensitive to the well-formedness of syllables in German. Therefore, they might follow language-specific constraints such as the branching rhyme principle during speech processing. On hearing a short lax vowel, they would assign a following consonant to the syllable that contains the vowel. In the reversal task, this would lead them to produce well-formed syllables (e.g., [zʊk.ro:], in the reverse order as [ro:.zʊk]).

In Slovak, no such phonological constraint exists; both [dʊ.grʊ] and [dʊg.rʊ] are permissible syllabifications. Whether the consonants [g] and [r] are assigned to a syllable onset or coda should by governed by phonotactic restrictions in Slovak. The [gr] cluster is phonotactically legal in Slovak syllable onsets (but not codas) and does not violate universal sonority-sequencing principles (see Rubach, 1993). Traditional accounts

---

2 German syllables have minimally two positions in the rhyme. A branching rhyme can be a tense or a long vowel (e.g., /ku:/ 'cow', /ʃɛ:dl̩/ 'skull'), or a diphthong (e.g., /brai/ 'porridge').

as well as Slovak orthographic rules about hyphenation at the end of a line in writing (which children are taught at school) suggest a syllabic division at morpheme boundaries whenever possible (e.g., Pauliny, 1979; Pravidlá slovenského pravopisu, 2000; Sabol & Zimmermann, 1994). If a division at morpheme boundaries is not possible, a syllable break should be made between two consonants (i.e., [dʊg.rʊ]). If this orthographic knowledge has an impact on how participants report that words are syllabified during speech processing, division between the consonants would be plausible (i.e., [dʊg.rʊ]). On phonological grounds, however, several solutions are permissible, and this could create a high degree of variation in syllabification among native speakers of Slovak.

The placement of syllable or morpheme boundaries can be further influenced by morphological, prosodic and allophonic information that might influence such syllabification processes. For example, consonant duration or aspiration of stops in German might lead German speakers to syllabify [zʊ.kro:] in the reverse order as [kro:.zʊ].

In two experiments, German native speakers and Slovak native speakers were tested to examine how they affiliate intervocalic consonant clusters (e.g., /kr, kl, kn, kv, ʃl, ʃv, ʃr, ʃn, pl, pr, tr/) after short lax vowels (e.g., /a, ɛ, ʊ, ɔ, ɪ/) in bisyllabic non-words. This data was then used in conjunction with previous word-spotting data to compute a correlation analysis. The reasoning is the following: If syllables are involved in speech segmentation, Slovak and German listeners might have been influenced by their syllabification preferences while participating in the previous word-spotting studies. Recall that segmentation at *gruka* in the sequence ***dugruka*** would require further segmentation in order to recognize the target word *ruka*. Such segmentation procedures could result in longer RTs in the syllable condition as compared to the single-consonant conditions (e.g., *gruka*), where no such 'double' segmentation would be necessary. If this is the case, there should be a positive and significant correlation between the proportion of responses with open syllables and the RT differences between the syllable and single-consonant conditions. This means that the higher the proportion of open responses (e.g., [grʊ.dʊ] on hearing [dʊgrʊ]) for a particular item, the larger the difference in reaction times in the word-spotting studies as a function of this segmentation. However, if alignment points for lexical

mapping processes do not hinge on syllabic structure or syllabification, the correlation analysis should not be significant.
Experiment 1 tested German speakers' responses on German material taken from a previous German word-spotting study (Hanulíková, 2008). In Experiment 2, Slovak native speakers were tested using the material from the earlier Slovak studies (Hanulíková et al., submitted). In the previous Slovak study, two sets of materials were used. In addition to the original recordings used in one experiment, the second study used cross-spliced material to manipulate stress information. Thus, while a sequence such as ***dugruka*** carried the primary stress on the first syllable in the first study, there was an additional main stress on the first syllable of the target word *ruka* in the second study. Because stress can influence syllabification (e.g., Bailey, 1978; Hoard, 1971; Titone & Connine, 1997), items from both these experiments were used in the syllabification study. This also allowed for direct assessment of the syllabification preferences for each of the previous studies.

1.1. EXPERIMENT 1

If German native speakers follow the maximal onset principle or if they use possible allophonic cues such as stop aspiration, they will more often divide a bisyllabic non-word into CV.CCV units (e.g., [zʊ.kro], hence producing [kro:.zʊ]). However, if they follow the language-specific branching rhyme principle, they will preferably create well-formed German syllables by closing the first syllable CVC.CV (e.g., [zʊk.ro], hence producing [ro:.zʊk]).[3] It is unlikely that speakers would attach the medial consonants to the first syllable (e.g., [zʊkr.o], [o:.zʊkr]) because /kr/ is not a permissible coda consonant cluster in German.

3 Alternatively, participants could follow the maximal onset principle and fulfill the requirements of a branching rhyme by producing an open syllable with a tense vowel. This would, however, create a mismatch between the perceived vowel quality and the produced one.

1.1.1. METHOD

Participants
Ten German native speakers, students at the Humboldt University in Berlin, volunteered for participation. They did not report any hearing problems or speech disabilities. None of them had knowledge of Slovak.
Materials
Eighty-eight bisyllabic nonsense items were created by splicing the material used in the German word-spotting experiment. This procedure was used in order to exclude lexical bias and possible pre-stored knowledge about syllable boundaries (e.g., Titone & Connine, 1997). The items were spliced in such a way that the last syllable was removed from each string, leaving a bisyllabic non-word. For example, the non-word *suckro* emerged from ***suck****rose*. This procedure was applied to all 48 target-bearing items from the word-spotting study. In addition, 26 real words and 14 non-words were chosen as fillers, which were removed from their preceding single-consonant or syllabic contexts (e.g., *rose* 'rose' from ***k****rose*). All splices were made at positive zero crossings. Note that this splicing method was necessary for the present purposes because no direct comparison with the previous experiments and material would have been possible if new recordings had been made. One experimental list was then constructed with a randomized order of items. Every participant heard all 88 items. Half of these items, namely those originating from target-bearing items (such as ***suck****rose*), were analysed.

Procedure
The participants were tested separately in a quiet room. They received instructions that on each trial they would hear a pseudoword or a real word. They were asked to divide these words into two parts and say them aloud in the reverse order, starting with the last part of the word (the word 'syllable' was avoided). They were informed that there would be only a short time for a response; therefore they should attempt to respond as fast as possible. Two examples were given in the instructions. The main experiment started after a short practice session with two further items. Participants heard the stimuli one at a time over headphones at a comfortable listening level.

The presentation of the stimuli was controlled by NESU (Nijmegen Experiment Setup), experimental software developed at the Max Planck Institute for Psycholinguistics. Each trial started with a 500 ms silence, after which the stimulus was presented. The time interval between the onsets of two successive trials was 3000 ms. The approximate stimulus duration was 500 ms, leaving 2500 ms as the response interval. The experiment was made short, so that no breaks were necessary and so that listeners could not use such breaks to reason about their strategies in the task. The reaction times were not measured. Subjects' responses were recorded on a tape using a Sony recorder and a Sennheiser microphone.

All responses were transcribed online during the experiment, and carefully inspected a second time using the recordings. The classification of the responses was determined according to the assignment of the first consonant of the intervocalic cluster to either the onset (first syllable open, CV.CCV, e.g., [zʊ.kro:]) or the coda (first syllable closed, CVC.CV, e.g., [zʊk.ro:]). If a consonant was assigned to the coda and to the onset (i.e., [zʊk.kro:]), such a response was classified as the closed syllable type. The proportion of such cases within the closed syllable responses is provided in brackets in Table 1. Note that the order of these syllables produced by the participants was always reversed; the actual responses here would be [kro:.zʊ], [ro:.zʊk], or [kro:.zʊk]. Errors include cases such as no response, no complete response, reversal of the phonemes instead of syllables, and deletion of intervocalic consonants. Segment substitutions or insertions were coded as errors only if they affected the critical clusters and the preceding vowels (e.g., [zʊp.rʊ] or [zak.rʊ]).[4] Thus, an open syllable response type (CV.CCV) is a response with /k/ assigned to the onset of the following syllable (hence, [zʊ.kro:]). Closed syllable response or CVC.CV is defined as a response with the /k/ assigned to the coda of the first syllable (hence, [zʊk.ro:]).

4 Note that segment substitutions might be due to the fact that the materials used in this task were non-words. Therefore, the number of misperceptions is likely to be higher than it would be with real words (see also Berg & Niemi, 2000, for similar problems).

1.1.2. RESULTS AND DISCUSSION

The mean proportion of responses for each type in Table 1 and Figure 1 shows that German speakers preferred to close the first syllable. A paired t-test revealed that the difference in the proportion of open syllable responses compared to closed syllable responses was significant by both participants (t1) and items (t2) ($t1(9) = 8.47$, $p < .001$; $t2(47) = 23.99$, $p < .001$).

Table 1: Mean proportion over participants (total number of responses given in parentheses), C = Consonant, V = Vowel.

		Response syllable type		
Group	**n**	**CV.CCV**	**CVC.CV [CVC.CCV]**	**Error**
German	480	7.5 % (36)	81.7 % (392) [8,7 % (34)]	10.8 % (52)
Slovak overall	1120	38.9 % (435)	35.6 % (399) [8% (32)]	25.5 % (286)
Slovak original	560	40.9 % (225)	33.9 % (190) [9% (17)]	25.2 % (145)
Slovak spliced	560	37.0 % (210)	37.3 % (209) [7% (15)]	25.9 % (141)

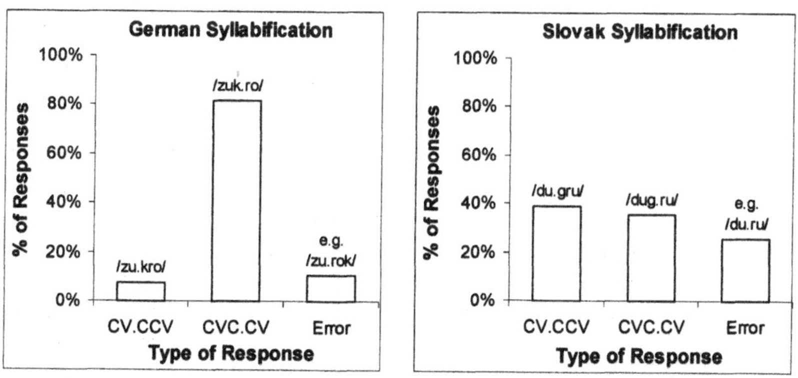

Figure 1: Proportion of responses in the syllable reversal task. C = Consonant, V = Vowel.

These results show that in the majority of cases German participants closed syllables with a lax vowel in conformity with the branching rhyme principle. The universal principle of maximizing the length of the syllable onset wherever possible was reflected only in a few cases, just as the use of allophonic cues such as stop aspiration. This result resembles the results of Schiller et al. (1997) on syllabification preferences in Dutch, a language with similar phonological restrictions to German. In that study, the production of open syllables was observed in only a few cases, similar to the present results. Schiller et al. (1997) further showed that open syllable responses might be more likely for syllables including the lax vowels /a/ and /ɔ/ than for syllables including /ɛ/ and /ɪ/. This is only partly consistent with the present results, as all open syllable responses occurred for syllables with the vowels /a/ and /ɛ/. It is important to note, however, that the materials used in Schiller et al.'s study differed from the present material not only in terms of language (Dutch vs German) but also in terms of items (e.g., word vs non-word, etc.).

However, the present results are not consistent with a syllabification study of intervocalic consonants in German using the syllable reversal task (Berg & Niemi, 2000). Berg and Niemi observed a clear preference for open syllables (e.g., in the nonsense word *vo.sta*). Several possible explanations could account for this contradictory result. First, Berg & Niemi (2000) used a relatively long response time window in their study (5000 ms). Even though the participants were required to respond quickly, the processing time was considerably longer than the time-out interval used in the present study (approximately 2500 ms). Second, the consonant clusters (e.g., Fricative + Stop) differed from the clusters used in the present study (e.g., Stop + Liquid). Third and more importantly, the material used in that study included short and long vowels in the first syllable, but no separate analysis was provided according to the vowel type. This information is important because long vowels correspond to a branching rhyme, and hence syllables with long vowels are well formed in German (i.e., they do not require an additional consonant). Syllables with lax vowels are not, and such syllables could thus trigger different responses. A direct comparison between my work and that study is therefore not possible.

To test whether the syllabification procedures shown by German speakers might have influenced the overall response latencies in the previous German word-spotting experiment (Hanulíková, 2008), a correlation analysis was conducted. First, the proportion of open syllable responses for each item was computed, i.e., the number of CV.CCV responses divided by the sum of both the CV.CCV and the CVC.CV responses. The question then is whether the difference observed in the word-spotting RTs between the prepositional and the syllable contexts as well as the difference between the non-prepositional and the syllable contexts were possibly influenced by the individual syllabification preference for a given item. Therefore, the proportion of syllabifications was plotted against the difference in RTs between those conditions (hence, for each item the RT in the syllable context was subtracted from the RT from either the prepositional or the non-prepositional context). There was a numerically positive but not significant correlation between the proportion and the RT differences between syllable and preposition ($R = .084$, $p = .57$). There was also a numerically negative but not significant correlation between the proportion and the RT differences between syllable and non-preposition ($R = -.14$, $p = .35$). Similar results were obtained using standardized scores (all correlations n.s.).
The correlation analysis hence suggests that there is no relationship between the syllabification preferences and the observed RTs. Note that this does not necessarily mean that syllabification preferences cannot influence the online processing of speech. The results merely suggest that the results obtained in the word-spotting experiments reflect operations of the PWC, and might not be influenced by the syllable structure. This also suggests that if there were additional allophonic or morpho-phonological patterns affecting the syllabic divisions, these would very likely be independent of the performance observed in the previous segmentation task.

1.2. EXPERIMENT 2

The second experiment examined the syllabification preferences used by Slovak native speakers. If Slovak listeners follow the maximal onset principle, they will more often assign the consonantal segments to the onset of the second syllable (e.g., *du.gru,* leading them to produce [grʊ.dʊ]). However, if listeners are influenced by their orthographic knowledge of hyphenation, they will prefer to close the first syllable with a consonant (e.g., *dug.ru,* leading them to produce [rʊ.dʊg]). Note that unlike in German, in Slovak both syllable divisions are possible as far as phonological well-formedness is concerned.

1.2.1. METHOD

Participants

Twenty students from Alexander Dubček's University in Trenčín as well as from the Komenský University in Bratislava volunteered for participation. They were all native speakers of Slovak. None of them reported any hearing difficulties or speech disabilities.

Materials

One hundred and eight Slovak bisyllabic words and non-words were created by splicing the material used in the earlier Slovak word-spotting experiments. As in Experiment 1, these items were spliced in such a way that the last syllable was removed from each string, leaving a bisyllabic non-word. For example, the syllable *ka* was removed from ***dugruka***. This procedure was applied to 56 out of 72 target-bearing items from both previous Slovak experiments (with the original material and the cross-spliced material).[5] In addition, 52 real words and non-words were chosen from the same material and removed from their preceding single-consonant or syllabic contexts (e.g., *ruka* 'hand' from *gruka*). These additional items served as fillers. All splices were made at positive zero crossings. Two experimental lists were constructed with a randomized order of items. On one list, there were 28 target non-words carrying the main stress on the first syllable and 28 cross-spliced target non-words with main stress on both syllables. Every participant heard 108 items. Only the 56 target items were analysed.

5 Note that to keep the experiment short, so that the participants did not think about syllabification strategies, only a subset of items was chosen, leaving out items with repeating consonant clusters.

Procedure
The procedure was identical to the one described for Experiment 1, except that the instructions were in Slovak.

1.2.2. Results and Discussion

As can be seen in Table 1 and Figure 1, there was no clear preference for either type of response. There was also a high number of errors (including cases such as no response and consonant deletion). First, overall responses were analysed. The difference between open and closed syllable responses was not significant by either participants ($t1(19) = .32$, $p = .75$) or by items ($t2(55) = .86$, $p = .40$).

In a second step, the responses to items were analysed as a function of the material from which these items were extracted, i.e., either from the word-spotting study with original material or from the study with cross-spliced material. In this analysis, the difference between open and closed syllable responses was not significant either for the original items ($t1(19) = .72$, $p = .48$; $t2(55) = 1.41$, $p = .17$) or for the spliced items ($t1(19) = .03$, $p = .97$; $t2(55) = .04$, $p = .97$).

The syllabification responses were then compared as a function of stress distinction on the second syllable. Thus, the proportions of syllable responses from the original material were compared with the proportion of syllable responses in the spliced material. If the main stress was provided on the second syllable, participants tended to produce open syllables less often ($t1(19) = 2.4$, $p = .03$; $t2(55) = 0.94$, $p = .35$), but there was no significant difference for closed syllable responses depending on stress ($t1(19) = 1.55$, $p = .14$; $t2(55) = 1.34$, $p = .19$).

The overall result shows high variability of responses. This is not surprising, as Slovak phonology allows both ways of syllabic division (*dug, du* and *gru, ru* are all well-formed syllables). In such a case, one would assume that the universal maximization of onsets would prevail. The results suggest, however, that Slovak speakers produced maximal onsets only half of the time. Almost equally often as producing maximal onsets, they closed the first syllable. It is possible that in such cases speakers were influenced by hyphenation rules, which suggest syllabic division between two consonants. However, they were not consistently applying either of these principles. A plausible explanation for these results is that Slovak speakers performed with greater variability due to a relatively low number of phonological constraints on permissible syllable structure as compared to German (concerning only the syllables used in the present experiments).

This could also explain why Slovak speakers exhibited a higher number of errors than German speakers ($t1(28) = 3.8$, $p = .001$; $t2(102) = 5.45$, $p < .001$; see Table 1). The high error rate could be due to misperceptions, greater uncertainty, or language-specific structural properties. Note that many of these cases included deletion of the intervocalic consonant /g/. Even though /g/ is not a possible syllable, it is an existing word in Slovak (the preposition *k* 'to'). If listeners recognized the preposition, they might not have parsed the input into syllabic chunks, but rather into viable chunks. Because *k* is a possible word in Slovak, it is also a viable parsing unit. If participants divided the speech input into viable strings, the uncertainty about the affiliation of the preposition would be due to the instructions, which required division into two parts. Participants reported two syllabic parts of the nonsense word, but did not report the preposition, because they did not consider it as part of the syllable. Alternatively, it could be that the uncertainty about syllabification led to the deletion without parsing the preposition as a meaningful unit at all. During a discussion after the experiment, the majority of participants asked what the correct syllabification should be. I therefore assume that the high error rate is due to the lack of explicit rules for syllable boundaries in the clusters used in this study (as they do not violate language-specific phonotactics). This uncertainty about syllable divisions is then also reflected in the higher error rate.

To assess whether the specific syllabification preferences might have contributed to detection latencies in the previous word-spotting experiments in Slovak, a correlation analysis was computed. The proportion of open syllable responses for each item was determined, i.e., the number of CV.CCV responses divided by the sum of the CV.CCV and the CVC.CV responses. To examine whether the observed differences in RTs between the prepositional and the syllable contexts as well as the non-prepositional and the syllable contexts were due to specific syllabification preferences, the proportion of syllabifications was plotted

against the difference in RTs between those conditions. Hence, for each item, the RT in the syllable context was subtracted from the RT from either the prepositional or the non-prepositional context. This procedure was applied for the RTs from the experiment with the original material, and separately for the experiment with the cross-spliced material.
For the original material, there was a numerically positive but not significant correlation between the proportion of open syllables and the RT differences between the syllable and both the preposition ($R = .16$, $p = .24$) and the non-preposition ($R = .21$, $p = .12$). For the spliced material, there was also a positive but not significant correlation between the proportion and the RT differences between the syllable and both the preposition ($R = .16$, $p = .24$) and the non-preposition ($R = .24$, $p = .08$). Similar results were obtained using standardized scores (all correlations n.s.). The results suggest that the effects observed in the Slovak word-spotting experiments were not driven by syllabification preferences.

1.3. General Discussion

This study shows that native speakers of German syllabify bisyllabic non-words in accordance with a language-specific constraint on prosodic output, namely the branching rhyme principle. Slovak listeners' syllabification is more variable and only partly consistent with the maximal onset principle. While segmental alignments within an individual syllable play an important role in linguistic syllabification theories, syllabification preferences seem not to determine segmentation of continuous speech. The syllabification strategies shown by the German and Slovak speakers in this study cannot account for the word-spotting data reported in earlier studies.
Two production experiments show how Slovak and German speakers syllabify intervocalic consonant clusters in nonsense words. German listeners followed language-specific phonological restrictions and, when syllabifying non-words, they produced well-formed German syllables (i.e., [ro:.zʊk] and not [kro:.zu]). As was predicted on phonological grounds, syllables with a lax short vowel attracted coda consonants to form branching rhymes (see also Schiller et al., 1997, for similar results with Dutch).

Slovak native speakers, in contrast, showed no such clear syllabification preferences. Slovak speakers seemed to follow the universal maximization of consonants (i.e., [grʊ.dʊ]), and they appeared to be influenced by hyphenation rules suggesting a syllabic division between two consonants in intervocalic position (i.e., [rʊ.dʊg]). Whether participants produced an open or closed syllable partly depended on stress information on the second syllable. Open syllables ([grʊ.dʊ]) were less often produced when the main stress was on the syllable [rʊ]; however, the results were significant only for participants and not for items. These results are thus partly in support of the stress principle in syllabification (Bailey, 1978; Hoard, 1971), according to which consonants are preferably attached to a stressed syllable (for similar results in English, see Titone & Connine, 1997; Treiman & Zukowski, 1990).

If the observed variation in Slovak syllabification was due to the nature of the material, i.e., nonsense words, then no such variation should be observed with real words. Using a questionnaire, Rubach (1993) presented native speakers of Slovak with real words. Participants had to indicate their preferred syllable division. The results showed a high variation if a syllable boundary was not signalled by phonotactic restrictions or clear morphemic boundaries. Moreover, this variation was observed even within individual speakers. Intervocalic consonant clusters were either assigned to the first syllable (e.g., *myd.lo* 'soap') or to the onset of the second syllable (e.g., *my.dlo*). Although items in this study were presented in their written form, the observed variability in syllabic division resembles the present results. The uncertainty about syllable division seems to apply independently of specific materials.

The goal of this study was not only to investigate syllabification, but also to consider an alternative explanation for the observed results in the previous word-spotting studies testing the Possible-Word Constraint. The present study investigated whether the way people assign individual speech sounds to larger units such as syllables might have influenced the segmentation of speech in the previous word-spotting experiments. In those experiments, a difference was observed between detection latencies in the Slovak prepositional context (such as *gruka*) and the syllable context (such as ***dugruka***), both of which are viable lexical parses. Syllables are possible words and prepositional consonants are existing words in Slovak. Therefore, no difference in detection times should have been observed. The present study revealed that the assignment of segments to individual syllables might not be the crucial factor affecting detection latencies in the syllable context as compared to single-consonant contexts. The difference between the prepositional context and the syllable context in the previous Slovak word-spotting experiment might be due to a stronger lexical support for a real word.

This conclusion is based on the lack of a significant correlation between the syllabification proportions and the detection latencies per item. Although the lack of a significant correlation does not fully exclude the possibility that syllabification does play some role in segmentation and word recognition, there are other proposals with strong empirical evidence. These do not rely on the assumption that specific syllable structure has a function in speech segmentation (e.g., Cutler et al., 2001; Norris et al., 2001; Titone & Connine, 1997). It is unlikely that listeners build up a syllabic representation before they decide at what point in the acoustic signal the lexical search can be initiated. As noted earlier, lexical access starts as soon as speech input is available. In addition, Norris et al. (2001) have shown that for the PWC principle, the language-specific constraints on syllables are not relevant. For example, as mentioned earlier, there was no significant difference in spotting an English target word in the two syllable contexts [dɛ] (with a lax vowel) and [dɑ] (with a tense vowel), although only the latter is a well-formed English syllable. Thus, it seems unlikely that in the previous word-spotting experiments German listeners had an advantage over Slovak listeners in terms of a segmentation cue provided by the syllable structure constraint (i.e., /zuk/ and not /zu/ is well formed in German while both /du/ and /dug/ are possible in Slovak). As Norris and colleagues suggest, any syllable independent of the language-specific constraints is viable in the segmentation process. Hence, spotting the target word (e.g., *Rose* 'rose') in the syllable context (***suck**rose*) in the previous German experiments was easy, not because of the branching rhyme constraint, but because of the PWC constraint. It appears that the viability of syllabic parses in general modulates word recognition and segmentation independently of the well-formedness of a specific syllable structure.

In addition to the PWC, however, there might also be acoustic cues to syllable and lexical segmentation. As the speech input unfolds over time, syllable or word boundaries might sometimes be predictable on the basis of the acoustic feature content and phonotactic restrictions on segment combinations (e.g., Lehiste, 1960; Nakatani & Dukes, 1977; McQueen, 1998). However, such cues are not systematically available in the speech signal and as mentioned earlier, they might only indirectly modulate competition of word candidates. Although listeners could have made use of allophonic cues present in both experiments alike, the fact that there was no relationship between syllabification patterns and lexical segmentation (as shown by the correlation analyses) led to the conclusion that syllabification did not affect lexical segmentation. Future studies might shed new light on this issue.

In summary, the results of this study show language-specific influences on syllabification preferences: Some linguistic theories of syllable structure (i.e., branching rhyme, specific to German) correspond to representations constructed by language users. In Slovak, however, less consistency in syllabification was observed. Despite these language-dependent preferences, syllabification does not seem to have played a crucial role in the segmentation and evaluation process of the speech signal in terms of the PWC.

For future studies, it would be useful to apply new experimental tools. Some researchers have argued that the syllabification task does not inform us about speech segmentation processes directly. Norris & Cutler (1985) point out that there are two distinct cognitive processes to be distinguished in speech processing: classification and segmentation. The former is involved in the assignment of some categories (e.g., syllables) to the speech input, and the latter is involved in segmentation and word recognition in running speech. An advantage of the syllable reversal task is, however, that it is possible to code the precise output, which provides insights into listeners' decisions about likely syllable boundaries. In order to reverse the syllables of a word, participants have to decide about syllable onsets. This search for a syllable onset resembles the online search for word onsets during speech comprehension. In this way, the likely segmentation is more explicit and straightforward. With this method, the specific syllabification response for an item can be correlated with the mean detection latency for that item in the word-spotting study.

Therefore, this task appeared appropriate for the present purposes and might partly help to determine perceptual processes (see also Content et al., 2001; Kolinsky, 1998; Pierrehumbert & Nair, 1995; Treiman & Kessler, 1995; Schiller et al., 1997).

However, an alternative approach would be the application of more direct methods to speech segmentation. In psycholinguistics, one of the central questions concerns a full understanding of the time course of cognitive processes. Many behavioural studies have shown that listeners use various cues to segment speech, and that the lack of or the presence of a specific cue influences the time needed for word recognition. What is less clear from these studies, however, is the time course of speech segmentation and word recognition. More recent approaches use methods that allow a better time resolution and permit the investigation of online segmentation. One such method is the measurement of event-related brain potentials (ERPs) using electroencephalography (EEG). This method provides online recording of certain aspects of brain activity with millisecond temporal resolution.

While there is only little available evidence from studies using ERPs, they suggest that ERP indices of speech segmentation can be seen within the duration of a syllable, if this syllable is word-initial (e.g., Sanders et al., 2002; Sanders & Neville, 2003). For example, ERP components such as the N100 and N400 have been suggested to indicate speech segmentation (e.g., Abla et al., 2008; Cunillera et al., 2006; Sanders et al., 2002).

Sanders & Neville (2003) investigated the role of syllable onsets in segmentation of continuous speech. ERPs were measured while participants listened to different types of sentences consisting of words or pronounceable nonwords. ERPs of word-initial syllables (in words and nonwords, e.g., ***bo**ttles, **bo**kkers*) elicited a larger N100 than to matched word-medial syllables (e.g., *to**ba**cco, do**ba**tty*). Although the syllables were controlled along various factors such as phonemic content, length, fundamental frequency, and amplitude, they were likely to differ due to spontaneous recordings. Therefore, an alternative explanation of the results could be that listeners used possible allophonic details to word onsets. However, the authors suggest that the N100 effect for word-initial syllables occurs independently of acoustic cues. Sanders et al. (2002) also recorded ERPs while listeners heard the same physical syllables as part of nonsense words embedded in continuous speech (e.g., *babupu, bupada,* *dutaba*). The authors again observed an N100 word-onset effect. The effect remained stable after participants learned the nonsense words through training and were again tested with the continuous speech. This suggests that transitional probabilities were sufficient to discover word onsets. In addition, the recognition of a word was indicated by the N400. This component seems to indicate not only online speech segmentation but also statistical learning (e.g., Abla et al., 2008; Cunillera et al., 2006; Sanders et al., 2002).

The ERP thus provides a promising tool for further studies on the role of syllables in speech segmentation. Most of the studies mentioned above use statistical-learning designs with controlled synthesized speech stimuli. Using a similar design, the differing role of syllables and consonants in speech segmentation could be addressed by teaching listeners a language that contains a limited number of single-consonant words as well as single-syllable and polysyllabic words (e.g., a simplified Slovak). If the recognition of words does not depend on the phonological characteristics of the previous context (i.e., vowel versus consonant), an early segmentation component should be elicited in both cases and the recognition of the following words should show a similar N400 effect. Such an outcome would challenge the PWC and the role of syllabic segmentation. Future studies combining both chronometric and electrophysiological methods will bring new insights into this issue.

ACKNOWLEDGEMENTS

For comments on earlier versions of the manuscript, I am grateful to James McQueen, Doug Davidson, Silke Hamann, Jenny Green, Kevin Russell, and two anonymous reviewers. All remaining errors are mine.

REFERENCES

Abla, D., Katahira, K., & Okanoya, K. (2008). On-line assessment of statistical learning by event-related potentials. *Journal of Cognitive Neuroscience 20*, 952-964.

Bailey, C. J. N. (1978). *Gradience in English Syllabization and a Revised Concept of Unmarked Syllabization*. Bloomington IN: Indiana Univ. Linguistics Club.

Berg, T. & Niemi, J. (2000). Syllabification in Finnish and German: Onset filling vs. onset maximization. *Journal of Phonetics* 28, 187-216.

Blevins, J. (1995). The syllable in phonological theory. In: J. Goldsmith (Ed.) *The Handbook of Phonological Theory*, 206-244, Cambridge (MA): Blackwell.

Brière, E. J. (1968). *A Psycholinguistic Study of Phonological Interference*. The Hague/Paris: Mouton.

Cholin, J., Schiller, N. O., and Levelt, W. J. M. (2004). The preparation of syllables in speech production. *Journal of Memory and Language* 50, 47–61.

Clements, G. N. (1990). The role of the sonority cycle in core syllabification. In J. Kingston, & M. E. Beckman (eds.) *Papers in Laboratory Phonology I*, 283-333, Cambridge: Cambridge University Press.

Content, A., Dumay, N. & Frauenfelder, U. H. (2000). The role of syllable structure in lexical segmentation: Helping listeners avoid mondegreens. In: A. Cutler, J. M. McQueen, & R. Zondervan (eds.) *Proceedings of the Workshop SWAP Spoken Word Access Processes*, 39-42, Nijmegen, The Netherlands.

Content, A., Kearns, R. K., and Frauenfelder, U. H. (2001a). Boundaries versus onsets in syllabic segmentation. *Journal of Memory and Language* 45, 177-199.

Content, A., Meunier, C., Kearns, R. K., and Frauenfelder, U.H. (2001b). Sequence detection in pseudowords in French: Where is the syllable effect? *Language and Cognitive Processes* 16, 609-636.

Cunillera, T., Toro, J. M., Sebastián-Gallés, N., Rodríguez-Fornells, A. (2006). The effects of stress and statistical cues on continuous speech segmentation: An event-related brain potential study. *Brain Research 1123*,168-178.

Cutler, A. (1993). Language-specific processing: does the evidence converge? In: G. T. M. Altmann, & R. Shillcock (eds.) *Cognitive Models of Speech Processing: The Second Sperlonga Meeting*, 115–124, Hove: Erlbaum.

Cutler, A. (1997). The syllable's role in the segmentation of stress languages. *Language and Cognitive Processes* 12, 839-845.

Cutler, A., Demuth, K., and McQueen, J. M. (2002). Universality versus language-specificity in listening to running speech. *Psychological Science* 13, 258-262.

Cutler, A., McQueen, J. M., Norris, D., and Somejuan, A. (2001). The roll of the silly ball. In: E. Dupoux (Ed.), *Language, Brain and Cognitive Development: Essays in honor of Jacques Mehler*, 181-194. Cambridge (MA): MIT Press.

Cutler, A. & Norris, D. (1988). The role of strong syllables in segmentation for lexical access. *Journal of Experimental Psychology: Human Perception and Performance* 14, 113-121.

Cutler, A., Mehler, J., Norris, D., and Seguí, J. (1983). A language specific comprehension strategy. *Nature* 304, 159-160.

Cutler, A., Mehler, J., Norris, D. G., and Seguí, J. (1986). The syllable's differing role in the segmentation of French and English. *Journal of Memory and Language* 25, 385-400.

Cutler, A., Mehler, J., Norris, D., and Seguí, J. (1992). The monolingual nature of speech segmentation by bilinguals. *Cognitive Psychology* 24, 381-410.

Cutler, A., Otake, T., and McQueen, J. M. (submitted). Vowel devoicing and the perception of spoken Japanese words.

Dumay, N., Frauenfelder, U. H., and Content, A. (2002). The role of the syllable in lexical segmentation in French: Word-spotting data. *Brain and Language* 81, 144-161.

Dupoux, E. (1993). Prelexical processing: the syllabic hypothesis revisited. In: G. T. M. Altmann, & R. Shillcock (eds.) *Cognitive Models of Speech Processing: The Second Sperlonga Meeting,* 81–114, Hove: Erlbaum.

Fallows, D. (1981). Experimental evidence for English syllabification and syllable structure. *Journal of Linguistics* 17, 309-317.

Frauenfelder, U. H. & Content, A. (1999). The role of the syllable in spoken word recognition: Access or segmentation? *Proceedings of the 2émes Journées d'Etudes Linguistiqu – La Syllabe,* 1-8, Nantes: Université de Nantes.

Frauenfelder, U. H. & Kearns, R. K. (1996). Sequence monitoring. *Language and Cognitive Processes* 11, 665-673.

Goslin, J. & Frauenfelder, U. H. (2000). A comparison of theoretical and human syllabification. *Language and Speech* 44(4), 409-436.

Grosjean F. & U.H. Frauenfelder (eds.) (1996). *A Guide to Spoken Word Recognition Paradigms. Language and Cognitive Processes* 11.

Hanulíková, A. (2003). *Der Erwerb der deutschen Coda durch slowakische Lerner: Eine empirische Studie.* Humboldt University Berlin: M.A. thesis.

Hanulíková, A. (in press). The role of possible words in speech comprehension. *Proceedings of the 2nd Postgraduate Conference in Linguistics,* Oxford.

Hanulíková, A. (2008). Lexical Segmentation in Slovak and German. Humboldt University Berlin: PhD dissertation.

Hanulíková, A. & Dietrich, R. (in press). Die variable Coda in der slowakisch-deutschen Interimsprache. In: M. Tarvas (Ed.) *Tradition und Zukunft der Germanistik,* Tallinn.

Hanulíková, A., McQueen, J. M., and Mitterer, H. (submitted). Possible words and fixed stress in the segmentation of Slovak speech.

Hoard, J. W. (1971). Aspiration, tenseness, and syllabification in English. *Language* 47, 133-140.

Hooper, J. B. (1972). The syllable in phonological theory. *Language* 48, 525 – 540.

Itô, J. (1986/1988). Syllable Theory in Prosodic Phonology. Ph.D. dissertation. New York: Garland.

Kahn, D. (1976). Syllable-based Generalizations in English Phonology. Ph.D. dissertation. New York/ London: Garland, 1980.

Kolinsky, R. (1998). Spoken word recognition: A stage-processing approach to language differences. *European Journal of Cognitive Psychology* 10, 1-40.

Lahiri, A. & Koreman, J. (1988). Syllable weight and quantity in Dutch. In: H. Borer (Ed.), *Proc. of the 7th West Coast Conference on Formal Linguistics,* 217-228, Stanford, CA: Center for the Study of Language and Information.

Lebrun, Y. (1966). Sur la syllabe, sommet de sonorité. *Phonetica* 14, 1–15.

Lehiste, I. (1960). An acoustic-phonetic study of internal open juncture. *Phonetica* 5(supplement), 5-54.

Liberman, I. Y., Shankweiler, D., Fischer, F. W. and Carter, B. (1974). Explicit syllable and phoneme segmentation in the young child. *Journal of Experimental Child Psychology* 18, 201—212.

Marslen-Wilson, W. D. (1987). Functional parallelism in spoken word recognition. *Cognition* 25, 71-102.

McClelland, J. L. & Elman, J. L. (1986). The TRACE model of speech perception. *Cognitive Psychology* 18, 1-86.

McQueen, J. M. (1998). Segmentation of continuous speech using phonotactics. *Journal of Memory and Language* 39, 21-46.

McQueen, J. M. & Cutler, A. (1998). Spotting (different types of) words in (different types of) context. *Proceedings of ICSLP 98 in Sydney (Australia),* 2791-2794, Rundle Mall: Causal Productions.

McQueen, J. M., Otake, T. and Cutler, A. (2001). Rhythmic cues and possible-word constraints in Japanese speech segmentation. *Journal of Memory and Language* 45, 103-132

Mehler, J. (1981). The role of syllables in speech processing: Infant and adult data. *Philosophical Transactions of the Royal Society* 295, 333–352.

Mehler, J., Dommergues, J. Y., Frauenfelder, U. H., and Seguí, J. (1981). The syllable's role in speech segmentation. *Journal of Verbal Learning and Verbal Behavior* 20, 298-305.

Mehler, J., Dupoux, E., and Seguí, J. (1990). Constraining models of lexical access: the onset of word recognition, In: G. Altmann (ed.) *Cognitive Models of Speech*

Processing: Psycholinguistic and Computational Perspectives, 236–262, Cambridge(MA): MIT Press.

Morais, J. & Kolinsky, R. (1992). In search of a paradigm for the study of speech perceptual codes. *Actas das I Jornadas de Estudo dos Processos Cognitivos da Sociedade Portuguesa de Psicologia, Lisbon,* 113-135.

Nakatani, L. H. & Dukes, K. D. (1977). Locus of segmental cues for word juncture. *The Journal of the Acoustical Society of America* 62, 714-719.

Norris, D. (1994). Shortlist: A connectionist model of continuous speech recognition. *Cognition* 52, 189-234.

Norris, D. & Cutler, A. (1985). Juncture detection. *Linguistics* 23, 689-705.

Norris, D., McQueen, J. M., Cutler, A., and Butterfield, S. (1997). The possible-word constraint in the segmentation of continuous speech. *Cognitive Psychology* 34, 191-243.

Norris, D., McQueen, J. M., Cutler, A., Butterfield, S. and Kearns, R. (2001). Language-universal constraints on speech segmentation. *Language and Cognitive Processes* 16, 637-660.

Otake, T., Hatano, G., Cutler, A., and Mehler, J. (1993). Mora or syllable? Speech segmentation in Japanese. *Journal of Memory and Language* 32, 258-278.

Pauliny, E. (1979). *Slovenská fonológia* [Slovak phonology]. Bratislava: Slovenské pedagogické nakladateľstvo.

Pierrehumbert, J. & Nair, R. (1995). Word games and syllable structure. *Language and Speech* 38, 77-114.

Pravidlá slovenského pravopisu [Slovak orthographic rules] (2000). Bratislava: Veda.

Pulgram, E. (1970). *Syllable, Word, Nexus, Cursus.* The Hague/Paris: Mouton.

Ramers, K. H. (1992). Ambisilbische Konsonanten im Deutschen. In: P. Eisenberg, K. H. Ramers, and H. Vater (eds.) *Silbenphonologie des Deutschen,* 246-283, Tübingen: Narr.

Rubach, J. (1993). *The Lexical Phonology of Slovak.* Oxford: Oxford University Press.

Sabol, J. & Zimmermann, J. (1994). *Komunikačný štatút prízvuku v spisovnej Slovenčine* [Communicative status of stress in standard Slovak]. Prešov: Filozofická fakulta Univerzity P. J. Šafárika.

Sanders, L. D. & Neville, H. J. (2000). Lexical, syntactic, and stress-pattern cues for speech segmentation. *Journal of Speech, Language, and Hearing Research* 43, 1301-1321.

Sanders, L. D., & Neville, H. J. (2003). An ERP study of continuous speech processing I. Segmentation, semantics, and syntax in native speakers. *Cognitive Brain Research 15,* 228-240.

Sanders, L. D., Newport, E. L., and Neville, H. J. (2002). Segmenting nonsense: an event-related potential index of perceived onsets in continuous speech. *Nature Neuroscience* 5, 700-703.

Sato, C. J. (1984). Phonological processes in second language acquisition: Another look at interlanguage syllable structure. *Language Learning* 34, 43–58.

Savin, H. B. & Bever, T. G. (1970). The nonperceptual reality of the phoneme. *Journal of Verbal Learning and Verbal Behavior* 9, 295–302.

Schiller, N. O., Meyer, A. S., and Levelt, W. J. M. (1997). The syllabic structure of spoken words: Evidence from the syllabification of intervocalic consonants. *Language and Speech* 40(2), 103-140.

Selkirk, E. O. (1982). The syllable. In: H. van der Hulst, & N. Smith (eds.) *The Structure of Phonological Representations*, 337-383, Dordrecht: Foris.

Titone, D. & Connine, C. M. (1997). Syllabification strategies in spoken word processing: Evidence from phonological priming. *Psychological Research* 60, 251-263.

Treiman, R. & Danis, C. (1988). Short-term memory errors for spoken syllables are affected by the linguistic structure of the syllable. *Journal of Experimental Psychology: Learning Memory and Cognition* 14, 145-152.

Treiman, R. & Kessler, B. (1995). In defense of an onset-rime syllable structure for English. *Language and Speech* 38, 127-142.

Treiman, R. & Zukowski, A. (1990). Toward an understanding of English syllabification. *Journal of Memory and Language* 29, 66-85.

Vennemann, T. (1982). Zur Silbenstruktur der deutschen Standardsprache. In: T. Vennemann (Ed.) *Silben, Segmente, Akzente*, 261-305. Tübingen: Niemeyer.

Vennemann, T. (1988). *Preference Laws for Syllable Structure and the Explanation of Sound Change*. Berlin: Mouton de Gruyter.

Vennemann, T. (1994). Universale Nuklearphonologie mit epiphänomenaler Silbenstruktur. In: K. H. Ramers, H. Vogel, and H. Wode (eds.), *Universale Phonologische Strukturen und Prozesse*, 7-54, Tübingen: Niemeyer.

Wiese, R. (1988). *Silbische und lexikalische Phonologie: Studien zum Chinesischen und Deutschen*. Tübingen: Niemeyer.

Wiese, R. (1996). *The Phonology of German*. Oxford: Clarendon Press.

Yip, M.C.W. (2004). Possible-word constraint in Cantonese speech segmentation. *Journal of Psycholinguistic Research* 33, 165-173.

Zwitserlood, P., & Schriefers, H., Lahiri, A., and van Donselaar, W. (1993). The role of syllables in the perception of spoken Dutch. *Journal of Experimental Psychology: Learning, Memory, and Cognition* 19, 260-271.

13

From production to perception and back: An analysis of two pitch accents

BARBARA GILI FIVELA

Abstract: An analysis of Pisa Italian speech material revealed the existence of specific pitch accents associated with linguistic functions. Two of these accents are investigated in this paper: a rising accent found in continuation contours, narrow focus and elliptic questions, and a rising-falling accent found in contrastive focus and questions with a strong flavour of disbelief. Two tests were performed both to verify the distinction of the two accents and to try to tease apart the contribution of their main phonetic characteristics to their distinction: a categorical perception test and an imitation test.

The results show that the two pitch accents are not perceived through categorical perception, although, in the imitation task, subjects appear to produce two different patterns, showing characteristics consistent with the pitch accents investigated. This suggests that the Categorical Perception paradigm may be not apt to be extensively used for intonation, giving results that appear to be too detached from the actual use of intonation observed in production data.

1. INTRODUCTION

In a recent paper, it was observed that according to some theories of intonational meaning, only categories of intonation seem to be the linguist's concern (Kohler, 2006). Linguistically relevant elements are expected to be discrete and categorical and, thus, linguists have to distinguish categorical modifications from paralinguistic variations, which are expected to be gradient. Nevertheless, intonation mainly deals with paralanguage, as it conveys expressive and attitudinal information, indicates the interactive structure, and communicates the speaker evaluation of events and the speech style. In fact, as Kohler (2006) observes, many communicative functions and meanings of intonation appear to be relevant, and only a few of them - such as sentence modality, accentuation, focus and phrasing - belong to the linguistic domain. Moreover, as clearly observed by Ladd (1996), intonation may also express different degrees of meaning associated with a linguistic unit. Thus, teasing the linguistic and the paralinguistic information apart may not be simple, especially when the meaning or the function of patterns is taken into account.

However, studies performed in different frameworks have referred to the function and meaning of intonational patterns and have proposed categories, or patterns, with which these functions and meanings are associated. For instance, different intonational categories have been proposed to be sufficient to differentiate statements and yes/no-questions[1] in Neapolitan Italian (D'Imperio and House, 1997); intonational patterns have been identified for yes/no-questions and wh-questions, confirmation seeking questions, types of focus, and continuation contours in various languages, such as English, Dutch, and Japanese (Cruttenden, 1986; Beckman and Pierrehumbert, 1986; Caspers, 1998); and intonation categories differentiate confirmation - seeking questions and information - seeking questions on the basis of the accessibility of information in Bari Italian (Grice and Savino, 2003). In some studies, even more general meanings are taken into account for distinguishing intonational events: discrete intonational patterns are found to be used for introducing new elements into the discourse, for committing to their presence in it, and for selecting them from background knowledge (Gussenhoven, 1984). To give some more examples, in English, different phonological units are suggested to differentiate new elements from salient ones, to indicate those linked to mutual beliefs, or to mark those elements to be interpreted in terms of the following information (Pierrehumbert and Hirschberg, 1990); in German, categorical choices are reported to convey meanings such as finality/knowing and openness/realizing (Kohler, 1987; 1991).

1 Yes/no-questions may be answered with 'yes' or 'no', while wh-questions (also called information questions, content questions or question - word questions) contain interrogative words and cannot be answered with 'yes' or 'no'.

In most of the work mentioned above, the proposal of a correlation between various functions or meanings and specific intonational patterns stems from the analysis of speech material, that is, auditory and acoustic analysis of speech productions; only in some cases have these observations and proposals been checked by means of perception experiments as well. However, categories hypothesized on the basis of production data may not be confirmed by perception experiments. For instance, on the basis of production data, Kohler (1987, 1991) checked the existence of three different patterns in German – patterns corresponding to different pitch characteristics, and expressing openness/realizing, unexpectedness/opposing and finality/knowing – but found a perceptual difference for only two of them, namely, for patterns corresponding to openness/realising and finality/knowing. This sort of observation has led some authors to point out that a semantic contrast is not sufficient 'proof' of a structural difference (Gussenhoven, 2006, 1999).

In the next section, an overview of the main methods used to define or check the existence of categories in intonation will be given. Data collection following some of the widespread methods will then be discussed with the main aim of pointing out mismatches in the results, and of arguing that, due to the complex and composite communicative role of intonation, some of the methods found in the literature may not be appropriate for checking intonational categories, or, at least, may not be suitable for deciding upon their existence in linguistic systems.

2. METHODS FOR THE CATEGORISATION OF TONAL EVENTS

Apart from studies using the IPO (Institute for Perception Research in Eindhoven) approach, proposals for categories in intonation usually stem from production data and, possibly, perceptual testing. According to the IPO approach ('t Hart et al., 1990), relevant pitch movements are defined through perceptual equivalence, by means of speaker intuitions of perceptual equality (i.e. by asking subjects whether two patterns are 'passable imitations'[2] of each other). For IPO, in fact, intonation features cannot be related to an intrinsic meaning while the semantics of intonation can be related to syntax in cases of ambiguity resolution.

However, in other frameworks, such as in autosegmental theories (Bruce, 1977; Pierrehumbert, 1980), intonation features do show relations with specific meanings. The intonation contour is seen as due to a result of interpolation between a sequence of L and H tone targets. These were first identified in speech productions, and were proposed to be (part of) pitch accents and edge tones, conveying both linguistic and paralinguistic meanings, and representing the phonological inventory in intonational systems (Pierrehumbert and Hirschberg, 1990; Ladd, 1996; Gussenhoven, 2004). For example, Pierrehumbert and Hirschberg (1990) propose that the meaning of an intonational contour is actually derived from its components: for instance, a high pitch accent (H*) corresponds to something that is new in the discourse, while a low phrase accent (L-) emphasizes separation from what follows.

If intonation is taken to convey different meanings and functions, the auditory analysis, or the auditory and the acoustic analysis, of speech productions is usually taken into consideration in order to evaluate the correlation between specific intonational patterns and different functions and meanings. Monologues, dialogues and various speech styles are considered, ranging from highly controlled speech to (more) spontaneous speech. Analysis pursuing linguistic goals mainly looks for invariant tonal events that can be related, independently of phonetic modifications, to specific functions and meanings.

Once the existence of different patterns has been proposed, there are a number of ways to try to show that these patterns are also perceptually different. The most widespread methods have been described in Gussenhoven's (1999; 2006) works. One of the methods used for testing intonational events is the Categorical Perception paradigm.

2 The usefulness of checking the perceptual equivalence of patterns, in terms of 'passable imitations' of each other, has recently been emphasised by Gussenhoven (2006) with reference to work by Odé (2005) on Russian.

2.1. THE CATEGORICAL PERCEPTION (CP) PARADIGM

Within the CP paradigm (Lieberman et al., 1957; Lieberman et al., 1967; Repp, 1984) the categorical perception of two patterns is confirmed when they are both identified and discriminated. In the identification test, subjects hear stimuli that represent a continuum of changes between the two patterns, possibly representing two phonological categories: subjects are asked to assign stimuli to either category. In the discrimination test, subjects hear stimuli – adjacent in the continuum used for the identify-cation task – and judge whether they are the same or they are different: the two main tasks used are AX (are X and A the same/different?) and ABX (or AXB – is X the same as A or B?) tasks. The presence of an abrupt shift in the association of stimuli to either category in the identification test (see
Figure 1, the S-shaped black line), and the presence of a high peak in the discrimination rate for the stimuli across the identification shift (see
Figure 1, grey line) make it possible to see whether there is categorical perception.[3] In this respect, for instance, cross-category stimuli are discriminated, and stimuli that are not at the identification shift, i.e. within-category stimuli, are expected not be discriminated. This is a good example of why perception shows invariance regardless of acoustic and articulatory variability. That is, the discreteness does not need to be in the signal, but rather is due to the way we perceive the signal, for instance, because we mediate our perception by means of our motor production mechanisms (Lieberman et al., 1957).[4]
The traditional CP paradigm is consistent with the idea of linguistic units, such as phonological units, as discrete elements. Nevertheless, CP is not found equally for all linguistic speech events.

---

3 Moreover, it has been proposed in the literature that reaction times are higher at perceptual boundaries, in particular with reference to identification results (Chen, 2003).

4 Nevertheless, the idea of the existence of (invariant) phonemes corresponding to a discretely differentiated phonetic space has also been interpreted as related to the existence of invariance/discreteness in the signal (see, for instance, the discussion in Port, 2008).

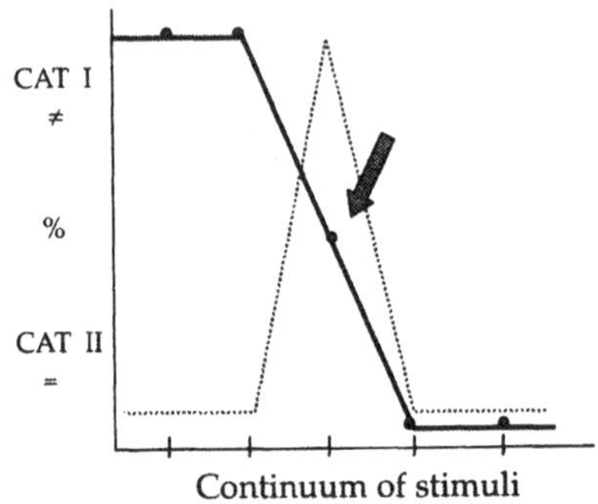

Figure 1: Schematic representation of ideal results of identification (black solid line) and discrimination test (grey dotted line) in case of categorical perception[5].

For instance, vowel categories have been found not to be as categorically distinct as reported for other linguistic categories. In Lieberman et al.'s (1957) terms, in fact, as perception is mediated by motor production, perception will be categorical whenever production is categorical. In this respect, /a/ and /u/ vowels are far less categorical than other linguistic units, such as /b/ and /d/, because of the articulatory processes involved in their production. In the case of vowels, in fact, discrimination results show discrimination plateaux rather than peaks; in this respect, an intonation event may be expected to give similar results, as intonation modulations relate to involve relatively long intervals, resembling more a vocalic than a consonantal event (Schneider et al, 2006). Moreover, it has already been observed that within-category differences can be perceived, exactly as different shades of a colour may be seen. Our way of dividing elements in different categories would only depend on how culture and language organize a continuum of variability (cf. The Whorf Hypothesis, Whorf, 1964), determining the compression of within-category differences and the separation of cross-category differences

5 The figure represents an ideal identification curve and discrimination curve consistent with the description of an AX type of discrimination test. In such a case, subjects are expected not to be able to discriminate within-category stimuli (in the case of the AXB or ABX task, the discrimination rate would be around 50% for subjects that are not able to assign stimuli to either A or B).

(Harnad, 1987). This should in principle allow a certain degree of within-category discrimination.
Further considerations may be made as to the degree of categoriality in subject perception in relation to cognitive aspects. Phonetic variability has been proved to have an impact subjects judgements (Clayards et al., 2007). In fact, if stimuli show a greater variance in distribution, as in the case of Voice Onset Time distribution in Clayards et al.'s (2007) study, subjects show a lower degree of confidence in judging the existence of a contrast: their response curve is found to be shallower as uncertainty increases. As the authors point out, this finding indicates the existence of a continuous assessing of the cue qualities in speech by listeners, who basically weigh the multiple speech cues. Moreover, there are other arguments in favour of a more 'cognition-oriented treatment' of categorical perception. As Niebuhr and Kohler (2004) show with a set of parallel identification and discrimination experiments on peak and valley alignment shifts in German, some of the tasks used in CP experiments may actually be 'perceptuo-cognitive tasks' and may challenge the idea that gradual perceptual changes are not consistent with the existence of phonological categories, and vice versa. As already mentioned, in their study on valley and peak contours, the authors perform both identification and discrimination tests. In the identification tests the authors presented their subjects with a context-stimulus sequence and asked them to judge whether they were a semantic match; in the discrimination task they presented pairs of stimuli and asked subjects whether they were the same or different. According to Nieburh and Kohler's findings, in the identification task subjects "project their perception of pitch patterns onto cognitive categories of semantic interpretation provided by a context-test sentence frame," that is, subjects would refer to prototypical realisations of a semantic set. Results show that there is a clear categorisation at either end of the continuum, with greater uncertainty in the transition between the ends. In the discrimination task, in contrast – which, as the authors state, is more related to perception – a difference between peak and valley results was found: in the valley series the perceptual differentiation is smaller – doesn't reach significance – and does not change across the continuum. According to the authors, perceptual decision was not as sharp as in the peak series because it depends on more than one cue. Additionally, some

of the cues correspond to periods in time rather than points, and, crucially, because the differentiation is linked in the vowel, with no clear landmark, rather than at the vowel onset. Thus, the lack of categorical perception appears to be mainly due to purely perceptual properties and is not taken as proof of the absence of phonological categories.

It may then not be surprising that the use of the CP paradigm for studying intonation has provided mixed results. For instance, it was used to demonstrate the existence of categorical perception for early and medial peak pitch accents in German (Kohler, 1987; 1991, and his subsequent work – for an overview, see Kohler, 2006) and for height contrast in Majorcan Catalan wh- and yes-no questions (Vanrell, 2006). However, as Gussenhoven (2006) recalls, Newport (1982) already observed that categorical perception is not a property of only linguistic contrast, but rather may also be a property of a "*class of acoustic stimuli that cross-cuts the linguistic-nonlinguistic distinction*"(Gussenhoven, 2006, p. 326) and "*may bypass the distinction the test is aimed to reveal, that between non-structural and structural phonetic differences*" (ibidem, 2006, p. 327).

Moreover, if the identification test is performed by referring to intonational meanings and functions, one could argue that categorical perception may become particularly difficult to obtain because of the difficulties implicit in the tasks used. In the identification test various tasks may be used. In addition to the already mentioned semantic match test, a forced choice corresponding to a semantic difference task may also be used. As shown by Gussenhoven (1999; 2006), the semantic difference task consists in asking for a categorical (or a gradient) judgement on the presence of a meaning or of its opposite. This is considered to be a difficult task due to the complex meaning intonation may have and the possible interpretations subjects may give (see Grabe, 1997, for discussion). When considering an identification task involving a linguistic distinction such as the one between questions and answers, or between yes-no- and wh-questions, the method may appear to be quite straightforward. Nevertheless, when considering linguistic meanings such as those related to focus, the issue may suddenly appear more problematic. On the one hand, focus may be clearly recognized as part of the linguistic set of meanings, at least considering that it may change the truth value of an utterance (e.g. the example by Rooth (1985): "OFFICERS may escort ballerinas" vs "Officers may escort BALLE-

RINAS," where the sentence has different truth values depending on which word is the focussed). On the other hand, focus may easily become part of the paralinguistic domain, involving degrees of emphasis rather than categorical changes of meaning/interpretation.

The Categorical Perception paradigm has been applied in both types of contexts – that is in relation to both focus and, say, sentence modality – with heterogeneous results even in cases that could appear more straightforward. As already mentioned, in studying Majorcan Catalan wh- and yes-no questions, Vanrell (2006) showed the existence of categorical perception for subjects who identified and discriminated two distinct patterns over a continuum of variation in pitch scaling. Different results with the categorical perception test have been obtained, for instance, in investigating the difference between statement and question interpretation for low and high boundary tones in German. Considering subject answers in relation to a continuum of pitch height variation, Schneider et al. (2006) report that a plateau rather than a peak was found in the discrimination test results. The authors observe that some criticism of the use of the CP paradigm for investigating intonation has already appeared in the literature, and perform a second experiment checking for the Perceptual Magnet Effect (Kuhl, 1991).[6] Apart from the fact that they found a perceptual magnet effect only for the statement category in German (and not for the question category), for the purposes of this paper it is relevant to note the difficulty in finding categorical perception even for features differentiating questions and statements.

An example related to focus was already mentioned when referring to Kohler's (1987; 1991) work on the lack of distinction between medial and late peaks for expressing openness/realising and unexpectedness/-opposing. Another example relevant for the purposes of the present

---

6 According to the Perceptual Magnet Effect hypothesis, each category has a prototype and the prototype and its neighbour stimuli should be more difficult to discriminate; on the contrary, the non-prototype and its neighbours should be easier to discriminate. Basically, Schneider et al. (2006) perform an identification task – with three possible answers – and, more importantly, a discrimination task performed after a goodness rating of the stimuli in terms of very bad or very good exemplars. This procedure enabled the authors to individuate the prototype for each category and to propose, in the discrimination task, pairs of stimuli that were not necessarily adjacent in the continuum.

paper is Ladd and Morton's (1997) use of the traditional CP paradigm to test categorical distinction of the pitch accents found in neutral statements and in emphatic conditions in English. In their CP experiment, the authors find no categorical perception, although subjects could categorically interpret stimuli at the extremes of the continuum. The authors conclude that a different meaning may be recognized without the need of categorical perception.

In a recent paper, Dilley (submitted) tests from a perceptual point of view two pairs of accents attested in American English (H* and H+L*, and L* and L+H*) by means of various experiments. For the sake of discussion, it is relevant to draw attention to the fact that by means of AX and AXB tasks, with no reference to the function of pitch patterns, Dilley shows that pitch accents are categorically perceived and subjects learn category exemplars. However, it is important to notice that in her discrimination test, the author pairs stimuli not adjacent in the continuum, increasing the step size in order to enhance the discrimination capabilities. Moreover, Dilley finds consistent proof of the existence of categorically different pitch accents by means of another relevant task for investigating categories in intonation, the imitation task.

2.2. THE IMITATION TASK

In the imitation task, first proposed by Pierrehumbert and Steele (1989) in their work on American English, subjects hear a continuum of stimuli varying for certain pitch characteristics and are asked to imitate the stimuli. Speakers are expected to produce instances of two discrete sets when they perceive two different categories; they are expected to imitate the continuum of variation when stimuli represent a gradual change in one specific pattern.

This method has been quite successfully used to demonstrate the existence of intonational categories, although some improvements with respect to its original version have been proposed in the literature. Gussenhoven (2006), for instance, proposes improving the task by having subjects imitate by 'correcting' non-acceptable patterns. More recently, Braun et al. (2006) have shown that asking subjects to imitate their own imitation may favour the implementation of a category rather than the accurate imitation of phonetic features. The above mentioned work by Dilley (submitted), to give another example, reports results based on the analysis of the second imitation by subjects who produced two imitations after each stimulus. However, the method appears to be useful for checking the existence of categories, as shown by various work on the imitation of patterns involving alignment and scaling characteristics of both peaks and valleys (Niebuhr, 2003; Redi, 2003 Dilley, 2007; Dilley and Brown, 2007). Moreover, Dilley and Brown (2007) recently used it to test the role of pitch range variation in the alignment of tonal targets. The authors asked subjects to imitate stimuli showing rising-falling, falling-rising and flat F0 contours across two target syllables, and found that the timing of peaks and valleys in subjects' imitations varied categorically according to the F0 levels of the two syllables in the stimuli. That is, pitch range manipulation affected the timing of peaks and valleys in production.

This method appears to be useful for testing the existence of categories in intonation, although, as suggested by one of the reviewers of this paper, it is hard to say which aspects of the stimuli the subjects concentrate on, and, as already observed in the literature, subjects may be differently skilled in (re-)producing their perception. According to the author of the present paper, the first observation is crucial if the experiment is run in order to point out which correlates the speakers reproduce, and the experimental design does not guarantee that only one correlate (at a time) is varied in the audio stimuli. However, the observation appears to be less relevant when the task is used in order to find out whether two discrete populations of productions may be found within speakers imitations; in this case results may be adequate even if the exact crucial correlate(s) remain unknown. As for the difference in skill subjects may show, various possibilities should be considered. First of all, speakers could lack the skill in the sense that they perceive categorically distinct events but cannot produce them as categorically distinct. In principle, among such subjects we may include both speakers that, say, perceive categories but produce gradual tonal modifications and speakers that perceive categories and produce whatever comes to their mind, probably because they are having trouble concentrating on the task. However, the former situation, as already observed by Dilley (2007), seems unlikely due to successful results for imitation tasks found in the literature (see references above); the latter appears more plausible, and it is unfortunately quite frequent (see the necessity of discarding subjects from the data set because of their inconsistent behaviour compared to other participants in, for instance, Dilley (2007) and the present work). Secondly, speakers may be skilled in imitating their percepts. In this case, though, speakers may be good imitators both when they perceive categories and produce categories, and when they perceive gradient variations and produce gradual changes. Nevertheless, they will also be good imitators if they hear a continuum of variation between two categories, as is usually the case in this type of test, and produce a gradient variation. Thus, in imitation tasks experimenters look for good imitators, imitators that are good enough to produce categories if they hear categories, under the assumption that the imitators should be so as to be able to produce gradient-like variation just because they hear a continuum of acoustic changes.

In the next sections, production and perception data collected in Pisa Italian will be described with the main aim of finding different sources of information on the possible distinction of pitch accent categories. A comparison will be made of an analysis stemming from production material, results obtained by means of categorical perception tests, and data collected with an imitation task, that is, data produced after a perceptual filtering. However, different correlates, i.e. alignment and scaling, will be separately manipulated to try to tease apart the contribution of the main phonetic characteristics of the pitch accents to their distinction.

3. PRODUCTION, PERCEPTION, AND PERCEPTION-PRODUCTION: AN ANALYSIS OF TWO PITCH ACCENTS

3.1. PRODUCTION DATA

An analysis of both read and semispontaneous speech, i.e. Map-Task dialogues,[7] showed which are the intonation contours typically used by

7 Map-Task dialogues are elicited by asking two speakers to reconstruct a path among some landmarks. One speaker, the instruction giver, has a map showing

Pisa Italian speakers to express specific linguistic functions. These contours have been analysed according to the autosegmental-metrical framework (Bruce, 1977; Pierrehumbert, 1980; Beckman and Pierrehumbert, 1986; for an overview, see Ladd, 1996). In this framework, the contour is accounted for by means of pitch accents, which are associated with tone bearing units, e.g. syllables and edge tones, such as phrase accents and boundary tones, which are associated with the edges of higher order prosodic domains, i.e. intermediate and intonation phrases, respectively. In Pisa Italian, three pitch accents, combined with different combinations of edge tones, turn out to be relevant for expressing the main linguistic functions (Gili Fivela, 2004), such as the contours of yes-no-questions, wh-questions, statements, and focus phenomena. The three pitch accents have been phonologically analysed as H*, H*+L[8] and H+L*. The first two of these will be further analysed in this paper.

The proposal of different phonological categories stems from the observation of the pitch accents in different functional contexts, where the accents constitute contours that convey specific functions. To give some examples, the H* accent is found in continuation contours, narrow focus and elliptic questions; the H*+L accent is found in contrastive focus and questions with a strong flavour of disbelief.[9] Due to the small number of different pitch accents relevant for the phonological description of Pisa Italian, in many cases contours are differentiated, in phonological terms, by the choice of the edge tone. Nevertheless, there are some cases in which the pitch accents, in fact, may all be followed by low edge tones, offering a tonal context suitable for direct comparison. The H* pitch accent may be followed by a low phrase accent in

a path among the landmarks drawn on it; the other speaker, the instruction follower, is given a map on which only the landmarks are shown, with no path. Landmark names are chosen consistently with the purpose of phonetic-phonological analysis, and some mismatches in landmark positions and names are introduced in order to encourage the verbal exchange (Anderson et al., 1991).

8 According to the proposal by Prieto et al. (2005), the specific – and contrastive – alignment properties of H* and H*+L may be more precisely accounted for by postulating a secondary association of the high tone.

9 The pattern was observed in the Map-Task dialogue, in 'object moves' (Grice and Savino, 1995).

statements when it occupies the nuclear position within an intermediate phrase that is early in the utterance (Gili Fivela, 1999); it is then particularly apt to indicate continuation. The pitch accent may also be used to express narrow focus, and, in the case of focus used to contrast different terms, it appears to be more suitable for syntagmatic contrast within the utterance (e.g. "X does that, Y does something else") rather than for paradigmatic contrast (e.g. "X does that," implying not Y, Z....). In contrast, the pitch accent phonologically analysed as H*+L followed by low edge tone(s) expresses narrow focus with a clear contrastive interpretation; it sounds more peremptory and conclusive than the H* accent, and it may therefore be found in utterance final position. Its peremptory and conclusive flavour may be pragmatically interpreted as a check of information.[10]

In production, the accents clearly have different functions, i.e. speakers choose the pitch patterns according to the context and the information they want to communicate. Nevertheless, it is clear from the description above that in some cases different patterns may be used to express the same function, perhaps with a difference in the degree of a meaning. As mentioned above, both H* and H*+L may express some kind of contrast[11], and in this case the attitude of the speaker and/or the position of the pattern in the utterance appear to be the main characteristics distinguishing them.

The pitch patterns are also clearly different regarding their phonetic characteristics (see Figure 2).

---

10 This observation stems from the analysis of Map-Task dialogues where the pattern is interpreted as a confirmation-seeking question when uttered by instruction followers: as they explicitly lack information in comparison to instruction givers - see fn. 7 - the utterance is actually interpreted as a question (as a conversational implicature (Grice, 1975; 1978), induced by the intonational pattern).

11 Notice that some of the investigations in the literature do not distinguish contrastive and narrow focus (Swerts, 2005).

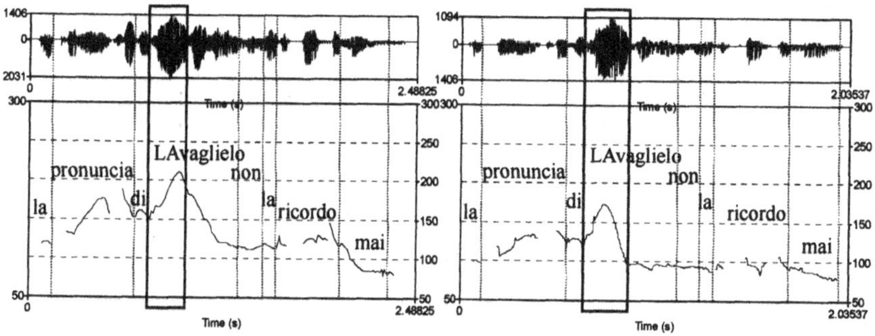

Figure 2: Fundamental frequency contour of the sentence *La pronuncia di lavaglielo non (la) ricordo mai* "The pronunciation of 'wash it for him' I never remember (it)", produced by a female speaker as narrow focus on the left dislocated phrase (utterance 'initial' H* on 'la-' – left panel), with a contrastive interpretation of *lavaglielo* (realised with an H*+L on 'la-' – right panel); the relevant syllable is highlighted by the square.

The H* and the H*+L are both characterised by a rise to the high peak that starts around the beginning of the accented syllable: in the H* accent, the rise end – the high peak – is aligned to the right end of the syllable (left panel in the Figure), while in the H*+L the rise ends earlier in the syllable and is followed by a fall, due to the presence of a low target[12] (right panel in the Figure). In terms of average F0 height and syllable duration, the H* target reaches the highest F0 values while, on average, syllable duration is greater for syllables bearing the H*+L accent than for those bearing the H* accent (Gili Fivela, 2005; 2006).

Thus, different pitch accents have been clearly recognized in speakers' productions in regard to their functions, meanings and phonetic forms. In the next sections, both categorical perception and imitation experiments aimed at finding out whether they really correspond to distinct categories will be described. All tests treat alignment and scaling

12 Gili Fivela (2006) argues that the starting point of the rise does not distinguish the two categories, which, however, are unambiguously differentiated by the choice of the starred tone together with the absence/presence of the trailing tone. Thus, the accents may be phonetically transcribed as involving a low leading tone target ([L+]H* and [L+]H*+L, respectively, where the phonetic feature in the transcription is highlighted by means of the squared brackets).

correlates separately, trying to find out whether the pitch accent differentiation may depend on both characteristics.

3.2. THE CATEGORICAL PERCEPTION TEST

As already mentioned, within the traditional Categorical Perception (CP) paradigm (Lieberman et al., 1957; Lieberman et al. 1967; Repp, 1984) two patterns are categorically perceived when they are both identified and discriminated.

In the following sections, the testing of the categorical perception of the patterns described above as H* and H*+L with this paradigm will be described.

An identification test had already been performed on H* and H*+L pitch accents in Pisa Italian (Gili Fivela, 2005). In particular, a semantic difference task was used to investigate the interplay of target alignment and scaling in the identification of the pitch patterns in Pisa Italian. Results showed that the F0 height of tonal targets affects subject judgements, and plays a role in the identification of the two pitch accents (see also Gili Fivela, 2006). The experiment is briefly summarised in the following, as the same stimuli have been used here for the discrimination task intended to investigate the categorical perception of the pitch accents, as well as for the imitation task.

3.2.1. STIMULI

Subjects were asked to listen to stimuli that had been manipulated to obtain a gradual shift from an H*+L accent (see Figure 2, right panel) to an H* L- pattern, i.e. an H* accent (see Figure 2, left panel) followed by a low phrase accent. The manipulation was carried out on the basis of mean latency and frequency values for the tonal targets[13] (Gili Fivela,

13 F0 inspection and detailed acoustic measurements showed that the two patterns differ for the syllable duration and both the alignment and scaling of the tonal targets (see section 3.1.; for details see Gili Fivela 2004; 2005). The manipulations described below relate to both the alignment and the scaling of the tonal targets, while no syllable duration was changed. Notice that the difference in F0 level

2004) by calculating the relevant interval to be covered to create a continuum between the two pitch accents.

The alignment of both the peak and the falling phase of an H*+L accent, realised on the penultimate syllable of the final word in the sentence *ho detto velava* 'I said veiled', was shifted forward in 8 steps of 15 ms, creating a continuum of alignment changes.[14] Moreover, for each step, the scaling of all the targets was shifted upward in 2 steps ('PR1' and 'PR2'): 13 Hz for the first low elbow, 17 Hz for the peak, and 6 Hz for the second low target (see Figure 3, left and right drawing, for alignment and scaling respectively).[15] The total number of stimuli was 27.

All stimuli manipulations were performed using PRAAT (developed at the Institute of Phonetic Sciences of the University of Amsterdam by P.Boersma and D.Weenink) and using PSOLA resynthesis.

---

found after the two pitch accents in the case of utterance initial position - see Figure 2 – in the present study is only encoded in the final low target F0 height. Thus possible influences on the perception of the postaccentual stretch (along the lines of Xu et al.'s (2004) findings) are not taken into account in the present study.

14 Thus the slope of the rising phase was changed gradually, creating a continuum of variation from the slope of one accent to the slope of the other accent. This was consistent with the acoustic characteristics of the two patterns – see Figure 2, where in addition to the different time scale, it is shown that the rise spans over the whole syllable in one case and over the beginning of it in the other. Thus the results definitely depend on the peak alignment and the consequential rising phase slope (for results on the peak-configuration shift with no rising phase slope variation, see Gili Fivela and D'Imperio (submitted)).

15 The step size was chosen in order to get a number of intermediate steps in alignment and in scaling that would be appropriate for observing the possible categorical shift and its possible interaction with scaling modification. In changing the step size, results for the identification and discrimination rates are of course expected to be different. Nevertheless, this is taken here as a possible limitation of the CP paradigm, as the data discussed in this paper show that, even if one could argue that no discrimination is found because of the choice of the size of manipulation step, say, in alignment, subjects do not appear to have trouble with the size of manipulation steps in the imitation task. As for the use of a hertz scale rather than a semitone scale, which may bring with it the risk that the differences considered here may be smaller and, crucially, too small, in perception, notice that the peak steps are 17Hz in this study, and positive results for categorical perception have already been reported in the literature with 15Hz steps of scaling variation (Vanrell, 2006).

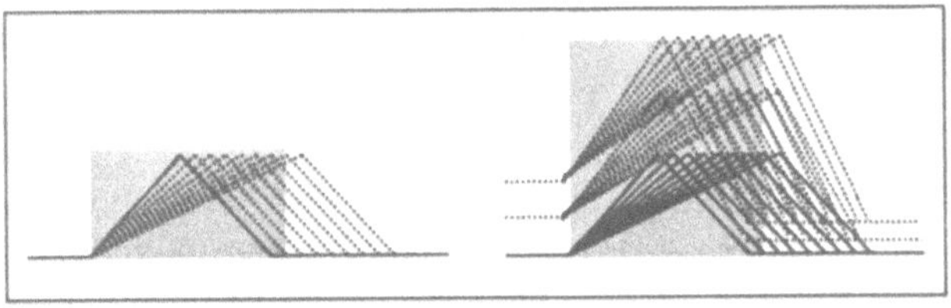

Figure 3: Schematic representation of the acoustic manipulations (grey area represents the nuclear syllable). From Gili Fivela (2005).

3.2.2. IDENTIFICATION TASK

Ten speakers of Pisa Italian listened to five repetitions of the randomized stimuli (for a total of 135 stimuli using the software Perceval - LPL, Aix-en-Provence), and judged whether they could represent a peremptory and conclusive correction or a neutral statement. It was made clear that the neutral statement option could also resemble a sort of correction, but only in case it was followed by other material – as a sort of motivation for the correction – that was closely linked to the preceding material from a prosodic point of view. Subjects were given these explanations and were then asked to answer 'yes' when they considered the stimulus appropriate to correct a possible preceding utterance in a peremptory and conclusive way ('does it correct a preceding utterance in a peremptory and conclusive way?'); they were asked to answer no otherwise. The task was thus quite complicated and the question subjects were asked was necessarily a composite one, involving a reference to both a function (expressing contrast) and a difference in the strength of the speaker's purpose (the peremptory and conclusive feature)[16] (for discussion, see Gili Fivela, 2005; 2006).

16 In a pilot experiment, subjects were asked to focus only on the function (the question was 'does it correct a preceding utterance?') and were not able to perform the task, while the composite question asked here allowed subjects to identify different pitch accents. On the contrary, the same question, as well as a good/bad-fit judgement in a question-answer context (see the semantic matching task mentioned in section 2.1.) did not give as positive results in the test of Pisa Italian contrastive vs broad focus falling accent (Gili Fivela, 2008). However, it may be the case that better S-shaped results would be obtained here with a question-answer context.

Figure 4 shows the mean of the answers given by the Pisa Italian subjects who took part in the experiment. As may be seen in the plot, subjects identify two accents although the graphs are not S-shaped as shown in case of the categorical perception. This is assumed to be due to the fact that the answers plotted in the graph relate to stimuli in which only one acoustic parameter was manipulated at a time, say alignment, while the other parameter, say scaling, was kept constant.[17] The best S-shaped trend is obtained for stimuli where the scaling information was intermediate between the two patterns – condition 'PR1'. The 'neutral' value for this correlate appears to favour a greater attention to alignment differences. However, the graph also shows that subjects were clearly identifying the stimuli with coherent correlates, i.e. the stimuli at the extreme of both the align and scaling continua (see circles in Figure 4), interpreting those stimuli as either contrastive or in agreement with the (coherent) alignment and scaling characteristics ('PR0' corresponds to the scaling characteristics of the contrastive interpretation, 'PR2' to those found in the H* L- pattern).

The ANOVAs performed on the data showed that alignment and scaling are significant in relation to the subjects' answers.[18] However, data also showed that scaling information interplay with alignment in the identification of the two accents, in terms of both 'when' and 'how precisely' they are identified. That is, the steps of alignment that (tend to) correspond to one category or the other vary depending on the scaling condition (i.e. the chance level is crossed on the second step for condition 'PR2' and on the sixth for 'PR0'). Moreover, the scaling characteristics of one pattern cause difficulties in the identification of the other one, and

17 Speaker judgements for the identification of stimuli which vary consistently for both alignment and scaling in fact show a more 'traditional' S-shaped plot (Gili Fivela, in prep.). Nevertheless, while the consistent manipulation of both alignment and scaling allows one to appreciate a more abrupt shift in subjects' answers, it does not permit the analysis of the specific role of alignment and scaling correlates, which was one of the goals of the present investigation.

18 Two- and one-way ANOVAs were performed on the data (see Gili Fivela (2005) for detailed results). The two-way ANOVAs with alignment and scaling steps as factors showed that they are both significant in relation to subject answers and there is no statistical interaction between the two ([$F(1334,8)=7.649$; $p<0.0001$] for alignment, [$F(1334,2)=20.453$;$p<0.0001$] for scaling, [$F(1334,16)=.438$; $p>0.05$] and for their interaction).

vice versa. In fact, the scaling characteristics of the broad pattern cause troubles in the identification of the contrastive accents even when the alignment characteristics give quite unambiguous information, i.e. the alignment is early in the syllable (the score is attested at about the chance level for steps '0,1' in the 'PR2' condition); similarly, the scaling characteristics of the contrastive pattern lower the identification rate of the broad pattern even when the alignment is late in the syllable (the score is attested between 0.3 and 0.45 for steps '6-8' in the 'PR0' condition)[19].

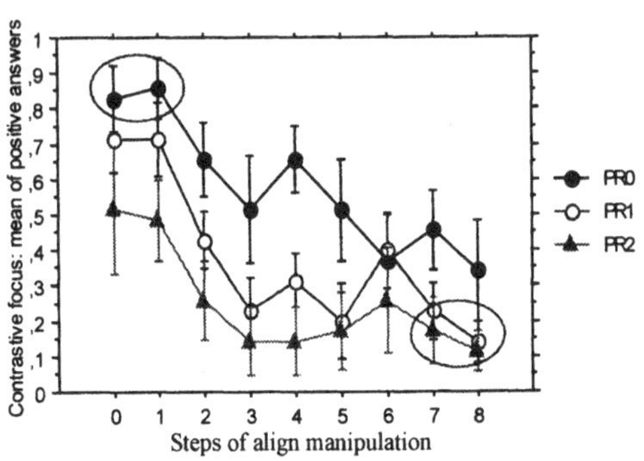

Figure 4: Mean and standard error of positive answers in favour of the contrastive interpretation in relation to stimuli manipulated for the peak (and following low) alignment – steps of manipulation on the x-axis – and for the target scaling – steps of manipulation in legend, represented by forms (Gili Fivela, 2005).

3.2.3. DISCRIMINATION TASK

The stimuli used for the identification task were then also used in the discrimination test. An AX test was performed by asking 10 Pisa Italian subjects to judge pairs of stimuli adjacent in the continuum used for the identification task. In the case of studies involving tones, discrimination appears to be easier if the second stimulus in the pair is higher in pitch

19 Plotting data per subject shows variation across subjects for the importance given to alignment or scaling variation (see the discussion in Gili Fivela (2006)). That is, most subjects show an identification shift according to alignment characteristics, whatever the target scaling is; others appear to do the opposite.

(Ladd and Morton, 1997; Vanrell, 2006). Thus, subjects listened to pairs of stimuli: AX, where X was either higher in pitch or had a later peak,[20] and AA pairs, as controls. Therefore, two series of AX stimuli were constructed: one series (henceforth, AXalign) for stimuli adjacent for steps of align manipulation, belonging to the same pitch value; the other series (henceforth, AXscaling) for stimuli adjacent for steps of scaling manipulation, showing the same alignment characteristics (for this latter series only two pairs of adjacent stimuli were possible). Subjects heard the pairs three times, in random order, and were asked to judge whether the stimuli in each pair were the same or different.

Discrimination test results show no positive discrimination peak (or plateau).

Figure 5 shows the mean of the subjects' answers in favour of 'different', calculated on the mean of all the answers given by subjects for each stimulus:[21] the left panel refers to answers for the AXalign series and the right panel for the AXscaling series. In the AXalign series, pairs of stimuli differed for alignment, and were kept constant for pitch scaling were not discriminated, i.e. they were mainly judged as 'same'. In the AXscaling, pairs of stimuli which differed for scaling and were constant for alignment characteristics were much more often discriminated, i.e. they were recognized as different in 0.6 to 0.8 of cases on a 0 to 1 scale. Two-way ANOVAs, with alignment and scaling steps as independent factors, showed that, for both the AXalign and AXscaling series, there was no significant effect of align or scaling steps, or of their interaction (AXalign series: [$F(7,168)=1.168; p>0.05$], [$F(2,168)=0.397; p>0.05$], [$F(14,168)=0.851; p>0.05$] for alignment steps, scaling steps and their interaction; similarly for the AXscaling series: [$F(1,126)=0.204; p>0.05$], [$F(8,126)=0.107; p>0.05$], [$F(8,126)=0.153; p>0.05$]). Thus, no discrimination peak is found for any continuum, although it is clear from the results that, when subjects discriminate, they do it on the basis of scaling characteristics, rather than alignment characteristics (see

---

20 Gussenhoven (2002) reports that delaying a peak may represent an alternative strategy to increase its height. Thus, in AX pairs, having X elements either higher or with later peaks appeared to be the most consistent choice.

21 Two subjects were discarded because they failed to recognize the AA pairs in more than 33% of cases.

Figure 5, left vs right panel).[22] Moreover, it has been proposed in the literature that reaction times are higher at perceptual boundaries (Chen, 2003). Chen's (2003) observation is related to identification results, while here reaction times were measured for the discrimination task in order to try to get further data in case – as expected from the literature – no real peak was found. Reaction times, measured from the onset of the trial, are shown for the AXalign series in Figure 6. As can be seen from the plot, reaction times cannot be related to any discrimination peak, although it is worth observing that they are somehow consistent with identification results.

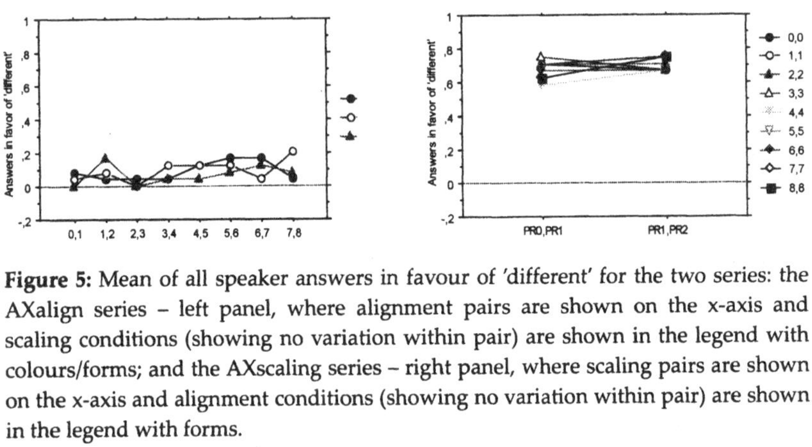

Figure 5: Mean of all speaker answers in favour of 'different' for the two series: the AXalign series – left panel, where alignment pairs are shown on the x-axis and scaling conditions (showing no variation within pair) are shown in the legend with colours/forms; and the AXscaling series – right panel, where scaling pairs are shown on the x-axis and alignment conditions (showing no variation within pair) are shown in the legend with forms.

Higher reaction times are found for stimuli at the intermediate scaling values ('PR1' condition). Moreover, higher reaction times are found for the pair 'al2-al3' in conditions 'PR1' and 'PR2': for these two conditions, in the identification scores, alignment step 'al2' appeared to be the 'transition' step towards lower identification scores and 'al3' was the step where the scores in identification reached the lowest values (see Figure 4). If reaction time cannot be taken here as an indication of the presence of a perceptual boundary, at least in categorical perception terms, it can

22 Contrary to what was observed for the identification results, plotting the data per subjects did not show interesting differences in comparison to pooling all subjects.

indicate a higher cognitive effort in the intermediate scaling condition 'PR1' and for steps 'al2' and 'al3' in alignment manipulation.

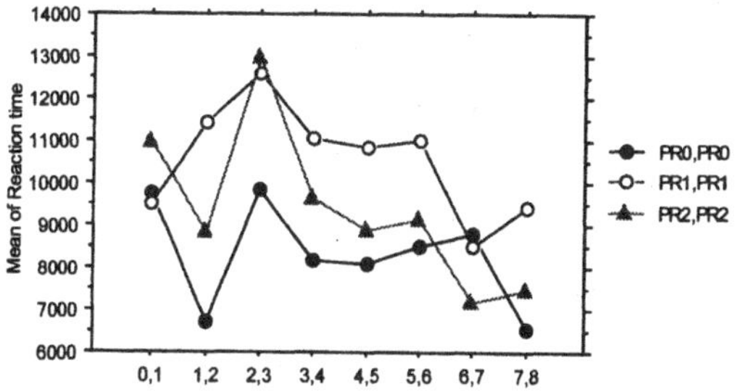

Figure 6: Mean of reaction times (RT) for the series AXalign. The alignment pairs are shown on the x-axis and the scaling conditions (showing no variation within pair) are shown in the legend with forms.

However, subjects did not show categorical perception for the H* and H*+L accents. Nevertheless, alignment appeared to play a significant role in relation to the subjects' identification scores, although it was influenced by scaling: subjects appeared to categorically interpret stimuli showing consistent correlates in terms of both alignment and scaling, that is, stimuli at the extremes of the continuum. However, discrimination results showed that subjects clearly perceived differences in F0 height, as shown by the (globally higher) discrimination score.

3.3. The perception-production test

3.3.1. Stimuli

The same stimuli used for the identification and discrimination tests were used for an imitation task. That is, speakers imitated the stimuli representing the gradual shift from an H*+L accent to an H* L- pattern, i.e. an H* accent followed by a low phrase accent (see Figure 2).

3.3.2. THE IMITATION TASK

The experiment was performed by asking three speakers of Pisa Italian to imitate three repetitions of audio stimuli played via headphones.[23]. The subjects – two females and one male - were seated in a sound-proof room, and were instructed to produce their best imitation of the randomized stimuli. However, between hearing the stimulus and imitating it, the subjects were also asked to perform a cognitive task: they were instructed to think of a number and to say it; after saying the number, they heard a beep, signalling that they could produce their imitation. The task of saying a number was chosen in order to increase the distance, both in chronological terms and in attentional terms, between the sound stimulus and the speech production.

Speakers' production were recorded and digitized at 22050 Hz. They were segmented and hand labelled by means of PRAAT, for the positions of segment boundaries within the syllable bearing the target accent (the penultimate syllable in the word *velava* 'veiled') and for tonal target positions. Latencies (between tonal targets and all segment boundaries) and F0 values at tonal target positions were calculated; latency measures were then normalized by dividing them by the duration of the reference unit, the syllable. Here only measurements concerning the high peak were considered as a diagnostic for checking the discreteness in speaker's imitations. As already mentioned, on average, the peak is earlier (at about the middle of the syllable rather than at the end of it) and lower in the contrastive H*+L accent than in the H* accent.

Figure 7 shows mean values of peak to syllable-offset normalized distance - left panels - and peak F0 values in Hz[24] (right panels) for all the

23 Preliminary results were presented during a seminar at Universitat Autonoma de Barcelona, Spain (May 2007).

24 One reviewer suggested the use of a semitone scale in order to account for pitch and register variations due to the presence of a male and two female subjects. However the goal of the present analysis and data discussion is to point out intra-speaker differences in production related to differences in stimuli characteristics rather than inter-speaker comparison. Thus hertz values are considered to suit the present discussion as well as semitones in terms of inter speaker/production comparison, although the plotted intra-subject production differences could be smaller in perception (for the hertz vs semitone scale, see also fn.15).

speakers imitations (three for each stimulus). The plots show normalised measures for stimuli varying in alignment (x-axis) and scaling (forms). As the figure shows, in fact the peak position with respect to the syllable offset changes according to the steps of alignment, independently of the F0 height of stimuli. Two way ANOVAs performed with align and scaling steps as factors shows that, for two out of three speakers, only alignment steps have a significant influence on speech productions; for the other speaker both alignment and scaling appear to have an influence.

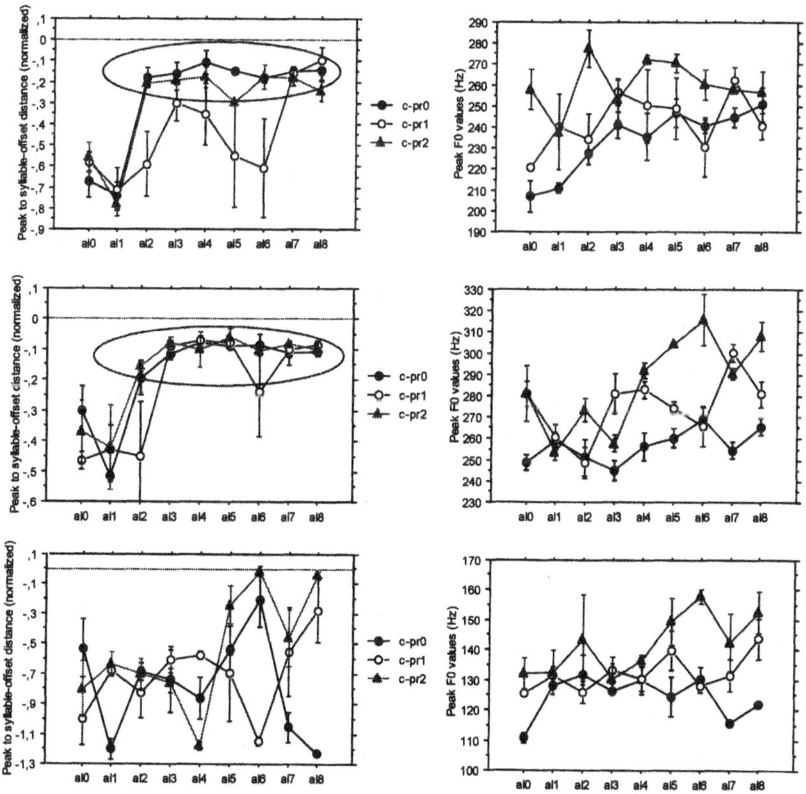

Figure 7: Peak to syllable-offset normalized distance and peak F0 values, left and right plots respectively. Speaker ILL, upper panels, speaker IL, middle panels, speaker NI, lower panels. Align (x-axis) and scaling steps (forms).

ANOVAs for speaker ILL's productions – upper panels in figure – show that only alignment steps have an influence on the peak position, with no interaction with scaling steps ([$F(8,54)=13.754; p<0.001$] for align steps, [$F(2,54)=7.171; p>0.05$], [$F(16,54)=1.682; p>0.05$] for scaling and interaction). The Fisher's post hoc shows that steps 'al0' and 'al1' are similar to each other and significantly different from all the others, and that steps 'al7' and 'al8' differ from 'al2', 'al5' and 'al6'. Similarly, for speaker IL (middle panels in the figure) only alignment steps have a significant influence on speech productions, with no interaction with scaling steps ([$F(8,54) =14.943; p<0.001$] for alignment steps, [$F(2,54)=2.129$; $p>0.05$], [$F(16,54)$-$=1.059$; $p>0.05$] for scaling and interaction). The Fisher's post hoc shows that steps 'al0' and 'al1' are similar and significantly different from all the others, and that step 'al2' differs from both of them and all the others. The results for speaker NI (lower panels in the figure) are less clear-cut. Both alignment and scaling characteristics appear to have an influence on his productions, and they also interact ([$F(8,54)=3.356$; $p<0.05$] for alignment steps, [$F(2,54)=6.597$; $p<0.05$], [$F(16,54)=6.106$; $p<0.001$] for scaling and interaction). The Fisher's post hoc shows that steps 'al0', 'al1' and 'al4' are similar and significantly different from steps 'al5', 'al6' and 'al8', while steps 'al2' and 'al3' differ from 'al6', and 'al2' also differs from 'al5'.

Data also show that speakers implement the tonal target at F0 heights that change slightly depending on the stimulus scaling (see Figure 7), panels on the right. Nevertheless, they also appear to be slightly positively correlated with the alignment characteristics (correlation, or determination, indexes are the following, for the three speakers: for ILL, $R^2=0.267$; for IL, $R^2=0.138$; for NI, $R^2=.286$) – see Figure 8. That is, the tendency is to maintain a lower height for smaller steps of alignment, in line with the characteristics of the H*+L accent.

Thus, speakers appear to produce two different patterns, and in their productions the peak position with respect to the syllable offset changes according to the steps of alignment in the audio stimuli; for two speakers this happens independently of the F0 height of the stimuli. The two accents under investigation consistently show a major difference in terms of alignment of the F0 peak, with the peak being earlier in the contrastive H*+L accent and later in the L+H* accent. However, data also show that speakers implement the tonal target at F0 heights that change slightly depending on the stimulus scaling, although data also suggest that they implement the peak at an F0 level that is consistent with the alignment characteristics. This latter result appears to be consistent with recent findings by Dilley and Brown (2007), who show that pitch scaling may be highly correlated to the identity of pitch accents, to the extent of affecting target alignment in speakers productions.

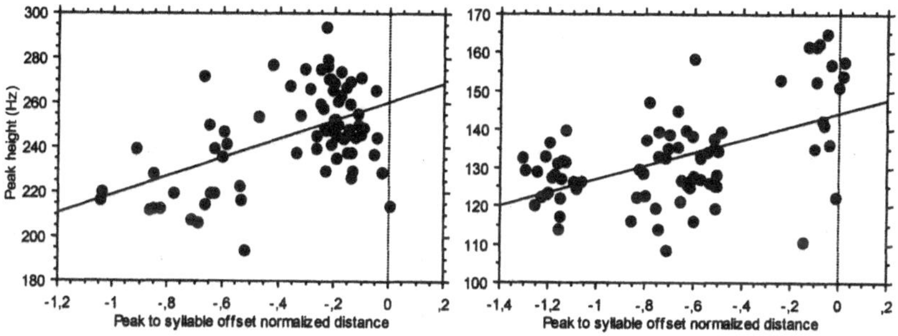

Figure 8: Bivariate regression plots: Peak F0 height and peak to syllable-offset normalized distance. Speaker ILL, left panel, and speaker NI, right panel.

4. DISCUSSION

The analysis of the Pisa Italian speech material revealed the existence of specific pitch patterns associated to functions and meanings that clearly belong to the linguistic domain. Different pitch accents, combined with other tonal events such as edge tones, have been found in read and semispontaneous speech in association to statements, different types of questions, and focus. In the autosegmental-metrical framework, tonal events are seen as conveying different meanings and as belonging to the speaker's phonological system. However, similarly to other phonological units, tonal events playing specific linguistic roles, including pitch accents, are expected to be discrete. In this respect they are different from other intonational modifications that are gradient in nature, and convey paralinguistic information such as the speaker's attitude. Thus, testing the existence of these phonological events would also require checking their perceptual properties, among which the discreteness related to their categorical nature is expected.

In order to verify the distinction between two pitch accents found in the Pisa Italian production data, the pitch patterns were considered in the most similar tonal environment, and two different types of tests were performed: a categorical perception test and an imitation test. The former clearly provides data on perception – although, as already observed by Niebuhr and Kohler (2004) in testing some intonational events, the discrimination task may be more properly considered as a purely perceptual test in comparison with the identification task, which requires some sort of cognitive process (see 2.1.); the latter guaranties production data, providing speech material produced through the speaker's own perceptual filter. However, both tests were forced, in a sense, since we tried to separately control the main temporal and frequency characteristics of the patterns under investigation. In fact, the two pitch accents found in Pisa Italian differ in many correlates, among which alignment and scaling of tonal events. Thus, apart from checking the perceptual discreteness of the patterns, an effort was made to tease apart the contribution of each of their main phonetic characteristics to their distinction. Thus, all tests separately treated alignment and scaling correlates.

The first test to be performed was the categorical perception test, composed of an identification and a discrimination task. The plot of identification results showed no S-shape, as it would have been expected for categorical perception. At first sight, the situation may not be surprising as subjects were asked to focus on a quite complex set of functional and paralinguistic features (they were asked to tease apart corrections from statements, being instructed to focus on the peremptory/conclusive feature of corrections with respect to statements in the corpus). Nevertheless, subjects were clearly identifying stimuli at the extreme of the continuum, those with consistent correlates: alignment and scaling turned out to be significant in affecting subjects' judgements, and, in particular, scaling information turned out to be relevant in the identification of the two accents, in terms of both 'when' and 'how precisely' they were identified. However, the discrimination task showed that no discrimination peak was found in subjects' perception. Subjects had to judge both stimuli adjacent for steps of alignment manipulation (belonging to the same scaling level) and stimuli adjacent for steps of scaling manipulation (showing the same alignment characteristics). Results showed no discrimination peak, but they also showed that stimuli differing in alignment were not discriminated while stimuli differing for scaling were discriminated. Moreover, reaction times, which could not be related to a discrimination peak, were somehow consistent with the identification results, being higher for answers corresponding to the acoustically most ambiguous stimuli. Thus, no categorical perception was found.

Nevertheless, in line with Kohler (2006) the categorical perception in intonation is taken here as "a special case and not essential for pitch categorization" (Kohler, 2006, p. 148). In fact, the lack of a clear S-shape plot of the results is taken to be due to the fact that stimuli, apart from those at the extreme of both alignment and scaling continua, were always ambiguous for at least one correlate. The situation resembles the one investigated by Clayards et al. (2007), that is, stimuli showed a greater variance in distribution, when considering the phonetic space given by both time - alignment - and frequency scale - scaling - as separately manipulated. An anomalous S-shaped curve may then correspond here to the lower degree of confidence in judging the existence of a contrast and to the shallower categorization function observed by Clayards and colleagues (see also fn.17). Moreover, the observations by Niebuhr and Kohler (2004) also fit this experiment. In their work, as already mentioned, Niebuhr and Kohler made the parallel testing of two series of stimuli and found similar identification results but different discrimination data for the two series. In the identification task, that was a semantic matching task - considered as a perceptuo-cognitive task - subjects were forced to "project their perception patterns onto cognitive categories of semantic interpretation" and performed similarly in the two series. On the contrary they performed differently in the discrimination task which, as the authors state, is "more closely related to perception". The authors suggested that the difference in discrimination was due to the lack of a prosodic-segmental link in the stimuli in one series. This lack caused two continua, an acoustic and a perceptual continuum, to be mapped one onto the other, offering no way for subjects to discriminate. The results of the CP test described in this paper consistently show that, by means of a semantic difference task - a "perceptuo-cognitive" task -

speakers identify two different tonal events although they do not discriminate pairs of adjacent stimuli – in the more properly perceptive task. Here, as well, it can be argued that the cues differentiating the patterns correspond to periods in time rather than points and, possibly even more importantly, the differentiation takes place in the vowel. Thus, here as well, it can be argued that the existence of phonological categories is not necessarily precluded by the absence of categorical perception. Moreover, both the identification and the discrimination tests deserve more comments.

The "perceptuo-cognitive" task, in Niebuhr and Kohler's terms, used in the present identification test was a clear metalinguistic task, requiring subjects to think about the specific possible meanings/functions associated to an utterance. Apart from the fact that participants appear to succeed in differentiating items on the basis of alignment and scaling, the reference to the meaning and functions conveyed by intonational patterns may definitely not be straightforward. In many cases, meaning and functions conveyed by intonation appear to have fuzzy boundaries and to be hard to delimitate, especially by means of metalinguistic tasks; moreover, small variations in intonation may actually be recognized as corresponding to slightly different nuances of the same meaning. Thus, at least when the difference between two patterns is not as easy to define as, say, a question vs statement difference, the forced choice in deciding for different meanings or functions appears to be highly difficult, probably even too subtle, to elicit abrupt shifts in subjects' answers[25].

Moreover, it may be a matter of debate that the meaning/functions indicated by the analysis of speech material is appropriate to induce subjects to project their perceived patterns on the expected semantic or functional category. For instance, the broad focus vs contrastive focus

---

25 The choice of semantic matching tasks, giving a context for reference, appears to be able to facilitate the subject decision and, in this specific case, it would probably have permitted to avoid the reference to paralinguistic aspects (i.e., the 'peremptory and conclusive' features). However, the choice of this more appropriate task did not prove to be sufficient to show the discreteness of the broad focus falling accent and the contrastive accent - see Gili Fivela (2008) and fn.16. It may then be the case that the choice of the identification task facilitates the successfulness of the test, although it does not determine a radical change in the results.

case appears to be quite problematic in this respect: while in producing speech speakers may clearly choose different patterns depending on the fact that they want to (peremptorily) correct a preceding utterance – exactly as they would decide to produce a different pattern for a question rather than a statement – in perception it may be hard to get clear results, as what sounds as a (peremptory) correction to one subject may not sound as a (peremptory) correction to another. The point is that the amount of variation is expected to be much greater than the one likely to be found for, say, the threshold between what sounds as a statement or as a question. In these terms, the difference in the two examples above - broad focus vs contrastive focus and statement vs question - apparently goes in the direction of a gradual (in the first pair) vs an abrupt shift (in the second pair), i.e. a gradient vs categorical difference. However, even if this was the case, should this difference be enough to deny the existence of different linguistically relevant intonational events for broad and contrastive focus?

Moreover, the discrimination test for intonation patterns also appears to be problematic. The comparison of pairs of stimuli appears to be too focused on the acoustic-perceptual properties of the stimuli to play a crucial role in deciding on the categoriality of intonational events and on their role in the linguistic system. In this respect, the choice of the size of step of manipulation appears to have a major impact on both the identification and the discrimination results: in identification tests it is expected to influence the steepness of the shift in subjects answers - which, crucially, is one of the characteristics pointing to categorical perception; in discrimination, the size of step of manipulation appears to be even more important as, being too short, it may be not perceptually detectable; being too big, it may correspond to globally higher discrimination scores, independently from the existence of category boundary[26]. Nevertheless, as the data discussed here show, even though subjects do not appear to discriminate stimuli manipulated for, say, alignment, they are able to produce an alignment difference between two patterns in the imitation task. Why should subjects be able to produce

26 Gili Fivela (in prep.) describes discrimination tests performed by pairing stimuli that were 2 steps of manipulation apart – thus not adjacent in the continuum – along the lines of the work by Dilley (submitted). Results consist of globally higher discrimination scores, with no discrimination peak.

two different patterns if the steps of alignment manipulation in the stimuli they hear are too short to be perceptually detectable?

The analysis of speakers' production of perceptually filtered material, elicited by means of an imitation task, offered data consistent with the idea that a lack in categorical perception does not imply the absence of two different categories. Results of measurements performed on speakers' imitation of audio stimuli show a bipartite distribution of subject productions. Basically, subjects appear to be far less sensitive to the presence of ambiguous correlates when they (re)produce speech: two out of three speakers produce two different patterns that show characteristics consistent with those of the pitch accents under investigation, even though listening to ambiguous stimuli. These results, then, point out that even though speakers perceive ambiguous correlates they seem to be able to associate them to two different and distinct patterns. Interestingly enough, speakers seem to refer to prototypical characteristics of the patterns: at least for two out of three subjects, the temporal alignment of the pitch accents produced appears not to be significantly influenced by the scaling of stimuli; on the other hand, at least to a certain extent, speakers implement their peaks at an F0 level that is consistent with the alignment characteristics of the prototypical pattern (although a small variation according to the stimulus scaling may be observed in the plots). Notice that the idea of subjects having quite precise reference patterns, for both scaling and alignment, is consistent with recent findings by Dilley and Brown (2007): they show that the relative pitch levels of syllables influence the timing of peaks and valleys[E1] in a categorical way, pointing to the existence of syntagmatic tonal features in the phonological representation.

Thus, the imitation results in this study appear to be qualitatively robust, although quantitatively limited, while the categorical perception data offer a composite picture, consistently with other findings in the literature. However, while the imitation task offers results consistent with observations on the actual use of intonational features, it does not solve problems related to the meaning or function associated to intonational patterns. Indeed, the production of two discrete sets of patterns, shown by the bipartite distribution of their acoustic analysis, does not inform about the meaning difference between the two patterns, the existence of two discrete categories of meanings, or the appropriateness of the assumed pattern-function or pattern-meaning correspondence.

Maybe the evidence for deciding on the role of intonational events in the linguistic system may come from neurolinguistic investigations, for instance by performing electromagnetic measures of neural activity.

An incursion in the neurolinguistics of intonation

In the literature, evidence is found for the existence of long-term language specific memory traces, acquired for the phonemes of the mother tongue and reflecting the native language phonology, even in pre-attentive tasks (Näätänen et al., 1997; Näätänen, 2001). These memory traces, predominantly found in the left hemisphere, at first include information on possible allophonic acoustic realizations (Jacobsen et al., 2004) that are later represented as one acoustic event (Näätänen, 2001). Consistently, neural data also provide evidence for categorical perception of segmental elements (see for instance Sharma and Dorman's (1999) work on categorical perception of Voice Onset Time, and Wolmetz et al.'s (2007) case study on the categorization of click/tones found, however, in the right hemisphere).

A possible solution to the problems pointed out in the present paper could then be searched in studies that focus on prosodic aspects, in particular on intonation, with the aim of finding out whether something similar to a phonological representation, or to long term memory traces, is also available for intonation events relevant for linguistic purposes, or, at least, whether it is possible to find different brain responses to linguistic and paralinguistic uses of intonation.

Although some works in the literature show that there is no language-categorical processing of complex tones (see Jacobsen's (2004) results stemming from a pre-attentive task), interesting indications may stem from other works, focusing on linguistic uses of prosodic information, and showing that it is possible to individuate specific brain responses in relation to prosodic processing. For instance, Astésano et al. (2004) use

ERPs[27] to investigate the prosodic processing and its relations with the syntactic and semantic processing. The authors were interested in finding evidence for on-line processing of prosodic modality and, in case of a positive result, they wanted to study the time course of the effect in comparison to the "well documented electrophysiological marker of semantic processing, the N400" (a negative ERP component peaking around 400 ms). However, for their purpose they manipulated the intonation contour of French statements and questions (basically differing in the direction of pitch variation: fundamental frequency rise vs. fundamental frequency fall) with the aim of creating a prosodic mismatch, i.e. an incongruity conveyed only by intonation. Thus, they focused on a context that [E2]may offer suggestions for the issues discussed here. The incongruous intonation was "created by cross-splicing the beginning of Statements with the end of Question" intonation, and vice versa, at the Noun Phrase/Verb Phrase syntactic boundary. Moreover, the authors orthogonally manipulated the semantic and the prosodic aspects in order to create four conditions for studying the relation between prosodic and semantic processing[28]. In different trials, they asked their subjects to focus on either the intonation contours or the semantics of the sentence, and to decide whether they were acceptable. The authors report data on 16 right-handed French native

---

27 Among the various ways of studying the electrical and magnetic activity both in temporal and spatial terms (Näätänen et al., 1994), Event-Related brain Potentials (ERPs) appear to be a useful technique for investigating issues similar to those discussed in this paper. ERPs are "small changes in electrical activity of the brain that are recorded from the scalp and that are brought about by some external or internal event" (Handy, 2005). The activity is recorded with a high time resolution (milliseconds) from a number of locations on the scalp. Thus ERPs may be employed to investigate cognitive processes, making inferences on their timing (observing the time course of the signals), degree of engagement (looking for their amplitude), and functional equivalence (in relation to the distribution across the scalp). For instance, ERPs may offer various types of information on the processing of auditory stimuli (Hillyard and Picton, 1987), ranging from single segments to sentences.

28 The four conditions were the followings: semantically and prosodically congruous; semantically congruous and prosodically incongruous; semantically incongruous and prosodically congruous; both semantically and prosodically incongruous.

speakers on a corpus of 240 sentences, built with the same phonological and syntactic pattern. Results show that a P800 component (a positive ERP component that they found around 800ms after the verb onset) was generated in case of prosodic mismatch, although only when subjects were asked to concentrate on the intonation contour. That is, the P800 was larger for prosodically incongruous than for prosodically congruous sentences, i.e. it was due to the pitch contour manipulation.

What is interesting to point out for the sake of discussion here, is that the authors argue that the P800 component is different from other components that are reported to be purely driven by prosody[29]. For instance, it is different from the Closure Positive Shift reported by Steinhauer et al. (1999), related to the perception of intonational phrase boundaries[30]. Discussing the nature of the difference is beyond the scope of this paper. Instead, it is relevant to report that the authors argue that a specific component appears to be associated to a re-analysis of a prosodic cue that violates the expected intonation contour.

Another point made by the authors is that the P800 component has a left parietal distribution, and this may be surprising with reference to the usual results on prosodic processing, preferentially found in the right hemisphere. The authors report that the lateralization may be task dependent, but they also refer to other works showing the relevance of the left hemisphere "in some aspect of prosodic processing". For instance, functional Magnetic Resonance Imaging (fMRI) suggests that pitch

29 Apart from being different from component elicited by other language related components, such as the P600. This component, for instance, is elicited by syntactic anomalies that may, as the authors state, have functional interpretations similar to the prosodic mismatch, and that have been reported as reflecting re-analysis or a more general integration of linguistic and non-linguistic information.

30 Of course the present 'incursion' in the neurolinguistic literature is not supposed to encompass all the relevant contribution to the field and does not offer the complete and composite picture of the pertinent findings. For instance, Eckstein and Friederici (2005), focussing on the relation between prosody and syntax, report a right anterior negativity effect as a purely prosodic effect due to the prosodic manipulation of the final word in subordinate clauses. To make another example, Roll et al. (submitted) report a weak positive effect (P600) in relation to a high left-edge boundary tone following mismatching non-assertive verb.

processing may be lateralized depending on its function, being left-lateralized in case of processing of tones in tone languages - having a clear linguistic function (e.g., Gandour et al., 2002) - and being right-lateralized for pitch cues such as voice quality (van Lancker, 1980).
Thus, specific properties, both in time and space, appear to identify the processing of "well-established" prosodic effects, such as those found in the comparison of contours indicating sentence modality (as in the case of the above mentioned question vs statement investigation). It would then be interesting to see whether similar specific properties may also be found for those intonational events that have been presented in this paper as possibly less clear-cut: those found in broad and contrastive focus. These aspects have been reported here as more difficult to pin down and, therefore, this difficulty is still expected in behavioural results; nevertheless it is possible that, in case of prosodic mismatch, brain responses turn out to be similar to those indicating a re-analysis of a prosodic cue that violates the expected intonation contour. This could suggest that the difference between the two patterns should be considered as a linguistically relevant difference, even though not categorically perceived.
A final point may be worth mentioning. Astésano et al. (2004) work also showed that the processing of semantic information was not influenced by prosodic information, while prosodic information was influenced by the semantic content of sentence. That is, when subjects focused on the semantics of the sentence, both the percentage of correct responses and the ERPs (N400 component) showed that there was no influence of the prosodic congruity of the sentence. On the contrary, when subjects focused on the intonation contour of the sentence, both the percentage of correct responses and the ERPs showed that there was an influence of the semantic congruity of the sentence. As the authors observe, "the semantic processing seemed to predominate over prosodic processing". This result may then suggest that asking subjects to focus on stimuli changing only for the intonation contour, apart from being obviously an artificial situation, is not representative of what speakers usually do. That is, coherent intonation correlates may be produced spontaneously by speakers and may be interpreted by listeners together with (or as a supplementary information with respect to) other information – the semantic information, according to these results. It may then be not

surprising that, in metalinguistic tasks, subjects have trouble in pinning the prosodic meaning or function down, as they usually interpret it together with other available information.

5. CONCLUSIONS

The difference between a narrow focus pattern and a contrastive focus pattern appears to be clearly exploited by speakers in production (see read and spontaneous speech material, described in 3.1.), may be quite clearly imitated by speakers listening to audio stimuli and imitating them (see 3.3.), but may not be categorically perceived, i.e. it does not correspond to an abrupt shift in identification aligned with a discrimination peak (see 3.2.). Results from the present study point out that, at least in testing some tonal events, categorical perception may not help in distinguishing structural and non-structural properties in intonation - as already observed by Gussenhoven (2006) – and, therefore, it does not appear to be suited for being extensively used for intonation purposes. On the contrary, a perception-production task, such as the imitation task, appears to more clearly reveal such structural properties, and to give results that are more consistent with observations on the actual use of intonational features and the existence of a grammar of intonation. Thus, the impact of the lack/presence of categorical perception of pitch patterns on the definition of intonational systems, and on the differentiation of their components, should be carefully evaluated and weighed on the basis of evidence stemming from other sources.

Thus, as Kohler (2006) argues, the perception of categories could actually be more important than categorical perception. In this respect, the capability of subjects to associate stimuli belonging to the extremes of the continuum to two different sets of functions could be enough to show that two categories are perceived in relation to intonation changes. In the present study, subjects identify two different patterns, although not through categorical perception, and this result is taken here as a perceptual confirmation of the existence of two intonational categories.

As already observed in the literature (see e.g. Kockanski, 2006: 104), the best evidence for intonation should be taken by means of a task that does

"not ask subject to think about the stimuli; it observes the subject's behaviour in a situation as close to natural conversation as possible". Thus the sources should mainly be those related to the use of intonation in contexts, and to the actual effects of intonational events on speech processing. In this respect, production data and not-purely-perceptual tests should be taken into account; moreover, it appears that interesting indications may also stem from neurolinguistic investigations.
Speech production is considered as a relevant source of data, especially when enabling the analysis of discourse, and interaction in general. This may show that tonal events, due to their specific meanings, may be used in contexts to elicit specific reactions. This is what happens, for instance, when speakers use contrastive patterns, clearly opposing their position to the other speaker's position, even though they officially lack (and cannot be sure about) the information they contrast. In Pisa Italian Map-Task dialogues, for instance, when instruction followers - lacking information on the reconstruction of the path, as only the instruction giver owns that information - realise a contrastive accent on an item, their phrase is interpreted as a confirmation question on the presence of that item, eliciting an answer by the information giver. Such a non-literal use of the contrastive pattern, inducing a sort of conversational implicature (Grice, 1975/1978), clearly points to the existence of a specific tonal event, with a specific meaning or function (that may also be used non-literally!), irrespective of possible problems speakers may have in categorically perceiving it as different from other patterns.
On the perception side, not purely perceptual tasks appear to offer evidence on the existence of intonational categories. Asking subjects to 'do' something related to what they perceive, or instrumentally analysing the effects of intonational events on speech processing appears to be a promising way of obtaining fruitful data. In this respect, imitation tasks such as the one described here, together with eye tracking studies, or, as discussed above, neurolinguistic investigations could offer the appropriate type of data.

ACKNOWLEDGEMENTS

I wish to thank an anonymous reviewer and O. Niebuhr, the second reviewer, for their very useful comments on a preliminary version of this paper. Thanks also to M. Roll for discussion on the use of ERPs for investigating intonation and suggestions on neurolinguistic studies on this issue.

REFERENCES

Anderson A., Bader M., Bard E., Boyle e., Doherty G., Garrod S., Isard S., Kowtko J., McAllister J., Miller J., Sotillo C., Thompson H., Weinert R. (1991). The HCRC map task corpus. *Language and Speech* 34 (4), 351-366.

Astésano, C., Besson, M., and Alter, K. (2004). Brain potentials during semantic and prosodic processing in French. *Cognitive Brain Research* 18, 172-184.

Beckman, M. & Pierrehumbert, J.B. (1986). Intonational structure in Japanese and English. *Phonology Yearbook* 3, 255-309.

Braun, B., Kochanski, G., Grabe, E., and Rosner, B.S. (2006). Evidence for attractors in English intonation. *Journal of the Acoustical Society of America* 119(6), 4006-4015.

Bruce, G. (1977). *Swedish word accents in sentence perspective*. Gleerup: CWK.

Caspers, J. (1998). Who's next? The melodic marking of question vs. continuation in Dutch. *Language and Speech* 41(3-4), 375-398.

Chen, A. (2003). Reaction Time as an Indicator of Discrete Intonational Contrasts in English. *Proceedings of EuroSpeech*, 97-100.

Clayards, M., Aslin, R.N., Tanenhaus, M.K., and Jacobs, R.A. (2007). Within category phonetic variability affects perceptual uncertainty. *Proceedings of the ICPhS*, Saarbrücken (Germany), 701-704.

Cruttenden, A. (1986). *Intonation*, Cambridge Textbooks in Linguistics, Cambridge University Press.

Dilley, L.C. (submitted). The role of F0 alignment in distinguishing intonation categories. *Language and Speech*.

Dilley, L. (2007). Pitch range variation in English tonal contrast: Continuous or categorical? *Proceedings of the ICPhS*, Saarbrücken (Germany), 1153-1156.

Dilley, L.C. & Brown, M. (2007). Effects of pitch range variation on F0 extrema in imitation task. *Journal of Phonetics* 4(35), 523-551.

D'Imperio, M. & House, D. (1997). Perception of questions and statements in Neapolitan Italian. In: A. Botinis et al. (ed.) *Intonation: Theory, Models and Applications*, Proceedings of the ESCA Workshop on Intonation, Athens (Greece), 251-254.

Gandour, J., Wong, D., Lowe, M., Dzemidzic, M., Satthamnuwong, N., Tong, Y., and Li, X. (2002). A cross-linguistic study of spectral and temporal cues underlying phonological processing. *Journal of Cognitive Neurooscience*, 14,7,1076-1086.

Gili Fivela, B. (in prep). *Perceiving and imitating: Testing categories in intonation.*

Gili Fivela, B., D'Imperio, M. (submitted). High peak vs high plateau in the identification of contrastive accents in Italian. *Submitted to TIE 2008 Conference*, Lisbon (Portugal).

Gili Fivela, B. (2008). Broad focus vs contrastive focus: Is there categorical perception in Pisa Italian? *Speech Prosody 2008*, Campinas (Brazil).

Gili Fivela, B. (2006). The coding of target alignment and scaling in pitch accent transcription, *Italian Journal of Linguistics* 18(1), 189-221.

Gili Fivela, B. (2005). La percezione degli accenti: il ruolo dell'allineamento e dello 'scaling' dei bersagli tonali, *Atti del Convegno AISV 2004*, 313-326.

Gili Fivela, B. (2004). *The phonetics and phonology of intonation: The case of Pisa Italian.* PhD dissertation, Scuola Normale Superiore, Pisa (Italy).

Gili Fivela, B. (1999). The prosody of left-dislocated topicalized constituents in Italian read speech. *Proceedings of the EuroSpeech* 1, Budapest (Hungary), 531-534.

Grabe E., Gussenhoven C., Haan J., Marsi E., and Post B. (1997). The meaning of intonation phrase onsets in Dutch. *Proceedings of the ESCA Workshop on Intonation, Athens, Greece*, 161-164.

Grice M. & Savino, M. (2003). Map Tasks in Bari Italian: Asking questions about given, accessible and new information, invited contribution to special issue "Intonation in Romance". *Catalan Journal of Linguistics* 2(2), 153-180.

Grice, H.P. (1975/1978). Logic and conversation. In P. Cole & J. Morgan (eds.) *Studies in the ways of words*, (reprinted 1989), 41-54, Cambridge University Press.

Grice, M. & Savino, M. (1995). Intonation and communicative function in a regional variety of Italian. In W.J. Barry & J. Koreman (eds.) *Phonus* 1, 19-32.

Gussenhoven, C. (2006). Experimental approaches to establishing discreteness of intonational contrasts. In: Sudhoff et al. (eds.) *Methods in Empirical Prosody Research*, 321-334, Berlin: de Gruyter.

Gussenhoven C. (2004). *The Phonology of Tone and Intonation*. Cambridge: Cambridge University.

Gussenhoven C. (2002). Intonation and interpretation: Phonetics and phonology. In B.Bel and I.Marlien (eds.) *Proceedings of the Speech Prosody 2002 Conference*, Aix-en-Provence: Laboratoire Parole et Langage, 47-57.

Gussenhoven, C. (1999). Discreteness and gradience in intonational contrasts. *Language and Speech* 42, 281-305.

Gussenhoven, C. (1984). On the grammar and semantics of sentence accents. Dordrecht: Foris.

Handy, T.C. (ed.) (2005). *Event-Related Potentials. A Methods Handbook*. The MIT Press.

Harnad, S. (1987). *Categorical Perception: The Groundwork of Cognition*. New York: CUP.

Hillyard, S.A. & Picton, T.W. (1987). Electrophysiology of cognition. In: F. Plum (ed.) *Handbook of Psychology Vol. 5 Part 2,* Bethesda MD: American Physiological Society

Jacobsen, T., Schröger, E., and Alter, K. (2004). Pre-attentive perception of vowel phonemes from variable speech stimuli. *Psychophysiology* 41, 654-659.

Jacobsen, T. (2004). Mismatch negativity to frequency changes: no evidence from human event-related potentials for categorical speech processing of complex tones resembling vowel formant structure. *Neurosciences Letters* 362, 204-208.

Kockanski, G. (2006). Prosody beyond fundamental frequency. In: Sudhoff et al. (eds) *Methods in Empirical Prosody Research*, 89-121, Berlin: de Gruyter.

Kohler, K. (2006). Paradigms in Experimental Prosodic Analysis: From measurements to function. In: Sudhoff et al. (eds) *Methods in Empirical Prosody Research*, 123-152, Berlin: de Gruyter,.

Kohler, K. (1991). A model of German intonation. *AIPUK* 25, 295-360.

Kohler, K. (1987). Categorical pitch perception. *Proceedings of ICPhS* 5, Tallin (Estonia), 331-333.

Kuhl, P.K. (1991). Human adults and human infants show a 'perceptual magnet effect' for the prototypes of speech categories, monkeys do not. *Perception and Psychophysics* 50, 93-107.

Ladd, D.R. (1996). *Intonational Phonology*, Cambridge Studies in Linguistics, Cambridge University Press.

Ladd, B. & Morton, R. (1997). The perception of intonational emphasis: Continuous or categorical? *Journal of Phonetics* 2, 313-342.

Lieberman, A.M., Cooper, F.S., Shankweiler, D.P., and Studdert-Kennedy, M. (1967). Perception of the speech code. *Psychological Review* 74, 431-461.

Lieberman, A.M., Harris, K.S., Hoffman, H.S., and Griffith, B.C. (1957). The discrimination of speech sounds within and across phoneme boundaries. *Journal of Experimental psychology* 54, 5, 358-368.

Näätänen, R. (2001). The perception of speech sounds by human brain as reflected by the mismatch negativity (MMN) and its magnetic equivalent (MMNm). *Psychophysiology* 38, 1-21.

Näätänen, R., Lehtokoski, A., Lennes, M., Cheour, M., Huotilainen, M., Iivonen, A., Vainio, M., Alku, P., Ilmoniemi, R.J., Luuk, J., Sinkonen J., and Alho, K. (1997). Language-specific phoneme representations revealed by electric and magnetic brain responses. *Nature* 385, 432-434.

Näätänen, R., Ilmoniemi, R.J., and Alho, K. (1994). Magnetoencephalography in studies of human cognitive brain function. *Trends in Neurosciences* 17, 389-395.

Newport, E.L. (1982). Task specificity in language learning? Evidence from speech perception and American Sign Language. In: E. Wanner and L.R. Gleitman (eds.) *Language acquisition: The state of the art*, 450 –486, Cambridge University Press.

Niebuhr, O. & Kohler, K. (2004). Perception and cognitive processing of tonal alignment in German. *Proceedings of the International Symposium on Tonal Aspects of Languages: Emphasis on Tone Languages (TAL)*, Beijing (China), 155-158.

Niebuhr, O. (2003). Perceptual study of timing variables in F0 peaks. *Proceedings of the ICPhS*, Barcelona (Spain). 1225-1228.

Odé C. (2005). Neutralization or truncation? The perception of two Russian pitch accents on utterance-final syllables. *Speech Communication* 47, 71-79.

Pierrehumbert, J. (1980). *The phonology and phonetics of English intonation.* PhD thesis, MIT (USA), published in 1988 by IULC.

Pierrehumbert, J. & Hirschberg, J. (1990). The meaning of intonational contours in the interpretation of discourse. In: P.R.Cohen, J.Morgan, and M.E.Pollack (eds.) *Intentions in communication*, 271-310, The MIT Press,.

Pierrehumbert, J. & Steele, S.A. (1989). Categories of tonal alignment in English. *Phonetica* 46, 181-196.

Port, R.F. (2008). All is prosody: Phones and phonemes are the ghost of letters. *Speech Prosody 2008*, Campinas (Brasil), 7-12.

Prieto, P., D'Imperio, M., and Gili Fivela, B. (2005). Pitch accent alignment in Romance: primary and secondary association with metrical structure. In: P. Warren (guest editor) *Language and Speech, Special Issue: Intonation in Language varieties* , 359-396, London: Kingston Press

Redi, L.C. (2003). Categorical effects in production of pitch contours in English. *Proceedings of the ICPhS*, Barcelona (Spain), 2921-2924.

Repp, B. (1984). Categorical perception: Issues, methods, and findings. In: N. Lass (ed.) *Speech and Language: Advances in Basic Research and Practice* 10, 243-335, Academic Press.

Roll, M., Horne, M., and Lindgren, M. (submitted). *Left-edge boundary tone and main clause verb effects on syntactic processing in Swedish embedded clauses-An ERP study.* Elsevier.

Rooth M. (1985). *Association with focus.* University of Massachusetts at Amherst:. Ph.D. dissertation.

Schneider, K., Linfert, B., Dogil, G., and Möbius, B. (2006). Phonetic grounding of prosodic categories. In: Sudhoff et al. (eds.) *Methods in Empirical Prosody Research,* 335-362, Berlin: de Gruyter.

Sharma, A. & Dorman, M.F. (1999). Cortical auditory evoked potential correlates of categorical perception of voice-onset time. *Journal of the Acoustical Society of America* 106(2), 1078-1083.

Steinhauer, K., Alter, K. & Friederici, D. (1999). Brain potentials indicate immediate use of prosodic cues in natural speech processing. *Nature Neurosciences* 2, 191-196.

't Hart, J., Collier, R., Cohen, A. (1990). A perceptual study of intonation. An experimental phonetic approach to speech melody. Cambridge University Press.

Van Lancker, D. (1980). Cerebral Lateralization of pitch cues in the linguistic signal. *Papers in Linguistics: International Journal of Human Communication* 13(2), 201-277.

Vanrell, M. (2006). A scaling contrast in Majorcan Catalan interrogatives. *Proceedings of Speech Prosody,* Dresden (Germany).

Whorf, B.L. (1964). *Language, thought and reality.* Cambridge (MA): MIT Press.

Wolmetz, M., Rapp, B., and Poeppel, D. (2007). Investigating the phonemic categorization capacity of the right hemisphere: A case study. *Brain and Language* 103.

Xu, Y., Xu, C.X., and Sun, X. (2004). On the temporal domain of focus. *Speech Prosody 2004,* Nara (Japan), 81-84.

FSC
www.fsc.org
MIX
Papier | Fördert gute Waldnutzung
FSC® C083411

Kolibri 360 GmbH
Ferdinand-Jühlke-Straße 7
99095 Erfurt, Deutschland
produktsicherheit@kolibri360.de

Druck:
CPI Druckdienstleistungen GmbH
im Auftrag der
Kolibri 360 GmbH
Ferdinand-Jühlke-Str. 7
99095 Erfurt